Into the Community

Nursing in Ambulatory and Home Care

Into the Community
Nursing in Ambulatory and Home Care

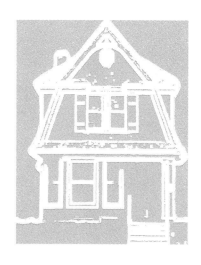

Joan C. Stackhouse, RN, MS

Consulting Home Care and Hospice Staff Nurse, Brevard, North Carolina

Clinical Specialist, Private Practice

Former Associate Professor, Rockland Community College, Suffern, New York

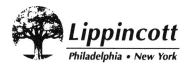

Lippincott
Philadelphia • New York

Acquisitions Editor: Susan M. Glover, RN, MSN
Editorial Assistant: Bridget Blatteau
Project Editor: Sandra Cherrey Scheinin
Senior Production Manager: Helen Ewan
Production Coordinator: Patricia McCloskey
Designer: Doug Smock

9   8   7   6   5   4   3   2   1

Library of Congress Cataloging-in-Publications Data
Stackhouse, Joan C.
    Into the community: nursing in ambulatory and home care/Joan C. Stackhouse.
        p.   cm.
    Includes bibliographical references and index.
    ISBN 0-397-55475-3 (alk. paper)
    1. Community health nursing.   2. Community health nursing—United States.   I. Title.
    [DNLM: 1. Community Health Nursing.   2. Ambulatory Care—nurses' instruction.   3. Home Care
    Services.   WY 106 S775i 1998]
    RT98.S76   1998
    610.73'43—dc21   97-36822
                                                                                              CIP

Care has been taken to confirm the accuracy of the information presented and to describe generally accepted practices. However, the authors, editors, and publisher are not responsible for errors or omissions or for any consequences from application of the information in this book and make no warranty, express or implied, with respect to the contents of the publication.

The authors, editors and publisher have exerted every effort to ensure that drug selection and dosage set forth in this text are in accordance with current recommendations and practice at the time of publication. However, in view of ongoing research, changes in government regulations, and the constant flow of information relating to drug therapy and drug reactions, the reader is urged to check the package insert for each drug for any change in indications and dosage and for added warnings and precautions. This is particularly important when the recommended agent is a new or infrequently employed drug.

Some drugs and medical devices presented in this publication have Food and Drug Administration (FDA) clearance for limited use in restricted research settings. It is the responsibility of the health care provider to ascertain the FDA status of each drug or device planned for use in their clinical practice.

♾This Paper Meets the Requirements of ANSI/NISO Z39.48-1992 (Permanence of Paper).

I wish to dedicate this book to my beloved family: Bill, my best friend, husband, and the treasure of my life; as well as our three children: Ginny, Charlie, and Paul, their spouses, and children.

Reviewers

William N. Ames, RN, BSN
Assistant Professor
School of Nursing
Elizabethtown Community College
Elizabethtown, Kentucky

Dennis J. Brown, RN, MSN
Acting Director of Nurses
Psychiatric Division
Texas Tech University Health Sciences Center
William P. Clements Jr. Unit
Amarillo, Texas

Marian D. Edmiston, BSN, MSN
Associate Professor
Coordinator of Allied Health Programs
Nursing and Allied Health
Delaware County Community College
Media, Pennsylvania

Renee S. Schnieder, RN, BSN
Faculty
Associate Degree Nursing Program
Southeast Community College
Lincoln, Nebraska

Preface

Into the Community: Nursing in Ambulatory and Home Care evolved from efforts to find a concise textbook. In 1995, I was writing a community health nursing curriculum for one of the associate degree programs of the State University of New York (SUNY) system. I searched for a small, clinically oriented text that included the basic theoretical components of community health nursing. I wanted a text that dealt with current issues and one that was pedagogically sound. Complaints to publishers' representatives regarding my inability to find such a text produced calls from acquisition editors to write such a book. I believe that *Into the Community: Nursing in Ambulatory and Home Care* fulfills my objectives.

Level of the Learner

This text can be used for all levels of nursing education in community health, such as ADN, generic BSN, and RN to BSN bridge programs. It is appropriate for MSN programs due to its strong clinical orientation, real case situations, and inclusion of advanced practice opportunities. It may also be useful for continuing education programs because of its concise format.

Organization of the Text and Chapters

The text is organized into the following four parts:

Part 1   Theoretical Foundations of Community Health Nursing
Part 2   Nursing Practice in Wellness Care
Part 3   Nursing Practice in Ambulatory Care
Part 4   Nursing Practice in Home Care

Each part contains four chapters focusing on various aspects of that part.

An extensive list of references and additional readings appears at the end of each part to enable students to easily access more detailed information contained in that part.

Each chapter contains the following features:

Key Terms: A strong emphasis is placed on understanding key terms and mastering the language of this discipline.

Learning Objectives:	These directives help the reader to focus on important chapter content.
The Nurse Speaks:	A real account by a community health nurse describing how he or she dealt with a situation related to the chapter content.
Clinical Application:	A critical thinking case study that enables students to work through a true case situation.

Figures, Tables, and Displays further elaborate on the chapter content.

A *Chapter Summary* completes each chapter for the student's convenience.

Several very useful tools for students and faculty are included in the *Appendices.*

Appendix A	Death and Dying Customs Among Religious Groups in the United States
Appendix B	List of Nursing and Related Resources
Appendix C	Toll-Free Directory
Appendix D	Sample Clinical Paths
Appendix E	Sample Standard High-Tech Care Plans

A *Glossary* conveniently defines many of the terms found in this text.

An *Instructor's Manual* is available and includes various teaching strategies such as learning games, critical thinking questions based on the case studies, and additional learning activities.

- Several enlarged figures and tables are presented for use as transparencies.
- A sample test bank of 100 multiple choice questions also is included in the Instructor's Manual.

It is the author's sincere wish that this text will prove valuable to both students and instructors.

Joan C. Stackhouse, RN, MS

Acknowledgments

I wish to thank all the nurses who told me their experiences as community health nurses. All the case situations in *The Nurse Speaks* and in the *Clinical Applications* in this book are based on true accounts, with some editorial changes to preserve confidentiality. In particular, I wish to thank my niece, Laurie Graaf, who supplied many of the case studies and whose photo appears at the start of Part 4. All of the following nurses make me exceedingly proud of our profession: Ann Marie Collins, Elaine Peneno, Donna Schweiter, Joyce Spencer, Pat Smith, Joan Shea, Laurie Graaf, Karen Hanusik, Lonnie Morris, Carmen Szabo, Ellen Witte, Deborah Bradley, Karen Woehler, Elaine Raday, Patricia Strys, Toni Babington, and Ruth Rykowski. Several other persons were very helpful in supplying information and deserve my special thanks. They are Richard vonRueden, Marie Clark, Denise McGraw and Pamela Potter Hughes, Sue Ann Eitches, Deborah Aggrey, Sandee Massey, and Ruth Mahtani Dearing.

My special gratitude goes to my sister-in-law, Sally Stackhouse, who rescued me from many computer glitches and whose marvelous computer skills and perseverance enabled me to produce this book more efficiently and on schedule.

Last but not least, I want to thank the editorial staff at Lippincott-Raven Publishers, especially Sue Glover, Senior Nursing Editor, who showered me with encouragement all along the way.

Contents

10
Mental Health Nursing in the Community   237

11
The Elderly and the Disabled: Major Consumers of Health Care   259

Part 1

Theoretical Foundations of Community Health

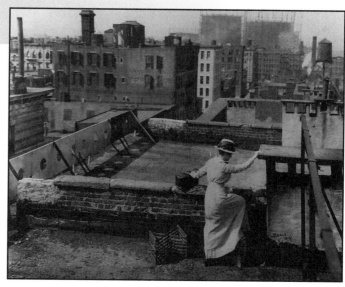

A visiting nurse from the Henry Street Settlement
Here an intrepid nurse crosses rooftops to visit residents on the Lower East Side about 1910. (Courtesy of Museum of the City of New York)

1

Community Health Nursing

Key Terms

advocacy
aggregates
autonomy
case managers
certification
client
community
critical thinking
cyberspace
disease prevention

e-mail
epidemiology
health promotion
herd immunity
holistic
humanistic
immune globulin
Internet
laptop computers
pandemic

passive immunity
primary prevention
public health nurse
secondary prevention
tertiary prevention
visiting nurse
voice mail
vulnerable populations
World Wide Web

Learning Objectives

1. Define "community health nursing."
2. Describe at least 10 characteristics of community health nursing.
3. Trace the history of community health nursing from Florence Nightingale to the present time.

4. Identify current opportunities and challenges in community health nursing.
5. Describe at least six factors regarding the future of community health nursing.

Characteristics of Community Health Nursing

Community-Focused and Client-Centered

Community health nursing occurs wherever people normally live their lives. It seldom occurs in institutions, but sometimes people in places such as group homes, halfway houses, or prisons are cared for by community health nurses. Although community health nursing is community-focused and usually community-based, it cannot be defined

---

DISPLAY 1-1
Beliefs Underlying Community Health Nursing

- Human beings have rights and responsibilities.
- Promoting and maintaining family independence is healthful.
- Environments have an impact on human health.
- Nurses can make a difference and promote change toward health for individuals, families, and communities. Vulnerable and at-risk populations, groups, and families need special attention, especially the aged, infants, and disabled, ill, and poor persons.
- Poverty and oppression are social barriers to achievement of health and human potential.
- Interpersonal relationships are essential to caring for others.
- Hygiene, self-care, and prevention are as important as care of the sick.
- Community health nurses can be leaders and innovators in developing programs of nursing care and programs for adequate standards of living.
- Community health nursing care should be available to all, not just the poor.

(Smith C, Maurer F [1995]. Community Health Nursing. Philadelphia: WB Saunders.)

---

by location. Community health nursing is a state of mind. See Display 1-1 for the beliefs underlying community health nursing.

Community nursing differs from hospital nursing in many more ways than the place where care is delivered. Hospital nurses care for patients. The term "patient" implies someone who is in a dependent, passive state in which a great deal of personal freedom is relinquished to receive care and to conform to hospital routines and regulations. On the other hand, community health nurses work with "clients" who usually live in their own homes and decide when they will bathe or take their medications and with whom they will share their bedrooms. Clients tend to seek health care on their own terms and exercise more autonomy about their care. Visiting nurses or home care nurses, as they are also called, may provide bedside nursing, but they work as guests in their clients' homes. This arrangement profoundly affects the character of community nursing care: it is much more collaborative, with a heavier focus on client and family teaching. The major goals for community health nursing are shown in Display 1-2.

DISPLAY 1-2
Major Goals for Community Health Nursing

- Care of the ill, disabled, and suffering in nonhospital settings
- Support of development and well-being throughout the life cycle
- Promotion of human relatedness and mutual caring
- Promotion of self-responsibility regarding health and well-being
- Promotion of relative safety in the environment while conserving resources

(Smith C, Maurer F [1995]. Community Health Nursing. Philadelphia: WB Saunders.)

Consists of Specialties and Subspecialties

The American Nurses Association (ANA) developed specific standards for this nursing specialty. As the name "community health" implies, a major focus is on health as opposed to disease. The three major dimensions of community health nursing practice are

1. Wellness care
2. Ambulatory care
3. Home care

Within these areas, several subspecialties have evolved. The ANA recognizes home care nursing itself as a highly specialized professional nursing practice worthy of national certification distinction. Within home care, there are further subspecialties—for example, hospice nursing. Expert hospice nurses can also seek special certification status issued by the National Board for Certification of Hospice Nurses.

A Holistic, Social Approach

Community nursing is holistic and deals with people within families and communities. People rarely exist in isolation. It is not enough to assess clients' physical, mental, and emotional states and call this holistic nursing; the nurse must also assess the social context in which clients live, including family, community, cultural, spiritual, and economic considerations.

The social approach is a chief characteristic of community nursing. In home care, nurses are heavily involved with their clients' families or support systems. The social context can be the client's family, geographic community, or aggregate. An aggregate is a group of people with specific health needs and concerns in common (Fig. 1-1). Examples of aggregates are clients with physical disabilities and persons with acquired immunodeficiency syndrome (AIDS). Sometimes the entire aggregate becomes the client, as in epidemiologic work with a pandemic or worldwide epidemic such as AIDS. Sometimes the geographic community becomes the client, as when a natural disaster or an environmental hazard occurs.

Prevention and Advocacy Focus

The branch of community nursing known as public health nursing has worked with the poor and underserved in society for more than 100 years (Display 1-3). Although ideally all nurses have a humanistic attitude and value the worth and potential of all persons, community health nurses have the strongest reputation for serving people who are poor and have little voice or knowledge about the services available to them.

Teaching about health promotion and disease prevention is one of the hallmarks of public health nursing. Principles of health are taught both to individuals and to groups. Disease prevention can be primary, secondary, or tertiary. Primary prevention includes all activities that prevent disease from ever happening. Secondary prevention focuses on early identification and treatment of disease. Tertiary prevention includes all efforts to promote rehabilitation and to avoid the long-term effects of disease.

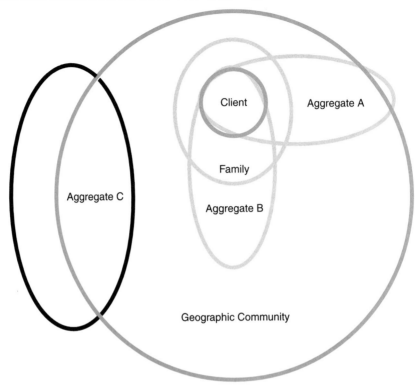

FIGURE 1-1
The relationship of communities and aggregates. The client is a breastfeeding mother.
Aggregate A: All breastfeeding mothers
Aggregate B: People in the community involved with La Leche League
Aggregate C: Persons who have breast cancer

DISPLAY 1-3
Commitments of Public Health

1. Patterning of an environment that promotes health
2. Promotion of healthy families
3. Equitable, just distribution of health care to all
4. A just economic environment to support health and vitality of individuals, families, and groups
5. Prevention of physical and mental illnesses as a support to the wholeness and vitality of individuals, families, and groups
6. Providing the greatest good for the greatest number—thinking collectively on behalf of human beings
7. Educating others to be aware of their own responsibility to move toward health, wholeness, and vitality

(Smith C, Maurer F [1995]. Community Health Nursing. Philadelphia: WB Saunders.)

Substantial Client and Nurse Autonomy

Community health nursing promotes client independence and responsibility. Client teaching of individuals or groups is a crucial function. Client responsibility must be promoted because community nurses are not available 24 hours a day like hospital nurses. Teaching is not merely distributing information but also assessing readiness to learn, motivating people to change, removing cultural barriers to learning, and evaluating whether learning has occurred and behaviors have changed.

No other branch of nursing provides as much nursing autonomy or accountability. Home care nurses do not have colleagues with them in clients' homes. Ambulatory clinics are usually managed by the nurses who work in them. Classes in health promotion and disease prevention are usually planned by the nurses who teach them (both formal and informal teaching).

Requires Collaboration and Critical Thinking

Strong collaboration with other health and social service professionals, as well as clients and families, is basic to community health nursing. Awareness of all community resources and how to access them are part of the required body of knowledge. Community health nurses were doing "case management" long before the term and the function became widely known. For example, since the 1960s home care nurses have been collaborating and coordinating the plan of care for Medicare clients who need additional services such as physical therapy, occupational therapy, speech therapy, social work, or home health aides. They are the ones who keep in close contact with physicians.

Community health nursing is complex and challenging. A community health nurse deals with persons of all ages and any variety of situations. It is not unusual for a nurse to visit a teenage mother struggling to care for a premature baby and on the next visit provide care for an elderly, dying client who is almost 100 years old. The Clinical Application case study at the end of this chapter was drawn from actual experience and demonstrates many of the characteristics of community health nursing. Critical thinking skills are necessary because of the many variables that confront community health nurses in complex situations (Table 1-1 and Display 1-4).

History of Community Health Nursing

Florence Nightingale's Holistic Approach

Florence Nightingale is known as the founder of modern nursing because she established the first training school for nurses at St. Thomas' Hospital in London. Earlier, she became famous for saving the lives of countless British soldiers during the Crimean War. Men were dying in great numbers from typhus and other terrible environmental conditions. Despite enormous resentment from military commanders and bureaucratic barriers, Ms. Nightingale and her nurses tackled the problems of sanitation and malnutrition. Because of her work, only 2% of the soldiers died; the prior death rate had been 40%. She returned to England a national heroine. This enabled her to proceed with her life's work of establishing nursing as an educated profession.

TABLE 1-1. Examples of Health Outcomes Related to Goals of Community Health Nursing

	Care of the Ill	Support of Development	Support of Relatedness	Promotion of Self-responsibility	Promotion of Healthful Environment
Person	Person learns self-management of diabetes mellitus	Teenage mother adjusts to newborn care	Retarded adult joins group for socialization	Adult child of alcoholic seeks counseling	Homeless person seeks shelter.
Family	Family cares for member with terminal cancer	Extended family decides how best to care for aging grandparents	Family with disabled child seeks out other such families	Family identifies preferences of members	Elderly couple improves safety in home
Group	Children with physical disabilities are cared for in school	Junior high school students explore responsibility regarding sexual activity	Several women in a residence start a sharing group	Women at a mother and children's center take on responsibilities in the center	Mothers Against Drunk Driving advocates laws against driving while intoxicated
Aggregate	Barriers are identified in a number of patients regarding failure to return for tests of cure after antibiotics	Worksite program regarding preretirement planning is established	*	Worksite program for counseling for health risk reduction is initiated	Curriculum is developed for schools regarding burn prevention
Community	A hospice program is initiated in a city	Regulations for safe day care are passed as county ordinance	A network of case management is established for discharged psychiatric patients	Crisis hotline is established	A waste recycling program is established

* By definition, aggregates are individuals or families with common characteristics who are identified as such by the community health nurse or other professional. If such clients become known to one another and develop a sense of belonging or support, the aggregate would become a group or community.
(Smith C, Maurer F [1995]. *Community Health Nursing*. Philadelphia: WB Saunders.)

Ms. Nightingale's approach was holistic. She emphasized prevention and taught families to care for their sick loved ones. In 1880, she described the role of the nurse:

Besides nursing the patient, she [the nurse] shows them [the family] in their own home how they can help in this nursing, how they can be clean and orderly, how they can call in official sanitary help to make their poor one room more healthy, how they can improvise appliances, how their home need not be broken up.

DISPLAY 1-4
The Inquiring Mind: Critical Thinking in Action

Throughout the critical thinking process, a continuous flow of questions evolves in the thinker's mind. Although the questions vary according to the particular clinical situation, certain general inquiries can serve as a basis for reaching conclusions and determining a course of action.

When faced with a patient situation, it is often helpful to seek answers to some or all of the following questions in an attempt to determine the most appropriate action:

- What relevant assessment information do I need and how do I interpret this information? What does this information tell me?
- What problems does this information point to? Have I identified the most important ones? Does the information point to any other problems that I should consider?
- Have I gathered all the information I need (signs/symptoms, lab values, medication history, emotional factors, mental status)? Is anything missing?
- Is there anything that needs to be reported immediately? Do I need to seek additional assistance?
- Does this patient have any special risk factors? Which ones are most significant? What must I do to minimize these risks?

- What possible complications must I watch for?
- What are the most important problems that we are facing in this situation? Do the patient and the patient's family see the same problems?
- What are the desired outcomes for this patient? Which have the highest priority? Do the patient and I see eye to eye on these points?
- What is going to be my first action in this situation?
- How can I construct a plan of care to achieve the goals?
- Are there any age-related factors involved and will they require some special approach? Will I need to make some change in the plan of care to take these factors into account?
- How do the family dynamics affect this situation, and will this have an impact on my actions or plan of care?
- Are there cultural factors that I must address and consider?
- Am I dealing with an ethical problem here? If so, how am I going to resolve it?
- Has any nursing research been conducted on this subject?

(Smeltzer S, Bare B [1996]. *Textbook of Medical-Surgical Nursing*, 8th ed. Philadelphia: Lippincott-Raven.)

In 1884, she also had some strong things to say about disease prevention:

Preventable disease should be looked upon as a social crime . . . It is much cheaper to promote health than to maintain people in disease . . . Money would be better spent in maintaining health in infancy and childhood than in building hospitals to cure diseases.

More than 100 years later, health planners finally reached the same conclusions.

Evolution of Visiting Nurse Societies

"Visiting nursing," "district nursing," and more recently "home care nursing" are all terms used to describe bedside nursing care delivered in the home by educated, professional nurses. Visiting nursing was begun in Liverpool, England, in 1859 by Mr. Rathbone, a wealthy Quaker businessman who had great concern for the health needs of poor people. After consulting with Florence Nightingale, he established a school to train nurses to nurse poor people in their homes. The effort was enormously successful and the movement spread.

In America, similar programs were established in Buffalo, Boston, and Philadelphia in the late 1880s. As in England, visiting nursing in the United States was first organized by philanthropic laypeople. The large influx of immigrants at that time resulted in overcrowded tenements and rampant health problems. Visiting nurse societies were first established in slum areas to care for the sick poor and to instruct families and neighbors in hygiene, nutrition, and the care of the sick. Such was the case of the Philadelphia Visiting Nurse Society initially. Because of the high quality of care they provided, these nurses were soon asked to care for the sick of all socioeconomic classes, and a fee for service was charged based on ability to pay. This practice spread, but as they evolved, visiting nurse groups varied greatly from place to place. There was no central organizing authority as there was in England. Depending on the sponsors, different services prevailed. This still exists to some extent, although the quality of service remains high. In some rural communities, school nursing, immunization programs, and other traditional public health nursing functions are performed by private visiting nurse societies if there is no nearby public health department.

Lillian Wald's Henry Street Settlement

An American nurse, Lillian Wald, coined the term "public health nursing." Florence Nightingale first used the term "health nursing," but Lillian Wald added the word "public" to emphasize that health should be available to everyone. As a young nurse of 26, her deep concern for the poor immigrants in New York City led her in 1893 to found the Henry Street Settlement House (see the photo at the beginning of Part I). The Henry Street House is still in operation and has provided health and social services for more than 100 years. A recent letter from the Chairman of the Board of Directors outlines 25 programs currently offered to women and children at risk. One example is a family-based HIV/AIDS program to help mothers with AIDS and to help prepare for the care of their children after the mother's death. Bereavement groups for the children are provided to help ease their fear and sense of abandonment.

Lillian Wald was a great nursing leader and social reformer. Establishing the specialty of public health nursing was one of her many accomplishments.

The Evolution of Public Health Nursing

The National Organization for Public Health Nursing was founded by Lillian Wald in 1888. Ten years later, the Los Angeles Health Department began hiring public health nurses (PHNs), and soon other health departments followed. Since then, public health nursing has been government-sponsored and tax-supported. Most PHNs work for health departments on a county, city, or state level. Their task is primarily health promotion and disease prevention, mainly working with groups. They do immunization and screening programs as well as formal and informal health education. In some locations where gaps in medical services exist, PHNs also perform personal services in facilities such as general medical clinics and women's health clinics. Some PHNs do epidemiologic work among high-risk aggregates. Maternal-child health programs include home visits to poor families or those with multiple problems.

The Evolution of Rural Nursing

Nursing services in rural areas evolved much more slowly. Sparsely populated areas may be served only in limited ways by some form of a state health department. County health departments provide various degrees of nursing service in most rural areas. Historically, the Red Cross and the Metropolitan Life Insurance Company assumed responsibility for the administration of rural nursing, which was privately funded until the 1940s, when health departments assumed this responsibility. The Frontier Nursing Service, founded in 1925 by Mary Breckenridge, was famous for delivering nursing service on horseback to isolated families in Appalachia. It is still delivering nursing care to disadvantaged or isolated families, sometimes by Jeep instead of horseback. The Indian Health Service provides care to Native Americans on reservations and for Eskimos. Work in camps of agricultural migrant workers also began during the past century and continues today.

There is no doubt, however, that nursing and medical services have not been readily available to most Americans living in rural areas. It is a surprise to many people that farming is rated the most dangerous of all occupations. The widespread idea that rural life is so healthy is a myth.

The Evolution of Community Health Nursing

During the 1970s, there was great interest in community life and in providing services to underserved communities throughout the United States. A wealth of sponsors of various affiliations began providing community social and health services. Many small storefront agencies and larger comprehensive agencies, as well as rural health centers, were established. The term "community health nursing" came into being. It is used by the ANA to include these various care settings and styles as well as the traditional care provided by visiting nurses and PHNs. Community health nursing is now an all-encompassing term that includes all the subspecialties of nurses who work in the community.

Current Practice Dimensions of Community Health Nursing

The present practice of community health nursing takes place in three dimensions: wellness care (health promotion and disease prevention); ambulatory care; and home care. Some community health nurses may work in all three dimensions in the course of a day, but most nurses work primarily in one of these fields. Employment opportunities exist primarily in one or another of these fields. Each of these dimensions is described in detail in Parts II, III, and IV of this text.

Employment Prospects and Educational Requirements

Nurses are aware that the nursing shortage is over, but even so, nursing was listed as second highest of the "15 Hottest Fields" in which to find employment (Greenwald, 1997). The projected growth of nursing jobs, according to the Bureau of Labor Statistics, is 473,000 between 1994 and 2005. However, some new graduates cannot find employment because of hospital staff reductions. The ANA has asked the Department of Labor to remove registered nurses from its shortage list.

However, employment opportunities exist for registered nurses in community health. Most openings are in home care agencies. The registered nurses may be associate degree or diploma graduates. They may be seeking a baccalaureate degree in nursing (BSN) while working. Some agencies hire only staff with BSNs or registered nurses who are working on their BSN. Certainly, leadership positions require a BSN or a master's degree in nursing.

There are also many job opportunities for registered nurses in ambulatory care. The educational requirements vary with the type of position. Nurses assisting in doctors' offices, emergency rooms, same-day surgical suites, outpatient departments, and some clinics may be required to be only registered nurses. Nurse practitioners who perform primary care should have a master's degree. Most public school systems now require school nurses to have at least a BSN. Health promotion and disease prevention work is done by PHNs employed by health departments. Most PHNs are required to have a BSN with a state-approved course in community health nursing. Some states hire registered nurses and enroll them in a course in community health nursing offered by that particular state. If the nurse completes the course and passes an examination, state approval for PHN status is granted.

Many nurses work as case managers for managed-care systems, and this trend will expand. Generally, experienced nurses with at least a BSN are sought for these positions, which require highly developed critical thinking skills.

As more and more hospitals merge and reduce their nursing staffs by closing patient care units, more nurses are leaving hospital work and moving into the community to work. This trend has been increasing since 1990. In 1995, more than 1,400 registered nurse positions were eliminated in New York City. However, by the middle of the decade, two thirds of nurses were still working in hospitals where only 40% of the beds were occupied. The movement of nurses into the community will intensify. In the coming century, the vast majority of nurses will be working in community health positions, reversing the nurse staffing patterns of the 20th century (Fig. 1-2).

Main Problems Affecting Community Health Nursing

Infectious diseases are a great concern to health-care workers. Historically, the fight against diseases such as tuberculosis has been within the domain of community health nurses. Pneumonia (4.4 million cases) and tuberculosis (3.1 million) are still the leading infectious causes of death in the world according to the World Health Organization in 1996 (Associated Press, 1996). Tuberculosis in the United States seemed well controlled until about 15 years ago, when a serious resurgence began.

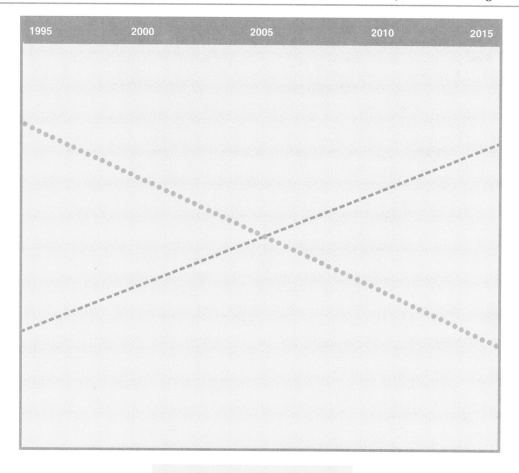

1995 2000 2005 2010 2015

% Hospital work ●●●●●●●●●●●●●●
% Community work ▬▬▬▬▬▬▬▬▬▬

FIGURE 1-2
The migration of nurses from hospitals to commmunity work.

Since 1992, the prevalence of tuberculosis has been declining again (CDC, 1997). A particular threat is the development of drug-resistant strains. The cure rate for drug-resistant tuberculosis is only 50%, and the disease is often fatal.

Health-care workers can use protective measures such as special masks and interview rooms with negative air flow that lowers transmission of the organisms. These measures are used with suspected cases. However, health-care workers cannot always protect themselves from infections transmitted by airborne droplets. Sharing the air with people who unknowingly have active tuberculosis is sometimes unavoidable. Fortunately, tuberculosis transmission usually requires frequent, close contact.

Also of great concern are other drug-resistant bacterial organisms such as *Staphylococcus aureus* and streptococcus A. Although not spread by airborne droplets, they nonetheless pose a threat to health-care workers. Conscientious adherence to universal precautions provides protection.

Although the use of combination drugs against AIDS has shown encouraging results, AIDS is still a fatal disease and therefore a grave concern to all health-care workers. Health-care workers who have an accidental needle stick with an HIV-contaminated needle are now immediately offered treatment with zidovudine (AZT), indinavir (Crixivan), and lamivudine (Epivir) when indicated (Gerberdine, 1996). As new drugs develop, latest protocols are available on the Internet at http://epi-center.UCSF.edu.com.

A vaccine is available to protect health-care workers against hepatitis B virus, a serious disease whose incidence is on the rise in the United States. The federal Occupational Safety & Health Administration requires that hepatitis B vaccine be made available free of charge by employers to all workers engaged in direct patient care. The vaccine is given in three injections for optimal protection. The second injection is given 1 month after the first, and the third injection is given 6 months later. The level of hepatitis B antibodies in the blood can be monitored to ensure adequate immunization against the disease. Sometimes postexposure protection is given in the form of hepatitis B immune globulin (HBIg). After an accidental needle stick from an infected client, HBIg can be given if the nurse lacks active immunity. Immune globulin provides passive immunity with antibodies produced by someone else. Passive immunity acts quickly but lasts only about 2 months and is not as effective as active immunity. It is better practice to be immunized with hepatitis B vaccine long before possible exposure to the disease. For example, many people do not realize that hepatitis B virus can survive in dried blood on bed linens at room temperature. Hepatitis B vaccine is now given to newborns to promote herd immunity. Herd immunity results in failure of the virus to spread when a high proportion of the population have antibodies against infection. Hepatitis A, B, and C infections are a lifelong contraindication for blood donation.

Current social problems such as crime and violence are reflected in Table 1-2, which shows the leading causes of death. Other social problems, such as addictions, homelessness, and teenage pregnancy, profoundly affect the work of community health nurses. Visiting nurses used to be safe in crime-ridden neighborhoods because they were recognized by their uniforms and nursing bags and were left alone by criminals

TABLE 1-2. Leading Causes of Death for American Adults Aged 15 to Over 65 Years

Age 15–24	25–44	45–64	65 and Over
Accidents (motor vehicle)	Accidents (motor vehicle)	Cancer	Heart disease
Homicide and legal intervention	Cancer	Heart disease	Cancer
Suicide	HIV	CVA	CVA
Cancer	Heart disease	Accidents	COPD
Heart disease	Homicide and legal intervention	COPD	Pneumonia and flu
HIV	Suicide	Chronic liver disease	Diabetes
		Diabetes	Accidents

CVA, cerebrovascular accident; COPD, chronic obstructive pulmonary disease; HIV, human immunodeficiency virus
(U.S. Bureau of the Census [1994]. *Statistical Abstract of the United States, 1994*, 114th ed. Washington DC: U.S. Government Printing Office)

who knew they served the sick. Today, nursing bags are a target for drug addicts seeking syringes and drugs. Visiting nurses no longer carry their distinctive black bags or wear uniforms for this reason; most do not even carry purses. In some high-crime neighborhoods or buildings, escorts are needed to provide safety for nurses.

Community health nurses may find themselves involved in situations of child or elder abuse, and must report these situations to the appropriate authorities and sometimes testify in court. Care of populations at risk such as the mentally ill, the chemically dependent, and the homeless usually falls within the domain of community health nursing. These populations are fragile and vulnerable to disease. Their situations can become incredibly complex and require enormous problem-solving skills, critical thinking, perseverance, and compassion from the nurse.

Despite these problems, community health nurses find their work deeply satisfying, some because of the diversity of clients and situations and others because of the autonomy and problem-solving challenges. Other nurses cite the relevance of this field to the problems of society as the reason they love community health nursing.

The Outlook for Community Health Nursing Into the 21st Century

A humorous forecast about the future is shown in Figure 1-3. It seems outrageous, but the following forecasts are not; in fact, they are already happening.

Anticipated Growth With Increased Autonomy and Accountability

The need for more nurses in community health is obvious; the field is expanding rapidly. For example, the total number of certified agencies providing hospice service nearly

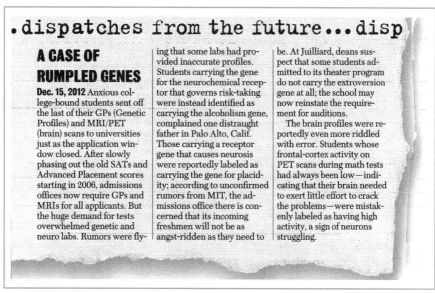

FIGURE 1-3
A humorous forecast of the future. (© 1997, Newsweek, Inc. All rights reserved. Reprinted by permission.)

tripled from 1989 to 1994, according to the National Association of Home Care's inventory of home care agencies. The number of privately owned (proprietary) agencies is increasing even more rapidly. Health-care reform will open more jobs for nurses in primary care and prevention. The shift from acute care to community care is estimated to create as many as 700,000 jobs in community health for nurses. According to *The Johns Hopkins Medical Letter* (1997), the home care industry is growing at a rate of 12% per year. Nurses will become more autonomous but also more accountable, particularly as they move into primary care and case management. Quality management programs will take on even greater importance because of the impact of cost-saving measures.

Expanding Certifications, Educational Needs, Competencies, and Subspecializations

The need for educational advancement will increase for community health nurses because of the complexity of their role. Good critical thinking skills are essential, and education promotes critical thinking. Display 1-5 lists the skills that will be needed by practitioners in the year 2005. Although some entry-level jobs will be available for associate degree and diploma school graduates, nurses will need to expand their education in the future. A BSN or higher will be the desired standard for community health nurses.

Voluntary certifications will carry even greater weight by verifying knowledge and

---

DISPLAY 1-5
Competencies Needed By Practitioners for 2005

Practitioners for 2005 should:
- Care for the community's health
- Expand access to effective care
- Provide contemporary clinical care
- Emphasize primary care
- Participate in coordinated care
- Ensure cost-effective and appropriate care
- Practice prevention
- Involve patients and families in the decision-making process
- Promote healthy lifestyles
- Assess and use technology appropriately
- Improve the health-care system
- Manage information
- Understand the role of the physical environment
- Provide counseling on ethical issues
- Accommodate expanded accountability
- Participate in a racially and culturally diverse society
- Continue to learn

(*Shugars DA, Bader JD, eds [1991]*. Healthy America: Practitioners for 2005, An Agenda for Action for U.S. Health Professional Schools. *Durham, NC: The Pew Health Professions Commission.*)

experience at generalist and expert levels. Certifications require many hours of experience before one can even sit for the rigorous examinations. Generalist certification is now available in community health, home health, hospice, and school and college nursing. Clinical specialists in community health and school nurse practitioner certifications are available with a master's degree. The end of the nursing shortage will mean more competition for job openings in community health, and certification and additional education will count heavily in securing employment and promotions.

Subspecialization within community health nursing will continue to increase. High-technology home care is an example. At present, special agencies provide infusion therapy or even only total parenteral nutrition to home care clients. Some nurses specialize in communicable disease nursing; some specialize even further and become tuberculosis nurses.

Multistate Regulation of Nursing Licensure

The National Council of State Boards of Nursing is studying the issues of multistate regulation and developing methodology. At present, boards of nursing in each state regulate the practice of nursing and issue nursing licenses according to respective state laws. Because nursing licensure laws vary from state to state, this is not an efficient system. New practice modalities and technologies are raising questions about compliance with state licensing laws. Community nursing practice is increasingly occurring across state lines, requiring multiple licensing, which is a cumbersome process.

In the future, multistate regulation will become more efficient and cost-effective. Features will include core standards for licensure in all states, a central database of licenses, and expedient processing of licensure applications. State-based authority and licensure linked to the state of residency are likely to be retained (Multistate Regulation Task Force, 1996).

Increasing Use of Technical Tools for Work and Research

The use of computers in health care is well established, but their full capabilities have just begun to be plumbed. Some home care agencies supply notebook or hand-held computers for use by home care nurses in the field. Programs to reduce the voluminous documentation needed in home care are being developed. Many community health nurses are "surfing the Internet" and finding a wealth of useful information on the World Wide Web. Cyberspace offers an open, unmoderated, global electronic forum to share ideas and discuss nursing issues on Nursenet (http://www.oise.on.ca/-jnorris/nursenet/nn.html). Several publications are on-line, such as *Computers in Nursing* (http://cin.lrpub.com/cin), *American Journal of Nursing* (http://www.ajn.org), and *Journal of Nursing Jocularity* (http://www.jocularity.com). The *Cumulative Index of Nursing and Allied Health Literature* (http://www.cinahl.com) is available for an annual fee. Table 1-3 lists more resources available on the Internet.

Nursing research will be needed as never before to ensure that quality care is being delivered and that client outcomes are satisfactory. Rapid changes in the health-care system and cutbacks in services in an effort to contain the astronomic costs of health

(text continues on p. 20)

TABLE 1-3. Hot Sites

To take advantage of the vast amount of health care information on the Internet, you need two essentials: A directory or search engine and a place to go; that is, the addresses of the best medical and nursing sites. The table below provides both.

Once you find your favorite Web sites, most Internet browsers will let you place a "bookmark" at each of those locations. You can then retrieve a list of these markers, allowing you to go directly to each site without typing in its address again.

Directories and Search Engines

Site	Address	Comments
AltaVista	http://www.altavista.digital.com	AltaVista is one of the fastest, most powerful search services, with a database of millions of Web sites and newsgroups.
CliniWeb	http://www.ohsu .edu/cliniweb/search.html	A search engine that categorizes sites by medical subject heading (MeSH) terms
Internet Sleuth	http://www.intbc .com/sleuth/medi.html	A search engine that lets you choose from two dozen medical databases with a single request form
Lycos	http://www.lycos.com	General purpose search engine
Matrix	http://www.slackinc.com	A searchable directory that reviews more than 1,000 medical Web sites
MedWeb	http://www.cc.emory .edu/WHSCL/medweb.html	MedWeb is one of the largest directories of health sites. You can find the subject you want by either using their search engine or by choosing key words to view lists of topics.
Yahoo	http://www.yahoo.com	General purpose search engine

Health Care Resources: Diseases and Specialties

Site	Address	Comments
ACLS Algorithms	http://www.cardiac.org/aclsalgr .html#algor	This offers a series of instructions on how to do advanced cardiac life support. By using hypertext links, it takes you step by step through all the branches of the ACLS algorithm tree.
American Diabetes Association	http://www.diabetes.org	This site covers pathophysiology and treatment, as well as details on different kinds of insulin.
Digital Anatomist	http://www1.biostr.washington .edu/DigitalAnatomist.html	This site offers an interactive anatomy atlas, with two- and three-dimensional pictures of various regions of the body. Each picture is linked to a wealth of textual information.
Drug Formulary	http://www.intmed.mcw .edu/drug.html	This Web page lets you enter the brand name of a drug and, within a few seconds, gives you a table showing the generic name, the formulation—tablet, oral suspension, etc.—dosage, and cost.
Nutrition	http://www.fsci.umn .edu/tools.htp	By typing a specific food into the search form, the site provides the amount of each nutrient contained in the food.

TABLE 1-3. *(Continued)*

Health Care Resources: Diseases and Specialties

Site	Address	Comments
PharmInfoNet	http://pharminfo.com	This site provides an alphabetic online formulary with links to articles from the *Medical Sciences Bulletin,* an online newsletter on drug therapy.
Psychiatry On-Line	http://www.priory.com/journals/psych.htm	An independent, peer-reviewed electronic journal
RxList	http://www.rxlist.com/	A searchable drug index that includes drug interactions for the most commonly used agents

Health Care Resources: General Clinical Sites

Site	Address	Comments
Centers for Disease Control and Prevention	http://www.cdc.gov	The CDC puts two journals online. *Morbidity and Mortality Weekly Report* (MMWR) and *Emerging Infectious Diseases.* You can also find extensive guidelines on infection control, immunizations, and hazardous substances.
Hospital Web	http://neuro-www.mgh.harvard.edu/hospitalweb.nclk	This site helps you to locate the Web sites of hospitals and medical organizations in the U.S. and around the world.
Laboratory Values	http://www.ghsl.nwu.edu/Norm.html	This online book gives normal lab values for blood, CSF, sweat, and urine, all in table form.
Online Clinical Calculator	http://www.intmed.mcw.edu/clincalc.html	The calculator lets you insert a patient's weight in pounds or his temperature in degrees Fahrenheit and then instantly converts it to kilograms and degrees Celsius. There are also electronic tools to quickly determine body surface area, body mass index, anion gap, and creatinine clearance.
Physical Exam	http://www.medinfo..ufl.edu/year1/bcs/clist/index.html	An online textbook offering basic instructions on how to take a complete history and do a physical, with diagrams
Virtual Hospital	http://vh.radiology.uiowa.edu	This site contains information on a number of medical specialties and includes teaching files, guidelines, patient simulations, and multimedia textbooks.

Health Care Resources: Nursing Sites

Site	Address	Comments
MedWeb: Nursing	http://www.gen.emory.edu/MEDWEB/keyword/Nursing.html	A list of hypertext links to upcoming nursing conferences, electronic publications, and professional associations

TABLE 1-3. (*Continued*)

Health Care Resources: Nursing Sites

Site	Address	Comments
Nursing and Health Care Resources	http://www.bath.ac.uk/-exxrw/nurse.html	A list of hundreds of Web sites, newsgroups, and mailing lists on nursing, alternative therapy, mental health, midwifery, and related fields
Nursing index	http://www.lib.umich.edu/tml/nursing.html	A well-annotated reference to nursing sites on the Web that cover career opportunities, discussion groups, organizations, and nursing research
Perioperative Nursing Resources on the Internet	http://www.aorn.org/nsgtoday/internet/links.htm	A good site to find OR nursing and general nursing information, including e-mail lists, research resources, and nursing organizations

Health Care Resources: Patient Education Sites

Site	Address	Comments
AIDS Pathfinder	http://www.nnlm.nlm.nih.gov/pnr/etc/aidspath.html	This site will point you to major collections of documents, organizations, and discussion groups on AIDS.
CancerNet	http://www.nci.nih.gov/hpage/cis.htm	This site is a service of the National Institutes of Health that contains hundreds of handouts on different cancers. Each comes in two versions: one for professionals and one for the public. Many are available in Spanish as well.
MedHelp International	http://medhlp.netusa.net/index.htm	One of the best patient handout sites. Its main library offers documents on hundreds of conditions and there are also specialized libraries on cancer, brain tumors, drugs, and mental health.
1-800 Numbers for Patient Support Organizations	http://infonet.welch.jhu.edu/advocacy.html	The phone numbers for patient support groups are often linked to related Web sites.

(Hutchinson D. A nurse's guide to the Internet. *RN Magazine*, January 1997.)

care demand close outcome monitoring and evaluation. We must ensure that limited funds are most appropriately used. Nursing research will increase in importance as the profession seeks to justify and demonstrate its value in a climate of decreased funding for all health care. Nurses must become computer-literate so they can use this valuable tool for research. In 1993 the National Center for Nursing Research (now known as the National Institute of Nursing Research) established priorities for research (Display 1-6).

Tools of the electronic age are helping to make the work of community health nurses more efficient. Voice mail, cellular telephones, fax machines, e-mail, and laptop computers are being used more and more in community nursing practice.

DISPLAY 1-6
Priorities Resulting From the Second Conference on Research Priorities in Nursing Practice, National Institute for Nursing Research

1—Community-based Nursing Models (1995)

Develop and test community-based nursing models designed to promote access to, use of, and quality of health services by rural and other underserved populations.

2—Health-promoting Behavior and HIV/AIDS (1996)

Assess the effectiveness of biobehavioral nursing interventions to foster health-promoting behaviors of different cultural backgrounds—especially women—who are at high risk for HIV/AIDS, incorporating biobehavioral markers.

3—Cognitive Impairment (1997)

Develop and test biobehavioral and environmental approaches to remediating cognitive impairment.

4—Living with Chronic Illness (1998)

Test interventions to strengthen resources in dealing with chronic illness.

5—Biobehavioral Factors Related to Immunocompetence (1999)

Identify biobehavioral factors and test interventions to promote immunocompetence.

(*National Institute for Nursing Research [1993].* Priorities Resulting From Second Conference on Research Priorities in Nursing Practice. *Bethesda, MD: The Institute.*)

Changes in the Health-Care System

Debate rages about proposed changes in health care in the United States. Proposals such as medical savings accounts are being piloted. States are experimenting with different models of home care, including these medical savings accounts. Uncertainty prevails about the kind of system that will emerge. The goal of universal health insurance remains important in an advanced nation where more than 40 million people have no health coverage. Financial constraints are a priority to reduce the increasing cost of health care. Managed-care systems have helped somewhat, but some form of rationing seems inevitable. Financial constraints will help drive the expansion of community nursing: expensive institutional care continues to be decreased, and home care is more cost-effective than hospital or nursing home care. For instance, the state of New York has a long-term care program to replace nursing home care. Called Nursing Homes Without Walls, its purpose is to reduce Medicaid costs. Clients on Medicaid at home receive all the available services of institutional long-term care if their cost does not exceed 75% of the cost of institutional care.

Financial constraints may cause ethical dilemmas for nurses if they are pressured to discharge clients from home care services because of lack of funding. Some managed-care programs limit the number of home nursing visits. See Chapters 2, 9, and 13 for more information about managed care.

Evolving Image and Political Power of Nurses

The image of nursing is poor in this country. Many archaic stereotypes prevail, such as ''doctors' handmaidens,'' ''pill pushers,'' and even ''bedpan carriers.'' A few years ago, a television program about student nurses was so demeaning and insulting that the National Student Nurses Association protested vigorously to the network and the program was canceled. As more nurses work in the community and in primary care, we hope that this image will improve. This will not happen, however, unless nurses work intentionally to promote the image of the profession.

Based on sheer numbers, nurses have great potential for political power. There are 2.3 million nurses in the United States, 83% of whom are working (U.S. Department of Health & Human Services, 1994). However, so many nurses are juggling jobs and family responsibilities that they say they have no time for political activity. Only a few are members of the ANA, their state nursing association, or even their local district association. These are the professional organizations that speak for nurses politically. If nursing is to be influential in the emerging health-care arena, nurses must seek to improve the public image and political power of the profession.

DISPLAY 1-7
Profile of the American People, the Year 2000

The total population of the United States will have grown to nearly 270 million people from 254 million in 1990. The rate of growth between 1995 and 2000 is expected to be the slowest in the nation's history.

Between 1990 and 2000, 6 million people will have migrated to the United States, primarily to the East and West Coasts.

The population will be older, with the median age being greater than 36 years (in 1975 it was 29 years). Persons 65 years and older will constitute 13% of the population; 4.6 million people will be older than 85 years.

There will be fewer children younger than 5 years of age (17 million, compared with 18 million in 1990).

Average household size will be smaller at 2.48 people (compared with 2.69 in 1985).

Racial and ethnic composition will be different. The proportion of whites will decline from 76% to 72% of the population. The proportion of blacks, Hispanics, and others (including American Indians, Alaska Natives, Asians, and Pacific Islanders) will increase to 28%. The Hispanic population will have grown at the fastest rate during the 1990s.

(Data from U.S. Department of Health and Human Services [1990]. Healthy People 2000: National Health Promotion and Disease Prevention Objectives. Summary Report. Washington DC: Government Printing Office.)

Display 1-7 shows a profile of the U.S. population in the year 2000. Health care, too, is changing in many ways. Organ transplants, the development of artificial body parts, advances in genetics, and new knowledge of the brain are examples of our expanding horizons. Greater awareness of the importance of spirituality and its effect on health is emerging from surveys and research studies. Dr. Herbert Benson, a professor of behavioral medicine at Harvard Medical School and the founder of The Mind/Body Institute, says, "Practicing medicine and conducting medical research for the past 30 years, I've learned that involving beliefs is not only emotionally and spiritually soothing, but vitally important to physical health" (Benson, 1997).

THE NURSE SPEAKS . . .
About the Spiritual Needs of a Client

Walt, age 68, had metastatic cancer of the prostate. When I first met him, his loving wife, and his son, I considered them to be an average family.

On subsequent visits, I noted that Walt continued to have severe chronic achy pain attributable to bone metastasis. Trilisate 1,000 mg t.i.d. had been ordered by his doctor because it is effective for bone pain. Walt seemed very lax about taking his pain medication, and I was puzzled. About my fourth or fifth visit, when I gently confronted him about this inconsistency, he confided, "I haven't been a good man. I haven't been honest and I haven't treated my wife right. I deserve this. I deserve to be punished for my life, and I believe that when I die God will punish me. I'm hoping this awful pain I'm having now will help when I die. Maybe God will be kinder to me because I've suffered."

I looked at him with all the tenderness I was feeling and said that I didn't believe God was harsh and punishing. We talked about God on that and subsequent visits. I conferred with our hospice chaplain and received guidance about talking with Walt. As we talked, Walt began to acknowledge the loving, forgiving, and merciful nature of God. Sometimes we prayed silently together. Of course I did not push a particular theology on him, but one day I asked him if he would like a member of the clergy to visit. He said he would like that but didn't think he deserved it. He added that although he had been raised a Catholic, he had not practiced his religion since childhood. With his consent, I made arrangements for a priest to come and also helped him talk to his family about his regrets. He apologized to his wife for not being a better husband and asked for forgiveness, which she freely gave him.

By this time he was feeling less pain and taking his pain medication as ordered. He was sleeping better as a result. His relationship with his family opened up and improved, and they were able to talk freely about many things. The priest visited several times. Walt said, "I feel restored. I feel God loves me and I can trust him about the future even when I die." Walt died a peaceful death about 3 weeks later.

It is so important that nurses be sensitive to the spiritual needs of their clients and encourage them to talk about their beliefs. We must be willing to make sure that appropriate spiritual care is offered to them.

Anne
HOSPICE NURSE

CLINICAL APPLICATION

A Critical Thinking Case Study About a Family With Multiple Problems

You are a PHN working for the department of health in a southwestern city. You receive a referral from a prenatal clinic to visit Maria Sanchez because she has missed appointments and has no telephone. You find her in her eighth month of pregnancy. She asks if you would check her rash "down there." She adds that the rash has been coming and going for years. On examination, you discover that Maria has active genital herpes; otherwise, her status appears healthy. The fetal heartbeat is 140 beats per minute, strong and regular.

The two-room apartment is crowded but clean. A young girl named Yolanda is playing on the floor. She does not move normally and on closer observation appears to be blind. Maria explains that Yolanda is 5 years old and has not been able to see since she was a baby. She adds that people told her that Yolanda's blindness was due to Maria's rash, but she never believed it. She adds that Yolanda has not been seen by a doctor for a long time because Alberto, her husband, has not been able to work and he is too proud to let her apply for help from the government.

Alberto is present but seems withdrawn and sullen. Although the couple tell you they came to the United States shortly after Yolanda's birth, neither has a very good command of English. Fortunately, you speak some Spanish. Alberto tells you he is a taxi driver but cannot drive anymore, which is why Maria missed her prenatal clinic appointments. He explains that he worked very long hours and saved extra money; their savings have been supporting the family since he became unemployed. He refuses to apply for welfare because people think those on welfare are lazy and he is not lazy. Ironically, the reason he cannot drive seems to be his eyes. From his vague description, it sounds like he may have a serious condition such as retinitis pigmentosa.

 and Think!

- What is this family's most immediate need?
- How will you address it?
- What will you do first?
- Would you call this primary, secondary, or tertiary prevention?
- What financial considerations might complicate this situation?
- How will you go about solving this complication?
- What will you tell the family when you revisit? Why?
- What information did you assume and forget to verify?
- Why is it ironic that Alberto has a vision problem?

Recognizing the danger of a newborn contracting herpes during a vaginal delivery, as well as the fact that Maria is in her eighth gestational month, you put in an urgent call to the clinic nursing supervisor and the obstetrician. You inform them that the previous child, Yolanda, no doubt contracted herpes during her delivery and it resulted in blindness. Prevention will safeguard the newborn. The cost of the necessary cesarean section and hospitalization is a big problem, because you assume the family has no health insurance and Alberto refuses to accept Medicaid. You had told the family you would visit the next morning because of the urgent need for a cesarean section. You had assumed they did not have medical insurance, and you need to verify this on your next visit.

Maria delivered a healthy baby boy by cesarean section. After you carefully explained that Medicaid is not the same as welfare and that many working people with low incomes receive Medicaid, Alberto agreed, with some reluctance, to accept Medicaid for the sake of his family's health needs. You also instructed him about the Office of Vocational Rehabilitation and the job retraining and employment help available. They will provide follow-up on his vision problem. You help Alberto set up an appointment after you explain to him that this is a service he helped pay for with his taxes.

The family has a serious transportation problem. You sit down with Maria and Alberto, review some bus schedules, and work on their transportation problems together. They agree that Alberto's brother and a friend in their building could be asked to drive them occasionally if they helped pay for gas and car upkeep. Maria will ride the bus to and from her house-cleaning jobs when she resumes them. Medicaid will provide transportation for important medical care.

 and Think!

- Who is the client in this case?
- Why didn't you refer the family's transportation and job training needs to a social worker?
- Define the other unmet needs of this family. How will you address them?

You visit daily for 3 days during the immediate postpartum period to monitor the mother and baby because Maria was discharged only 48 hours after delivery. She requires a great deal of health teaching and information about community resources, so you decide this family needs weekly visits for a few weeks. The whole family is the client and they have learned to trust you, which is why you do not make a social worker referral. You provide information about a food bank in a nearby church because you see that money is in short supply and that Maria is motivated to cook nutritious meals for her family once she understands the importance and has the resources. You refer her to the women's health clinic for her herpes and for contraception. You gently teach her about the chronic nature of her herpes and the risk to future newborns. One day she says they have decided that she will have a tubal ligation.

"Yolanda will probably always be with us as our baby. It's enough for us. This way we won't have to worry about making other babies blind," she explains.

Yolanda has many needs. You arrange for her to be seen in the pediatric clinic. You call the local society for the blind and learn that they accept children her age for training to function with blindness. They admit both her and Alberto for therapy. Through the school system, you learn that physical therapy is available for her if her parents apply. They are pleased with these opportunities for her. They also respond to your teaching regarding her need for special attention from them in light of the newborn's invasion of her world. Yolanda proudly helps Maria take the baby for his check-ups and immunizations at the free well-child clinic run by the local health department.

 and Think!

- Refer back to the characteristics of community health nursing at the beginning of this chapter and identify the characteristics that are demonstrated in this case. This situation turned out well. What are some of the obstacles you might have encountered?
- Many health departments are cutting back on services for financial reasons. What do you think the outcome would have been for this family if nursing visits were limited to just two or three or if clinic services were unavailable?

Chapter SUMMARY

This chapter described the characteristics of community health nursing, a nursing specialty with subspecialties. It is community-focused but not entirely community-based. It deals with clients who exercise more independence than hospitalized patients, and it deals with them in a social context that includes families, groups, geographic communities, or aggregates. Community nursing emphasizes advocacy, health promotion, and disease prevention. The three levels of prevention were defined. The complex and collaborative nature of community nursing was described, as well as the need for critical thinking.

The history of community health nursing was traced from Florence Nightingale to the evolution of the term "community health nursing" since the 1970s. The present practice of community nursing occurs in three basic dimensions

1. Wellness care (health promotion and disease prevention)
2. Ambulatory care (treatment as well as wellness care)
3. Home care (treatment delivered to homebound clients)

Current employment opportunities and educational requirements were discussed. The roles of case managers and primary care providers were described, and the magnitude of the shift from hospital nursing to community nursing was discussed.

The problems currently affecting community health nurses include safety issues such as the risk of contracting serious infectious diseases (drug-resistant tuberculosis, *Staphylococcus aureus*, streptococcus A, and HIV/AIDS) and the risk of working in high-crime neighborhoods. Community nurses may also deal with social problems of high-risk populations such as the mentally ill, the chemically dependent, and the homeless, as well as family violence.

The field of community health nursing is expected to grow, with increasing autonomy and accountability for nurses. Competencies, certifications, and education requirements are of increasing importance. The day-to-day work of community health nursing is increasingly dependent on the computer and other electronic tools, and the need for nursing research remains strong. Managed-care systems, advances in technology, new knowledge of the brain and genetics, and the importance of the spiritual dimension will affect community health nursing powerfully as we enter the new century. Further changes in the health-care system are expected to occur with a priority on curbing costs. More nurses must be involved in improving the public image and political influence of the profession if nursing is to have a strong impact on the future direction of health care.

A list of references and additional readings for this chapter appears at the end of Part 1.

2

The System and Financing of Health Care in the United States

Key Terms

Aid to Families with Dependent Children (AFDC)

American Public Health Association

block grants

Blue Cross, Blue Shield

capitation

case management

case managers

client outcomes

consensus

cost containment

cost shifting

defensive medicine

deficit budgets

Department of Health & Human Services

diagnostic related groups (DRGs)

district nursing

duplication of coverage

entitlement programs

escalating costs

fee-for-service

free market approach

gag rules

gatekeeper

Health Care Financing Administration (HCFA)

health-care rationing

health-care system

health departments

Health Insurance Portability & Accountability Act

health maintenance organizations (HMOs)

indemnity insurance

infant mortality rates

insurance premiums

Kaiser Permanente program

laissez-faire

laparoscopic surgery

legislature

lifestyle behaviors

long-term care insurance

malpractice insurance

managed-care systems

managed competition

maximum reimbursement

Medicaid

medically indigent

medical savings accounts (MSA)

Medicare

mortality rates

National Committee for Quality Assurance (NCQA)

national health plan

point-of-service riders (POS)

preexisting conditions

preferred provider organizations (PPOs)

primary provider

private sector

proprietary agency

prospective payment

public health agencies

public sector

quality assurance

quality management

rationing

regulatory power

retrospective

shared risk

Social Security

third-party payment

underinsured

universal coverage

utilization review

welfare approach

welfare-oriented system

working poor

World Health Organization (WHO)

Learning Objectives

1. Outline the private and public agencies that make up the community health system.

2. Relate the U.S. Department of Health & Human Services to the U.S. Public Health Service, the Centers for Disease Control & Prevention, and local health departments.

3. Identify the greatest potential problem that threatens international health.

4. Explain why U.S. health care is called both wonderful and terrible.

5. Compare the U.S. health care system with that of other industrialized nations.

6. Define universal coverage.

7. Trace the history of a national health-care plan in the United States.

8. Describe nine causes of rising health-care costs.

9. Compare and contrast Medicare and Medicaid.

10. Define managed care, gatekeeper, capitation, case managers, health maintenance organization, preferred provider organization, and point-of-service riders.

11. Compare traditional fee-for-service indemnity insurance with prospective-payment managed-care plans.

12. Explain how managed-care plans work.

13. Describe three major components of the Health Insurance Portability & Accountability Act of 1996.

14. Identify future legislative needs that have top priority with the American people.

15. Explain the issues involved with Medicaid block grants to states.

The Community Health-Care System

The community health-care system consists of many types of agencies. Some agencies are government-sponsored, such as local and state health departments. Others, such as home care agencies, are sponsored by private and public hospitals, health departments, or nonprofit community agencies such as visiting nurse societies, or are proprietary (privately owned) companies. These agencies were developed in response to local needs but have little centralized planning. Ambulatory care is offered in a wide variety of forms and settings and is discussed in Part III of this text. Part II discusses the various programs to promote health and prevent disease.

Public health agencies were developed as a subgroup of community health and are government-sponsored. County or city health departments are responsible for the public health in a specific area, be it rural, suburban, or urban. Financial support for these agencies comes from local, state, and federal taxes (Fig. 2-1). Each state has some form of a state health department, although they often differ. In many states, the health department exercises strong regulatory power over both private and public health care, sets standards for health planning, and engages in policy determination. Nongovernmental insurance companies are also involved with regulation oversight of health care.

The Department of Health & Human Services is the top federal agency responsible for the health of the nation. This agency consists of many divisions, including the U.S. Public Health Service (Fig. 2-2). Founded in 1798, the U.S. Public Health Service is directed by the assistant secretary for health and is responsible for the following agencies:

1. Agency for Health Care Policy and Research
2. Agency for Toxic Substances and Disease Registry

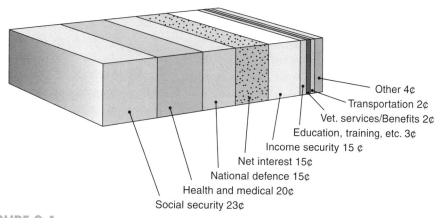

Other 4¢
Transportation 2¢
Vet. services/Benefits 2¢
Education, training, etc. 3¢
Income security 15 ¢
Net interest 15¢
National defence 15¢
Health and medical 20¢
Social security 23¢

FIGURE 2-1
Where your federal tax dollar will go, FY 1998. (Tax Foundation calculations based on projections from the Office of Management and Budget.)

3. Alcohol, Drug Abuse and Mental Health Administration
4. Centers for Disease Control and Prevention
5. Food and Drug Administration
6. Health Resources and Service Administration
7. Indian Health Service
8. National Institutes of Health

The Centers for Disease Control and Prevention is the primary source of information on communicable diseases and is a vital resource for health-care workers (Display 2-1).

The World Health Organization (WHO) was established by the United Nations in 1948 to direct and coordinate international health work. This proactive organization emphasizes prevention, adequate primary care, maternal-child health, nutrition, control of infectious diseases, environmental health, occupational health, and injury prevention. Many American nurses work outside the nation on international health projects. Some nurses volunteer for short-term projects; others work for the Peace Corps, church missions, or other private groups for a long period.

The biggest potential problem for global health is the burgeoning population growth in Third World countries. China has enforced a "one-child-per-family" policy to help curb population growth in that country. This law has caused havoc and heartbreak for many families in China and has failed to stop the population increase. Some people believe that the only solution to the population problem lies in a global, unified approach with effective contraception.

Problems in the U.S. Health-Care System

Emphasis on Acute Care Instead of Prevention

Health care in the United States is both wonderful and terrible. It is wonderful because of our superb biotechnology and expert acute-care treatment. This highly advanced

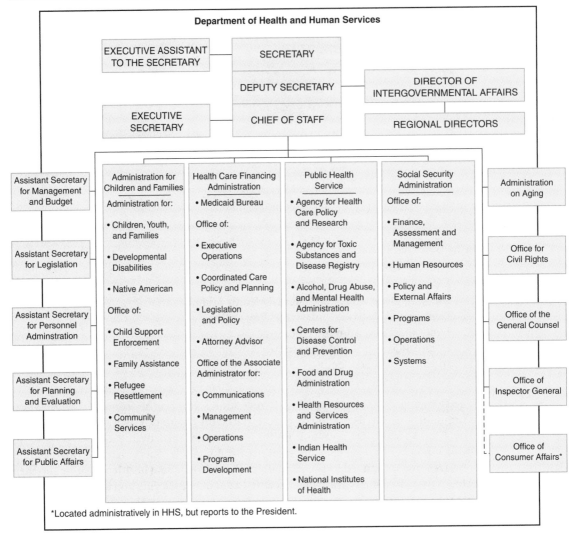

FIGURE 2-2
Organizational chart for the U.S. Department of Health and Human Services (HHS). (Smith CS, Maurer F [1995]. *Community Health Nursing.* Philadelphia: WB Saunders.)

system of care enables us to keep premature, 1-pound babies alive in neonatal intensive care units. However, the United States ranks 20th in the world in its infant mortality rate, long considered a major indicator of the health of a nation's children. Although the death rate for newborns has fallen in the United States, in 1990 it was still 9.1 per 1,000 births, almost double the rate in Japan. In 1993, our infant mortality rate dropped to 8.4 per 1,000 births (USDHHS—PHS—CDC, 1996), still extremely high for an advanced nation. The death rate among African-American newborns was 18.6 per 1,000 births, demonstrating an effect of unequal access to prenatal care in our country. In several other countries, prenatal care is free, making it more accessible to everyone and decreasing the

Scope of Services for Centers for Disease Control and Prevention (CDC)

NATIONAL CENTER FOR CHRONIC DISEASE PREVENTION AND HEALTH PROMOTION

To prevent death and disability from chronic diseases and promote healthy personal behavior

NATIONAL CENTER FOR ENVIRONMENTAL HEALTH

To prevent death and disability due to environmental factors

NATIONAL CENTER FOR HEALTH STATISTICS

To monitor the health of the American people, the impact of illness and disability, and factors affecting health and the nation's health-care system

NATIONAL CENTER FOR INFECTIOUS DISEASES

To prevent and control unnecessary disease and death caused by infectious diseases of public health importance

NATIONAL CENTER FOR INJURY PREVENTION AND CONTROL

To prevent and control nonoccupational injuries, both those that are unintentional and those that result from violence

NATIONAL CENTER FOR PREVENTION SERVICES

To prevent and control vaccine-preventable diseases, human immunodeficiency virus infection, sexually transmitted diseases, tuberculosis, dental diseases, and the introduction of diseases from other countries

NATIONAL INSTITUTE FOR OCCUPATIONAL SAFETY AND HEALTH

To prevent workplace-related injuries, illnesses, and premature death caused by trauma; toxic chemicals, dusts, and radiation; musculoskeletal and psychological stressors; noise; and other occupational hazards

EPIDEMIOLOGY PROGRAM OFFICE

To provide domestic and international epidemiologic, communication, and statistical support and to train experts in epidemiology

INTERNATIONAL HEALTH PROGRAM OFFICE

To strengthen the capacity of other nations to reduce disease, disability, and death

PUBLIC HEALTH PRACTICE PROGRAM OFFICE

To improve the effectiveness of public health delivery systems in health promotion and prevention

(CDC, Atlanta.)

need for costly neonatal intensive care units. Even though an infant's stay in a neonatal intensive care unit may cost up to $200,000, some argue that we cannot afford universal prenatal care, which is one of the best ways to prevent premature births! This is an example of how the health-care delivery system in the United States overlooks the importance of prevention and promotes unequal access to care (Fig. 2-3).

However, a system that places greater emphasis on health promotion and disease prevention is emerging. Kaiser Permanente, a health maintenance organization (HMO), has a program to prevent premature birth that includes frequent prenatal visits, nutrition counseling, and advice on how to recognize the signs of premature labor. The client is at the center of all decisions. This HMO system has decreased the number of premature deliveries and neonatal intensive care days. Each day of premature infant care costs 10 times that of each day of full-term newborn nursery care. Hospital cost savings in one metropolitan area alone translated into more than $1 million a year (Iglehart, 1994a).

High Health-Care Costs and Underserved Populations

Although large segments of our population have no medical insurance coverage, the cost of health care per person in the United States is more than double that of other nations in the Organization for Economic Cooperation and Development, a group made up of the United States and 14 other nations (Spradley & Allender, 1996). It is well known that prevention saves money, and in the United States inadequate attention to disease prevention and health promotion has caused enormous health-care expenses. Preventive measures are not usually covered by insurance companies, and it seems that

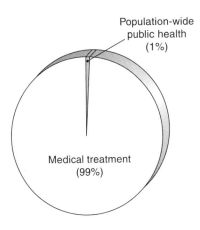
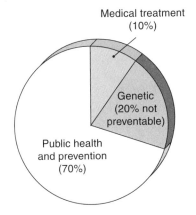

Percentage of health expenditures supporting population-wide public health vs. medical treatment

Percentage of early deaths that could be prevented by population-wide public health approaches vs. medical treatment

FIGURE 2-3
The pie chart to the left shows the lack of health expenditures supporting public health. The pie chart on the right shows the importance of prevention and public health. (Adapted from the Public Health Foundation [1994]. *Public Health Chartbook.* Washington DC: Public Health Foundation.)

health-care delivery is controlled primarily by these insurance companies. The primary question most often asked is how many days of care are covered for payment, not how many days of care the client needs. Fortunately, appreciation of the cost-saving value of preventive services is growing.

Health-Care Systems in Other Countries

The laissez-faire philosophy and free market approach to health care that exists in the United States is uncommon in other countries. Among developed nations, only South Africa has the same approach to health care. France, Japan, Canada, Germany, and Australia have a welfare-oriented approach that offers free health care to all needy people. Great Britain and Scandinavia have a comprehensive approach, offering free health care to everyone, regardless of economic status. This approach has been criticized because it leads to high taxes and often to long waiting periods for elective care, such as surgery (Roemer, 1991). As a result of this criticism, a second layer of private health care has been growing in Great Britain, with increased use of private physicians and clinics and privately paid insurance to cover health-care costs. Great Britain has always placed more emphasis on organized community-based care than the United States and has an excellent district nursing system, initiated by William Rathbone and Florence Nightingale.

Like the United States, other countries are also struggling to restructure their health-care systems. They all face the same fundamental issues of escalating costs and efforts to balance prevention and treatment. Some countries, such as Great Britain and Germany, are seeking a government-directed solution. Others, such as the United States, are looking toward private enterprise and a free market solution.

The National Debate Regarding U.S. Health-Care Policy

A National Health Plan

A government-directed national health plan was first proposed by President Theodore Roosevelt in 1912. Years later, President Harry Truman unsuccessfully proposed a national health plan. In 1993, President Clinton proposed a plan for comprehensive health-care reform. Although it too was rejected, it has affected the system. Fearing government-mandated reform, the system is doing much to reform itself and help reduce its unreasonable costs. The debate about a national health plan continues, and citizens have not reached a consensus about whether health care should be administered privately or by government, and how it should be funded. One member of Congress who favored a national unified health plan said she doubted that one would work in the United States because the country was too vast and too diverse. Who and what would be covered has also been an issue for great debate. The proposed cost of a governmental or public sector solution has been a major barrier to approval by Congress. States vary in their approach to health-care reform. However, it seems clear that managed care and competition, dominated by the private, business sector, are here to stay.

Universal Coverage

Philosophically, Americans cannot agree whether universal health coverage is a right or a privilege. According to the Census Bureau in 1991, 14% of the U.S. population, or 35 million people, had no health insurance at all. Five years later, in 1996, that number had risen to 41 million uninsured Americans. Many more people are underinsured. Most people receive health insurance as an employee benefit. Those who are unemployed or self-employed and those whose employer does not provide health insurance must purchase it privately, and insurance premiums are very expensive without the benefit of group rates. The working poor and children are most severely affected, but potential loss of health insurance coverage is a deep concern for everyone. Hawaii's state plan provides universal coverage, but Hawaii, as an island, is unique in many ways. Other states' officials are studying that plan to see if it can be applied elsewhere.

In 1994, the last year for which data are available, one in every seven children under age 18 had no health insurance coverage. These are generally the children of the working poor, who earn just a little too much to make their children eligible for Medicaid but not enough to purchase expensive health insurance if their employers do not provide it. The problem of uninsured children is a major one that ought to be solved in the near future.

Those who oppose a national health plan argue that it will diminish personal freedom to chose one's physician, will lead to health-care rationing, will reduce the quality of care received, and will inhibit medical advancement. Supporters of a national health plan claim that these things are already a reality because of managed care and other efforts to cut the high cost of health care in this country. Rationing of health care based on inability to pay has long been in existence; Oregon has been experimenting with rationing of costly, high-technology procedures. Supporters of a national health plan maintain that quality-control programs can be built into any system. The American Public Health Association has called for "Health Care For All" by the year 2000. The American Nurses Association supports some form of a national health plan, particularly universal coverage. Some other health provider organizations, such as the American Medical Association, oppose a national health plan.

Who Should Regulate the Health-Care Industry?

Opposition to governmental control and regulation is strong in the United States, one reason why President Clinton's health plan and any form of national health insurance have been rejected whenever proposed. A free market system has reigned, but more and more control over care is moving from health providers to insurance providers.

Computerization of the Health-Care System

In the current system, there is widespread confusion about the multitude of insurers, duplication of coverage, and gaps in coverage because more than 1,500 insurance groups or managed-care companies are involved in health care in the United States. Use of a single national health card and insurance form has gained favorable attention as a way to reduce some of this confusion. A central processing system is being developed for use of a health card, like that of a bank card. "Smart Cards" can store up to eight pages of data. These cards and the information they provide will help coordinate care across local, state, national, and international boundaries (McAlindon, 1995).

Using information technology, a client's health records can be retrieved and compared. Information systems to assist in nursing administration and clinical nursing care are also available. *Informatics* is the use of computerized knowledge that mimics the information-gathering process of the expert nurse, thereby assisting in nursing care. Increased access to client information by means of computerized information systems is making confidentiality even more important. Computerized health data systems will eventually make health care more efficient, more cost-effective, and less fragmented.

Why Health-Care Costs Are Increasing

As already mentioned, one reason for the excessive cost of health care in the United States is the inadequate effort and resources given to health promotion and disease prevention. The costly incentives of a retrospective fee-for-service (FFS) system is another. There are many other reasons for escalating costs. Since the 1970s, prevention has been given increasing attention, and the growth of managed care has reduced the expensive FFS system. However, costs continue to escalate.

Our society has *more elderly people living longer* than ever before. The elderly are the major consumers of health care in this country. *Costly entitlement programs* such as Medicare and Medicaid have helped them to live longer; so have *advancing medical knowledge, sophisticated care, and expensive technology*. For example, magnetic resonance imaging machines provide marvelous diagnostic data never before available to medical science. However, each test costs about $1,000, and the machines themselves cost well over $1 million. New procedures such as laparoscopic surgery may appear to lower costs because they are less expensive, require shorter hospital stays, and allow people to return to work in a few days. However, procedures such as laparoscopic cholecystectomies have actually driven total costs up, because many people are having the laparoscopic surgery who previously chose to have their cholelithiasis treated conservatively to avoid the uncomfortable, conventional, more costly surgery.

Salaries of health-care workers have increased to match inflation and to meet the demand of shortages. Nurses' salaries increased significantly during the 1980s, when there was a major shortage of nurses. Salaries of physicians and nurses in the United States are double those of similar professionals in Great Britain.

The *high malpractice awards* by courts or settlements by insurance companies have encouraged people to sue for malpractice. Stiff penalties should be assigned for frivolous suits. It is not just the high cost of malpractice insurance that is driving an increase in health costs; *the covert costs of the practice of defensive medicine and nursing* are enormous and result in much waste.

Although many women in other countries deliver their subsequent babies vaginally after a first cesarean section, American obstetricians have been fearful of the risks related to potential uterine rupture. Therefore, most American women have repeat cesarean sections unnecessarily for subsequent births. According to David M. Lawrence, M.D., the chairman and chief executive officer of the Kaiser Foundation Health Plan and Hospitals, the oldest HMO in the nation

> The average number of women in the United States who have all subsequent deliveries cesarean section is roughly 95%. In contrast, through very careful work in our Southern California region, Kaiser Permanente has demonstrated that upwards of 75% of women can deliver their babies by normal vaginal delivery after a prior cesarean section. That is an enormous savings in terms of improved quality of care and cost" (Lawrence & Schaeffer, 1996).

Unhealthy lifestyles contribute heavily to escalating health-care costs. Obesity, with its concomitant health problems, is increasing in the United States. The effect of addictions on health is so enormous that it is impossible to measure. Lung and cardiovascular diseases among smokers have been recognized for some time, and now we are beginning to recognize the costly effect of secondhand smoke. Alcohol and other drug addictions are tremendously costly to Americans in many more ways than financial. Most automobile accidents and violent crimes occur while the actor is under the influence of alcohol or another drug. There are incredible costs for treating the increasing violence in this country, especially with massive gunshot wounds. The acquired immunodeficiency syndrome (AIDS) epidemic is robbing society of young lives after a long, debilitating, expensive illness during the prime of their lives. Newer, more promising combination medication regimens for AIDS cost up to $20,000 a year. Teenage or drug-addicted mothers, with little or no prenatal care, produce low-birthweight babies who may need neonatal intensive care and years of ongoing care for chronic or congenital conditions.

Methods of Health-Care Financing

Health care is funded in various ways in the United States. Self-payment of health care still exists but is becoming increasingly difficult because of the extremely high costs of hospitalization, medical services, diagnostic tests, equipment, and medications. Sources of third-party payments are privately purchased insurance (indemnity) plans, managed-care plans, employer-provided health plans, Medicare, and Medicaid. Title XX government grants, donations, and charitable agencies are other payment sources.

Blue Cross and Blue Shield are the best-known and oldest health insurance companies. They have been nonprofit plans. Many of the "Blues" are now reorganized as managed-care plans. Plans such as Aetna or Travelers are commercial stock companies. Metropolitan Life and Prudential are owned by their policyholders. Self-insured health plans, offered through businesses, unions, and other employment groups, are growing.

Medicare is a federally sponsored and administered program for persons over age 65, those declared disabled, and those with end-stage renal disease. Medicare spending is growing at a rate of 10% a year. Medicare A is tax-supported and pays for hospitalization and home care. Until recent Medicare reform, that fund was expected to become bankrupt shortly after the turn of the century. Medicare B is funded by clients' premiums. Custodial care, which is exactly what many elderly and disabled people need to be able to stay in their own homes, is not paid for by Medicare.

Medicaid is a government-sponsored, state-administered program for the medically indigent, including those on public assistance. To be eligible for Medicaid, one must have very few assets and an income of less than $3,000 to 4,000 per year, depending on the state. Medicaid costs are split between the state and the federal government. Medicaid, unlike Medicare, pays for custodial care.

Although Medicaid was originally established to provide benefits to the poor, most Medicaid money has gone to pay for long-term nursing home care for elderly clients, most of whom were middle-class or even well-to-do. The common—and formerly legal—custom of giving gifts or transferring funds to family members reduced personal assets sufficiently to qualify these people for Medicaid. After that, their expensive nursing home care costs were paid by Medicaid. A law passed in 1996 made this practice illegal and imposes a heavy fine and imprisonment on those caught transferring assets to become eligible for Medicaid. About a third of nursing home residents have faithfully used up all their personal assets to pay for their long-term care needs before becoming Medicaid recipients and did not transfer their money to their families.

The next largest group receiving Medicaid benefits are disabled clients, many of whom need personal care at home or in long-term care facilities. These two groups become medically indigent after spending down any personal resources to pay for their care. Total Medicaid spending has more than doubled in just the past 10 years.

Medicare and Medicaid HMOs

About 12% of Medicare clients are already enrolled in Medicare HMO programs, and the number is rapidly increasing (Fig. 2-4). These HMOs are run by companies who receive the clients' premiums for Medicare B in exchange for providing supplemental health-care services. For several years, many senior citizens have been purchasing extra Medigap insurance policies to supplement their Medicare insurance. Now they often select Medicare HMO plans instead, but with mixed results. Some Medicare HMOs are excellent; some are not. Some people have transferred back to Medigap insurance plans when expected care from an HMO was not forthcoming. Other people have been very pleased with their HMO. For example, respite care may be provided for up to 80 hours annually when the family caretaker needs help. Some Medicare HMOs supply medications, eyeglasses, and hearing aids not covered by traditional plans. Freedom from paperwork has great appeal to many people. However, later, when expensive health-care benefits are desperately needed, some Medicare HMOs are very limited in what they provide. More about Medicare and Medicaid is found in Chapters 9 and 13.

Cost-Containment Measures

Until recently, health care in America was dominated by an FFS delivery system. It is widely recognized that FFS is a major reason why health care is so expensive in this country. In a FFS system, there is little incentive for cost containment or preventive measures to reduce care. Providers' incomes are dependent on the amount of care delivered, be it the number of office visits to a physician, the number of hospital days

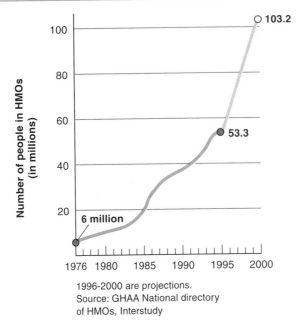

FIGURE 2-4

A medical revolution. From 1976 to 1995, HMO membership has risen nearly tenfold. (© 1996, Newsweek, Inc. All rights reserved. Reprinted by permission.)

1996-2000 are projections.
Source: GHAA National directory of HMOs, Interstudy

of care, or the number of home visits by a nurse. Fees are set by the provider. Sick clients require more care and bring in greater revenue, reducing the incentive to prevent illness. People have preferred the FFS system because they tend to ignore preventive medicine and seek care only when they are sick. Clients like the maximum amount of care they receive when they are sick. Under the FFS model, they can seek out expensive specialty services as they desire. Neither clients nor providers have incentives to limit care.

A Prospective-Payment System with Managed Competition and Managed Care

Recognizing the high cost of the FFS system and the negative impact the high cost of health care is having on the entire U.S. economy, there has been a move toward reform with prospective-payment systems (PPS). Insurance companies led the way with a rapid increase in competing managed-care systems in the 1980s and 1990s. Control of the amount of services with prepaid fees charged by providers has been the basis of managed care. Health-care providers, such as hospitals or physicians, share the financial risks of waste, creating a powerful incentive for cost containment and reduction of waste. In fact, managed care has halved the inflationary cycle of health-care costs.

Definitions of managed care vary. Generically, it includes a variety of organizational structures and health-care programs that all use strategies to control the cost of, access to, and use of services within a provider network. There is a single point of entry to health care through a primary provider, who may be a physician or a nurse practitioner. This person is the gatekeeper to specialists and further health care. A gatekeeper can also be a case manager hired by the insurance provider. The gatekeeper reviews the appropriateness of services such as visits to specialists, x-rays, laboratory tests, and other expensive diagnostic and treatment procedures. The goal of the gatekeeper is to achieve cost containment by preventing unnecessary services and using the least-costly providers of services while ensuring adequate quality of care. Case management is discussed in detail in Chapter 12.

Types of Managed-Care Plans

Forms of managed care have been in existence for some time under different names. *HMOs* were first established during the first half of this century in California by Kaiser Permanente. HMOs are a type of prepayment plan in which money is paid in advance for comprehensive services, including primary, secondary, and tertiary preventive services. The term "health maintenance organization" implies that prevention and wellness programs are offered (they are, but in varying degrees). Efforts are made to keep costs down; clients appreciate this, because then the prepayment premiums remain as low as possible (Display 2-2).

In some areas of the country, HMOs have been very successful; in others, they have not been successful at all. A major reason for this is the quality of the physicians hired by HMOs and strong resistance by physicians in private practice. There has been peer pressure against working for HMOs, so many top-quality physicians have not wanted to do so. Physicians working for HMOs receive a set salary, which can limit the amount they can earn.

In most HMOs, clients can use only physicians hired by the HMO. The same is true for home care and other service agencies. This is creating great hardship for small home care and other health agencies who traditionally delivered excellent care so that their clients returned to them again and again for service. Now those same clients must use agencies affiliated with their new HMO, and many smaller visiting nurse agencies are in jeopardy of closing. Responding to criticism regarding lack of freedom to see the physician of one's choice, some HMOs permit clients to purchase, for an extra premium, a point-of-service rider that allows them to go to any physician they want.

DISPLAY 2-2
Amount of HMO Money Spent for Client's Medical Care*

Nonprofit plans have spent an average of 91 cents of every dollar.
For profit plans have spent an average of 79 cents of every dollar.
  HMOs generally spend 17% of premiums they collect on:

* Marketing
* Administrative expenses and costs for managing care:
    Case managers
    Utilization review personnel
    Data management specialists

A general estimate; individual HMOs vary.

Preferred provider organizations (PPOs), another popular form of managed care, contract with physicians and other health providers to work for discounted fees. Clients then pay a small copayment. They pay more to see a provider outside the network, which they are free to do. PPO members are also free to see specialists without being referred by a gatekeeper. If they seek health care outside the PPO, members must pay 20% of the cost themselves.

Managed-care companies save money by setting up networks that help reduce waste through quantity merchandising and management. They negotiate fees competitively with physicians and other health providers. They practice capitation, the prepayment of a fixed amount per patient. Actuarial data are used to determine the average yearly cost of comprehensive services, including all three levels of prevention, for a given population. The capitation rate is then set for that population. All health-care costs for that population must be taken from the pool of money that accumulates. The company makes a profit if the expenses of the population are less than the accumulated money in the pool. Again, this provides a strong incentive to keep costs down.

Eventually, capitation will be used across the whole continuum of health-care services throughout the United States. It is already being used that way as a pilot project in the Carondelet Health System in New Mexico, a nursing HMO (see Chap. 12). Capitation is also being piloted in home care agencies and in mental health agencies in various places throughout the United States.

Diagnostic related groups (DRGs), which have been used for several years for hospital reimbursement, are a form of capitation. DRGs were developed in the recognition that hospital care is the most expensive aspect of all health care. DRGs were developed by Medicare and have transformed hospital care, resulting in shorter hospital stays, lower patient counts, closure of many hospital nursing care units, reductions in nursing staff, and an end to the nursing shortage. For each of the 467 diagnoses, preestablished, fixed reimbursement fees are allowed for each day spent in the hospital. If patients spend fewer days in the hospital or receive fewer services than the DRGs allow, the hospital makes extra money. The opposite is true if patients stay longer than the DRG allows, unless unavoidable complications require a longer stay.

In short, patients with brief hospital stays produce revenue for the hospital. This has led to very early discharges and has created a great deal of public criticism. Some patients who were discharged early suffered complications and problems related to inadequate follow-up care in homes that were not conducive to healing and recuperation. However, overall patient outcomes have been satisfactory, even if early discharge is often inconvenient for patients and families. Serious problems resulting from ''drive-by deliveries''—in which mothers and newborns were required to be discharged within 24 hours of birth—have been corrected in some states by laws that mandate 48-hour hospital stays and follow-up home visits by community health nurses.

Utilization Review Programs and Quality Assurance

To ensure both quality and quantity, client care is monitored by utilization review and quality assurance programs. Utilization review programs were designed to ensure that appropriate care is received and unnecessary care is avoided. Insurance companies' utilization review programs are moving away from oversight, inspection, and regulation because of the new shared-risk status, in which the financial risks of waste are shared by health-care providers and insurance companies. Each hospital has a utilization review committee, as do home care agencies. Many nurses work in utilization review programs across the nation. Quality assurance programs exist to ensure that quality care is not sacrificed to cut costs. More about quality management programs in home care can be found in Chapter 16.

Public concern about quality reductions in health care by managed-care organizations has led many states to pass laws to protect consumers enrolled in HMOs (Display 2-3). The National Committee for Quality Assurance collects data on health plans and has launched a "quality compass" project.

Hospital and Managed-Care Mergers and Networks

Hospitals have suffered financially in recent times; many operate with deficit budgets. In response to this problem, mergers and hospital closings are occurring. Managed-care companies are uniting into conglomerates, such as the 1997 merger of U.S. Health Care and Aetna. The resulting staff downsizing may increase operating efficiency, but the process is difficult for everyone.

The Role of Nursing in Cost Containment

Quality of care must be maintained during this cost-containment process, and nurses must prove their worth to the system. There has been a great deal of waste and duplication in health care in the past. Nurses can do much to reduce waste with careful use of supplies and equipment and more efficient time management. Good documentation ensures maximum, fair reimbursement from third-party payers but is a

---

DISPLAY 2-3
Key Actions Taken by States in 1995 and 1996 to Protect Consumers Enrolled in HMOs

- 18 states prohibited "gag rules" in provider contracts that limit physician–patient communication.
- 17 states required managed-care plans to provide a range of new types of information to enrollees and prospective members.
- 28 states set standards for length of maternity stays.
- 19 states joined California and New York in maintaining that HMOs provide direct access to obstetricians/gynecologists.
- 6 states joined California in establishing stronger utilization review criteria.
- 10 states passed legislation to ensure access to emergency care.
- 2 states (New York and New Jersey) adopted regulations that give those states some of the strongest managed-care consumer protection laws in the nation.

(Source: Families U.S.A. Foundation, a consumer advocacy group. Washington DC, 1997.)

great drain on nurses' time. A good topic for nursing research would be how to reduce unnecessary paperwork. Reducing paperwork would also lead to greater job satisfaction for nurses. Computer literacy will be a basic qualification for all nurses in the very near future.

Recent Laws Affecting Health Care

The Health Insurance Portability & Accountability Act of 1996

Effective in July 1997, this law safeguards health coverage for people who change or lose their jobs. Also known as the Kassenbaum-Kennedy Health Reform Act, it bars insurers from denying coverage to workers who change employment status. Exclusions for preexisting conditions are sharply curtailed as well. An estimated 21 million Americans previously denied coverage for preexisting conditions will receive coverage under this bill. An additional 4 million people who stay in jobs they dislike for the sake of health insurance now can change jobs without losing their health-care coverage. This bill does not help people who cannot afford or are not offered health insurance by their employers.

This bill also endorses the use of medical savings accounts (MSAs), which are tax-sheltered, high-deductible insurance plans. Clients establish MSAs as savings accounts from which money is withdrawn for medical expenses as needed. Naturally, clients search carefully for the most cost-effective, highest-quality health care so as not to waste their money. These accounts continue to build, tax-free, until the client reaches age 65; money may be withdrawn for other uses before age 65, but the withdrawals are then taxed. As an experiment, 750,000 people will use MSAs for a 4-year period. Current MSA members are self-employed or employees of small businesses (Brider, 1996, p. 67). Critics say MSAs are likely to siphon off younger, healthier people, pushing up insurance rates for sicker, older, needier people; critics estimate that Medicare costs would increase as much as $15.2 billion by the year 2002 if MSAs were widely adopted (Sheils, 1996).

Long-Term Health-Care Insurance

As mentioned earlier, Medicaid will no longer be an option for middle-class or well-to-do people to pay for their nursing home care. The most serious threat to the financial security of older Americans and their families is the cost of long-term care, which can run $35,000 to $60,000 a year. An increasing number of people are buying special long-term care insurance policies to prepare for this eventuality. However, these policies are usually too costly for middle-class people. The Health Insurance Portability & Accountability Act of 1996 makes these premium costs tax-deductible (up to $2,500 a year), and the benefits are collected tax-free, up for to $170 per day for care either at home or in a long-term care facility (Display 2-4). This includes the much-needed custodial care not covered by Medicare.

Only 5% of the population needs nursing home care for a long period; in fact, the average time spent in a nursing home is 3 years. However, most frail, elderly people

DISPLAY 2-4
Tax Deductions for Long-Term Care Insurance

At Age:	You Can Deduct:
40 or younger	$200
41 to 50	$375
51 to 60	$750
61 to 70	$2,000
71 or older	$2,500

do need custodial care in their later years at home. Because most women now work, and women are the traditional caregivers, daughters are less likely to be able to assume all the care for elderly parents, as was the pattern in previous generations.

Uninsured Children in the United States

Various bills are being discussed by Congress to deal with the serious problem of uninsured American children (an estimated 10 million). In April 1997, a bipartisan bill (S525) proposed that 43 cents in federal taxes be added to the sale of each package of cigarettes. Two thirds of the tax was to go toward health insurance for children and one third toward reducing the federal deficit. Although opposed vehemently by the tobacco industry, this bill was a meaningful step toward solving two very serious problems in this country. In addition to providing health insurance to millions of uninsured children, it would have curbed the number of youths who become addicted to cigarettes (Fig. 2-5). Prevention of smoking by young teenagers, which often results in lifelong addiction, would be a major cost savings to the health-care system. This proposal was sacrificed for political reasons during negotiations to develop a balanced budget by the year 2002. Many people believe that political pressure from the powerful tobacco lobby was a reason.

Several states are suing the tobacco lobby to recover tax money spent treating sick smokers. Tobacco firms are discussing a settlement with these states as evidence mounts regarding the serious health risks of smoking. Part of the settlement money could be used to provide health care to the millions of uninsured children of the working poor who are not covered by Medicaid.

Welfare Reform

In 1996, President Clinton signed the Personal Responsibility and Work Opportunity Reconciliation Act, a welfare reform bill that provides block grants to states so that each can determine how welfare monies should be spent. The law allows states to withhold welfare and Medicaid from low-income legal immigrants and sets a 5-year limit on cash welfare benefits. Each state must decide the length of time (up to the 5-year

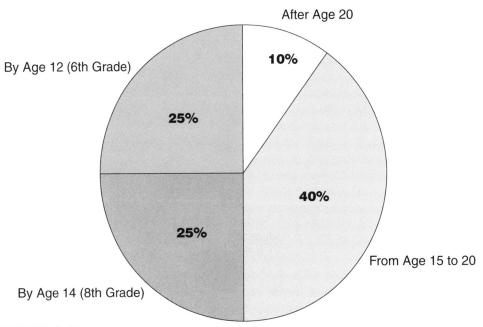

FIGURE 2-5
Tobacco use begins early. (Source: Department of Health and Human Services' High School Senior Survey.)

limit) recipients should be able to receive cash benefits, the number of hours of work or training that should be required in return for receiving cash benefits, whether able-bodied single adults should receive any welfare benefits at all, and whether help should be provided for legal immigrants.

Some health officials worry about the effects of this welfare bill, fearing a resurgence in tuberculosis and other infectious diseases if poor immigrants can no longer receive welfare benefits and access to health care provided by Medicaid. States such as California and New York, with very high populations of legal immigrants, are particularly vulnerable (Fig. 2-6). Limits on welfare cash mean that mothers receiving Aid to Families with Dependent Children will be required to go to work and leave their children in day-care centers.

The health risks of these welfare changes remain unknown. If adequate training, jobs, and quality child care are forthcoming, the reforms could prove beneficial to everyone.

Medicare Reform

The changes in Medicare approved in 1997 will slow the growth of Medicare but are inadequate for the long term. Although they prevent Medicare A from going bankrupt by the year 2002, as was generally predicted, more drastic measures are needed before the 70 million baby boomers retire and become eligible for Medicare. (Medicare A is

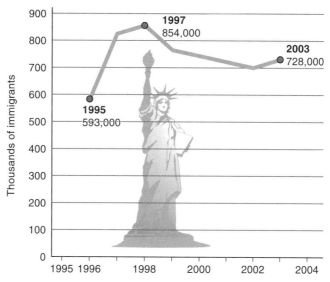

FIGURE 2-6
U.S. legal immigration: projected number of legal immigrants. Does not include refugees, asylum, adjustments, and a few other types of admissions. (Source: Statistics Division, U.S. Immigration and Naturalization Service.)

tax-supported and covers hospitalization and home care. Medicare B, which is supported by premiums paid by clients and is more financially secure, reimburses visits to physicians and other ambulatory care.) One suggestion for salvaging Medicare A is to transfer the payment of home care benefits from Medicare A to Medicare B. However, senior citizen groups oppose this because it will lead to more expensive premiums for clients. Another suggestion is to increase Medicare premiums for wealthy people.

Medicare issues are complex and have many political undertones. It is impossible to predict what changes will finally be made. These are politically explosive issues, so politicians prefer to delay their decisions as long as possible. For the present, Medicare savings will come mainly from reducing payments to hospitals and other care providers. A bipartisan national commission needs to start work soon on reaching long-term solutions; otherwise, it is predicted that the nation's entitlement programs (Medicare, Medicaid, and Social Security) will cause another downward spiral of deficit spending by the year 2008 (Associated Press, June 4, 1997a).

THE NURSE SPEAKS . . .
About Work for a Primary Provider of Managed Care

work in a primary care doctor's office. Agnes S. has been a patient of our office for many years and continued with us when we joined a managed-care organization. She had a variety of minor ailments over the years, but mainly episodes of hiatal hernia inflammation and chronic low back pain. She came in fairly often and also went to see other doctors because we would get reports about her from various specialists from time to time. When we joined managed care, we thought she would probably transfer to a FFS provider because she wouldn't want to have limits set on specialist care. So it was a surprise when she called for another appointment about 5 months ago.

At this appointment, Agnes came in complaining of severe headaches and stiff neck occurring four or five times a week. Doctor diagnosed tension headaches based on her symptoms. He prescribed use of ice packs, neck massage, and Fiorinal as needed when the pain was unrelieved by over-the-counter medications. I taught her progressive muscle relaxation exercises and meditation to help prevent the headaches. He agreed to have me teach her these techniques and talk to her about doing daily exercise such as walking to boost her endorphin levels. He offered to send her to a gynecologist to have her hormone levels checked due to her age (48) and new data that suggest a correlation between varying hormone levels and headaches. She refused the referral, saying she didn't want to see a gynecologist.

Five weeks later, Agnes returned, saying nothing had helped and she wanted to be referred to a headache specialty center in a nearby city. Doctor repeated the information about estrogen, but she adamantly refused to see the gynecologist. She also admitted that she was too busy to try meditation and "that other stuff you told me to do." Agnes was not subject to allergies, so they were ruled out as a cause of her headaches. Doctor felt the symptoms were still indicative of tension headaches and was reluctant to make a referral for expensive specialist care. Anyway, the headache specialty center she mentioned is not part of our managed-care network. We informed her that she would have to pay privately if she went there, and this made her extremely angry.

All her lab work was normal. When I called to tell her about her lab results, I asked if she had decided to go to the headache specialty center, and she again became very angry. She said she couldn't afford to go there. She added that she planned to sue the doctor "for every penny he's got" if his diagnosis for her headaches was wrong. She added that her brother was an attorney and this was not an idle threat.

Doctor decided to refer her to a neurologist in our managed-care network. He told me about another physician in town who performed an inadequate primary work-up on a patient with headaches and failed to refer this patient to a specialist. The patient turned out to have a brain tumor! "I'd bet anything that Agnes is having tension headaches, but we'd better refer her to a neurologist, just in case," he added.

The neurologist reported that he ordered an MRI of her head and put her on daily doses of amitriptyline, a tricyclic antidepressant that also helps suppress headaches and other chronic pain. The MRI was negative. The neurologist diagnosed tension headache. Agnes has not been back to our office, so we are unsure whether her headaches have ceased.

All this is so expensive. We're supposed to be saving the system money. I wish Agnes had listened to this doctor and had done what he suggested. It's as if she wants a quick fix from somebody else and doesn't want to take any responsibility to do the things herself that would help her.

Mary Lou
OFFICE NURSE

CLINICAL APPLICATION

A Critical Thinking Case Study About an Elderly Couple Needing Respite Care

Y ou are a home care nurse. One morning you receive an urgent call from your grandmother's friend in the Midwest stating that your grandmother is in trouble and needs your help. She severely injured her back the previous night while lifting your grandfather from the bathroom floor where he had fallen. The friend adds, "Your grandfather falls a lot at night. You know your grandfather is rather unbalanced, both physically and mentally, since his stroke last year. He expects your grandmother to wait on him hand and foot, and she feels very guilty if she doesn't do it. He's very stubborn and doesn't remember things. Right now he's calling her to fix his break-fast and she can hardly move, she's in such pain!"

You request a 2-week leave without pay from your job to go help them (the Family and Medical Leave Act guarantees your right to take this leave). You hurriedly arrange with the supervisor to parcel out your home care clients to other nurses and leave for the airport.

 and Think!

- What will you do first in this situation?
- What additional information do you need?
- How will you go about gathering this information?

T he situation is not good. You arrange for your grandmother to be seen medically, and x-rays reveal a fractured vertebra. She is instructed to rest her back, mainly in bed, for the next 6 to 8 weeks and not to lift or carry anything. An elastic lumbosacral support is ordered to protect her back while she is out of bed. Motrin is ordered to reduce the inflammation. Ice or heat application is suggested to reduce the pain as well.

Your grandfather seems to be the bigger challenge. You discuss with your doctor the possibility of hospitalizing him for 3 days so that he would be eligible for 100 days of Medicare benefits in a long-term care facility. The doctor is sympathetic but says your grandfather's condition is stable and he can find no indication to warrant hospitalization. He adds that he doubts that Medicare would pay for nursing home care for him because he requires only custodial care, not skilled nursing care. You are not surprised by the doctor's response because you already assessed that your grandfather does not meet Medicare's criteria for home care services.

 and Think!

- Describe Medicare criteria for home care services (see Chap. 13). Would your grandfather be eligible for service if he required physical therapy?

- What options can you suggest for your grandfather's care after you leave in 2 weeks?
- What additional assessments must you make regarding your grandfather?

You assess that your grandfather's condition is indeed stable. He walks well without assistance; in fact, he likes to take an afternoon walk in the neighborhood. He has never been known to wander off and always is oriented to time, place, and person. However, he is somewhat forgetful, resistant to change, and very insistent that his routines are not disturbed in any way. Your grandparents have been married for 55 years and he has always been very demanding. Your grandmother has prided herself on taking such good care of him and doing everything for him. She even helped him get dressed. Now she is very frail. Aside from her back condition, it is unlikely that she can care for him in the same way for much longer. You are the only family member they have. Neighbors in the senior citizen complex where they live are friendly but are also frail and elderly.

You realize that your grandfather best meets the criteria for assisted living. He can walk to the dining room and other activities but needs minor assistance with dressing and other activities of daily living. You phone a nearby facility and are told that no room is available at present but one opens up every month or so. Your grandfather's name will be put on their waiting list. The cost is $60 per day, which would have to be paid privately. You realize that this would mean a drastic adjustment for your grandfather, but it would solve the problem of his care so that your grandmother can heal.

You have been told that your grandparents receive only Social Security payments; they do not receive a pension, because your grandfather was self-employed. They live frugally and have some savings, which are sacred to them. When you approach them about using some of their savings to hire household help or to pay for assisted living, they both recoil. When they learn the cost, they are shocked. "What will happen to us when it is all used up?" they ask. You explain that they would then become eligible for Medicaid to pay for the care they need (Medicaid pays for custodial care).

You constantly tell your grandparents separately and together that your grandfather must become more independent because your grandmother cannot continue to wait on him. If he cannot do so, then the only alternative is for him to move to the assisted-living facility. You repeatedly remind your grandparents of their need to use their savings for additional help when you leave. They finally agree and reveal the amount of money they have in the bank. Based on the meager amount, you begin the process of applying for Medicaid for them.

 and Think!

- How would you feel saying these things to your grandparents and probing their financial situation?
- Do you see some role conflict in this situation?

- What would be your next step if your grandparents did not accept your professional advice?
- What would be the benefits of having a home care nurse from a local agency involved in this case?
- Explain the difference between custodial care and skilled nursing care. What procedures define the latter?
- If household help were hired, what kind of help would your grandparents need?
- When does someone need to be present, and specifically what duties are to be done?
- How can you ensure that the helper will remember what to do each day?
- How will you evaluate the caregiver?

Skilled nursing care means procedures and assessments that only a licensed professional nurse can perform. You find the names of nursing proprietary agencies in the telephone book and call to arrange for personal care aides for 16 hours a day (midnight to 8 a.m. and 10 a.m. to 6 p.m.) A 24-hour live-in aide may have been less expensive, but their tiny, one-bedroom apartment makes that impossible. Also, you want the aide to be awake to help your grandfather when he gets up to go to the bathroom during the night, because that is when he is apt to fall. A certified personal care aide (PCA) has less training (30 hours) than a home health aide and is less expensive. Your grandparents can bathe and dress themselves with minimal assistance. They need help with meal preparation and shopping, light housecleaning, and laundry. However, they need more than housekeeping services. PCAs are trained in personal care and body mechanics to help move patients. You write out the job description for each aide in detail and post it on the refrigerator so that the aides and your grandparents can refer to it. The nighttime aide is to do laundry, prepare breakfast, and clean up before she leaves. The daytime aide will prepare the other meals, shop, and tidy up the house. You will arrange to have them begin working the day before you go home so that you can go over their job description with them. You will call your grandmother frequently to evaluate their service and may revisit if there are problems. The aides' work will also be supervised by their agency. If your grandfather learns to avoid falls at night and to get up independently if he should fall, the nighttime PCA can be dismissed. Before leaving, you teach these strategies to him and the PCA and have her reinforce these strategies with him daily.

Chapter SUMMARY

The community health system in the United States comprises a variety of public and private organizations and health-care providers. Governmental or public agencies are headed by the Department of Health and Human Services, which has four major divisions, including the U.S. Public Health Service. It, in turn, has several branches, including the Centers for Disease Control and Prevention, whose primary responsibility is surveillance, prevention, and control of infectious diseases.

The U.S. health-care system has many serious problems, even though spending on health care is double the amount per capita than that of any other nation. Uneven distribution of care is a major problem, as well as inadequate attention to prevention. Proposals for a national, comprehensive, government-controlled health plan have been repeatedly rejected by Congress, although many Americans still favor some form of universal health coverage.

For years, health-care financing in the United States was dominated by the costly, retrospective FFS system, which had no incentives to curb costs. Recently, a prospective-payment system, in which a fixed fee is paid to cover all health care during a given period, has reduced the inflationary cycle of health care. These managed-care programs, such as HMOs and PPOs, are growing rapidly. Nevertheless, most health care is still paid for through traditional FFS third-party payers: Medicare, Medicaid, indemnity or traditional health insurance, or self-payment.

Managed-care systems offer all health care for a prepaid amount per period (usually 1 year). HMOs are growing most rapidly and have gatekeepers or case managers to prevent unnecessary care. In PPOs, providers agree to charge discounted fees when they join the system. Clients of PPOs are generally freer to see specialists or go outside the system to see physicians of their choice for extra fees.

Additional reasons that health care in the United States is so expensive are as follows:

1. More people living longer.
2. Costly entitlement programs (Medicare and Medicaid)
3. Cost of biomedical technology and sophisticated care
4. Increased salaries of health-care workers
5. High malpractice awards by courts
6. Covert costs of defensive medicine
7. Unhealthy lifestyles (eg, obesity, lack of exercise, addictions)

The U.S. health-care system is undergoing the greatest transformation in its history, with mergers or closings of many institutions and agencies. In all these changes, nurses have a vital role in cost containment and a strong need to prove their worth to the system.

Recent laws, such as the Health Insurance Portability & Accountability Act of 1996 and the welfare reform bill of 1996, seriously affect health care. Priority issues that must be addressed in the near future are the 10 million uninsured children in the United States and the need for serious Medicare reform.

A list of references and additional readings for this chapter appears at the end of Part 1.

3

Legal, Ethical, Cultural, and Spiritual Considerations

Key Terms

advance directives
ANA Code for Nurses
beneficence
code of ethics
cultural assessment
cultural relativism
dominant culture
double-blind study
equity
ethical dilemmas
ethnic foods
evaluative judgment
executive branch
Federal Register

fidelity
forced choice ranking
habeas corpus
judicial branch
legislative branch
lobby
mandatory policy
nonmaleficence
Occupational Safety and
    Health Administration
    (OSHA)
ordinances
personal space
Roe vs. Wade

spiritual assessment
state board of nursing
state jurisdiction
statutes
stereotype
subcultures
terminal values
torts
values
values clarification
veracity
world view

Learning Objectives

1. Define public health laws.
2. Describe the difference in public health laws regarding the control of tuberculosis and the control of acquired immunodeficiency syndrome (AIDS).
3. Explain the pros and cons of those differences.
4. Identify the genesis of three types of public health laws.

5. Explain the laws derived from legislative, executive, and judicial branches.
6. Identify the laws that regulate nursing licensure and practice.
7. Describe at least six specific legal responsibilities of community health nurses.
8. Explain the relationship of values, ethics, laws, and culture.

9. Perform a values clarification exercise to identify and clarify your values.

10. Define an ethical dilemma.

11. Identify at least eight major categories of decision making that can result in ethical dilemmas for nurses.

12. Use the resources described in this chapter to resolve an ethical dilemma.

13. List the major ethnic groups in the United States.

14. Identify several culture subgroups other than ethnic groups.

15. Explain the problems that result from variations of meaning of concepts regarding health, illness, and suffering.

16. Perform a cultural assessment.

17. Perform a spiritual assessment.

18. Practice the relaxation response.

Legal Considerations

Many laws affect community health nursing. Nurses must be aware of how public health laws come into being and how they can have a voice in influencing legislation.

Public Health Laws

Over time, laws have been developed that govern health promotion and disease prevention. These laws, however, often differ in regard to the health needs of the community and those of the person. For example, a person with active, communicable tuberculosis who is noncompliant with treatment poses a threat of spreading tuberculosis to the general public. In some states, the law permits local health officers to force that person into treatment, even if incarceration is necessary. Another example is a person who is HIV-positive and very sexually active. Current laws in those same states protect that person's confidentiality rights and do not permit enforced restriction of sexual activity, despite the threat of communicability.

Why is there such a difference in policy between these two infectious diseases? One reason may be historical. Public health laws about tuberculosis have existed for a long time and were passed in an era when patients' rights were not so highly valued. Another reason may be ethical. Tuberculosis treatment stops the spread of the disease and cures the illness. However, the spread of the HIV infection will not necessarily be stopped, nor will it be cured, by prohibiting sexual activity. According to current knowledge, its eventual outcome is AIDS and death. Is it fair, therefore, to force someone into treatment?

Patient confidentiality is highly valued today. Enforced testing is apt to lead to breaks in strict confidentiality. Given the great fear about and stigma of AIDS, it is believed that a mandatory testing and treatment policy would serve only to drive the disease underground, making it more difficult to control in society. Instead, a voluntary, free testing policy has been put into effect with double-blind, confidential test results. In addition to the free and confidential testing, an educational program has been instituted to encourage the use of condoms and to notify all sexual contacts to come for testing. Although AIDS is still not considered curable, it has been found that combination treatment with zidovudine (AZT) and protease inhibitors can delay the onset of active disease. Already, some optimists are using the term ''cure'' for AIDS clients who respond favorably to this rigorous treatment regimen.

Sources and Types of Federal, State, and Local Laws

The various types of laws and their sources are sometimes confusing to the average person. The Constitution of the United States contains most of the federal (national) government's legal basis for congressional action in health care in Article 1, Section 8. States retain legal powers not delegated to the federal government. Many public health laws are under state jurisdiction. States differ significantly in their public health laws; some are much more regulatory than others. *Local* laws, called ordinances, are passed by cities, towns, or counties. Like state laws, they can be more specific or restrictive than, but never inconsistent with, the laws from the larger authority (the state or national government).

The three branches of the federal government are *legislative, executive*, and *judicial*. Each branch exists on state and local levels as well, and each can be a source of public health laws. Legislative branches vote and enact statutory laws. Judicial branches, such as the U.S. Supreme Court or state supreme courts, enact judicial or common laws by court decision (for example, the Roe vs. Wade decision that made abortion legal by action of the U.S. Supreme Court). The executive or administrative branches enact laws to regulate certain functions. In each state, a board of nursing regulates nursing licensure and practice by order of the state's administrative branch. State and local health departments of health exist by administrative law, as does the U.S. Department of Health and Human Services on the federal level.

How Nurses Can Influence Public Health Laws

Nurses can and do work to lobby and affect public health laws at all levels of government. It is very important for community health nurses to be knowledgeable about proposals that relate to health. Federal and state proposals for public health regulations must first be published in the Federal Register or state register and be available to the public. Studies, public commentary, and public hearings follow, offering an opportunity for input from citizens. Community health nurses should monitor these registers to learn about proposed laws; in this way, they can have input into the final draft. Regulations are refined depending on the reactions of the public and the decisions of the committees that study the laws. Once a proposed law appears in the Federal Register, more study may be conducted before the final regulations are prepared for printing. Once published in the Code of Regulations, however, the force of the law is behind the regulation, and changes in practice will be mandated.

The American Nurses Association (ANA), state nursing associations, and local district associations have legislative committees where nurses join together to be more effective in monitoring and influencing public health laws. Information about public health laws can be found in many public libraries and law libraries.

Legal Responsibilities of Community Health Nurses

The two sets of laws that have the most direct impact on nursing are each state's Nurse Practice Act and torts of malpractice. The first defines the scope of nursing practice allowed in each state. The second deals with legal wrongs committed by nurses, whether from improper discharge of professional duties or failure to meet appropriate standards

DISPLAY 3-1
The Legal Risks of Community Health

Some of the more commonly encountered risks include:

RISKS RELATED TO AUTONOMY

You're alone in the field, and you're expected to make on-the-spot decisions, but your clinical manager should be only a phone call away if you need help. Know the chain of command and your agency's policies and procedures for dealing with emergency and nonemergency situations. For example, what should you do if a client's condition is deteriorating and you can't get in touch with the physician for new orders? What if a client develops an adverse reaction to a drug? What if you suspect elder abuse or neglect? Failing to take the proper action could leave you open to charges of negligence.

RISKS RELATED TO PATIENT EDUCATION

Client education is a vital part of nursing care, but it can also be legally risky: the client might claim he or she was harmed because your teaching was inadequate. You can protect yourself by making sure you address all points the patient needs to know and assessing how well your client is learning. For example, have the patient return demonstrations of procedures. Then document everything you've taught the client, how you assessed learning, whether a family member was present, and what handouts you left behind. Include copies of these handouts in the client's chart.

RISKS RELATED TO EQUIPMENT

If you don't know how to use or troubleshoot certain equipment necessary for a client's care, tell your manager and ask to be assigned to a different client. Otherwise, you could be liable for negligence if the client is harmed. Then get the education you need to expand your skills. If you are familiar with the equipment and can accept the patient, review agency policies and procedures for dealing with equipment malfunctions.

RISKS RELATED TO DELEGATION OF AUTHORITY

When a home health aide is assigned to one of your clients, make sure he or she has been adequately prepared to give the type of care your client needs and that the care falls within the aide's scope of practice. Review the care plan with the aide so he or she understands what's expected, when you're to be called, and what should be documented. Also consider how safe it is to delegate a task. Is the client too unstable or is the care too complex for the aide to perform a certain task? Does the aide feel confident performing it? Remember, you could be liable if the aide makes any errors in carrying out the delegated task.

RISKS RELATED TO TRANSPORTATION

Nurses and clients are not protected by their agency's insurance when they transport clients in their own automobile, should an accident happen.

(Adapted from Calfee B [1996]. NSO Risk Advisor. *Trevose, PA: Nurses Service Organization)*

of care, that results in harm to another person. In addition to adhering to prescribed scope of practice laws and meeting appropriate standards of nursing care, involvement with other laws is common in community health (Display 3-1).

The most important public health laws are those designed to protect the rights of the public. These include patients' rights, such as informed consent, confidentiality, right to privacy, and right to limit or refuse care. The right of habeas corpus says that a person may not be held against his or her will unless that person is a threat to self or society. Regulations requiring reporting of suspected child or elder abuse, compliance with Occupational Safety & Health Administration (OSHA) standards, and securing advance directives from home care clients are common examples of nurses' legal responsibilities.

Ethical Considerations

Laws are generated externally for the good of society as a whole. Ethics are generated internally and govern our behavior by our personal code of ethics (Display 3-2). A code of ethics is derived from personal values. Sometimes groups or professions develop a code of ethics to govern decision making and behavior. Our values are the things we hold most dear, the issues and ideas we believe to be most worthy. Our values are

---

DISPLAY 3-2
MORAL Model for Ethical Decision Making

M "Massage" the dilemma. Identify and describe the issues in the dilemma. Consider the opinions of all the major players in the dilemma, as well as their value systems. This includes clients, family members, nurses, physicians, clergy, and any other interdisciplinary health-care members.

O Outline the choices. Examine all the choices, including those less realistic and conflicting. This stage is designed only for considering choices and not for making a final decision.

R Resolve the dilemma. Review the issues and choices, applying the basic principles of ethics to each choice. Make a decision and select the best choice based on the view of all those concerned in the dilemma.

A Act by applying the selected choice. This requires actual implementation; the previous steps had allowed for only dialogue and discussion.

L Look back and evaluate the entire process, including the implementation. No process is complete without a thorough evaluation. Ensure that those involved can follow through. If not, a second decision may be required and the process must start again at the initial step.

(Adapted from Thiroux J [1977]. Ethics, Theory, and Practice, Philadelphia; McMillan; Halloran MC [1982]. Rational ethical judgements utilizing a decision making tool. Heart and Lung 11[6]; 566–570; Guido GW [1995]. Legal and ethical issues. In Yoder-Wise P. Leading and Managing in Nursing. St. Louis: Mosby.)

powerful, deeply ingrained influences that govern how we choose to act. Values endure and give purpose to our lives. They are the criteria by which we make decisions, even when operating on a subconscious level. Although values are enduring and provide stability, they can change with experience.

Values Clarification

Many people are unaware of their values. Values clarification exercises such as in the following list can help you identify your personal and professional values.

1. Write a personal obituary containing all that you would like people to say about you when your life is over.
2. Write a reference or personal evaluation about yourself as you would like to be known professionally.
3. Fold a paper in three parts and write in each part one of your three top values, the ones you hold most dear or believe in most dearly. Then relinquish one of these values by tearing it off the paper and discarding it. This is difficult to do if you take the exercise seriously. Then discard a second value in the same manner. Some people find this nearly impossible, indicating the powerful nature of values. If you play the game honestly and seriously, the remaining value is your terminal value, the one most influential and cherished. As this exercise indicates, there is a hierarchical quality to values, but sometimes our most important values are so important to us that it is painful to choose among them.

Forced choice ranking is another way to determine which values hold greater importance than others. Even people who hold the same basic values, such as a group of community health nurses, might prioritize things differently. Some situations cause our personal values to be in conflict. When two strongly held values of the same rank occur in conflict, an ethical dilemma occurs.

Ethical Decisions and Dilemmas

Ethics deals with moral decisions regarding right and wrong. An ethical decision is an evaluative judgment; these are often recognized as ''shoulds'' and ''oughts.'' These days, community health nurses are frequently faced with ethical decisions about limited allocation of resources. Other ethical principles with potential for dilemmas are confidentiality, autonomy, beneficence (doing good), nonmaleficence (preventing harm), equity, justice, respect for others, fidelity, and veracity (telling the truth).

Many conflicts arise regarding nonmaleficence. Common problems confronting community health nurses occur when clients' choices conflict with what nurses know will promote their health. This is a conflict between autonomy and nonmaleficence. Often community health nurses must deal with limited funds or resources for poor people or an inadequate number of allowable nursing or home health visits to provide quality care. These conflicts involve the principles of equity, justice, allowed allocation of resources, and nonmaleficence.

Ethical codes guide behavior and decisions. The ANA's Code for Nurses sets standards, guides nursing practice, and helps in decision making. Nurses cope by conferring with one another or with clergy or other community resource people. Agencies have ethics committees that assist in negotiating decision-making dilemmas (see Display 3-2 for a framework for ethical decision making). The Patient Self-Determination Act of 1990, which affects the ethical decisions of health-care providers, is described in Chapter 16.

Cultural and Spiritual Considerations

Values and culture are closely related; in fact, values are derived from culture. Culture is defined as "the accepted beliefs, values, and behaviors that are shared by members of a society and provide a design or 'map' for living" (Spradley & Allender, 1996). In the United States, we have the dominant American culture as well as the culture of various ethnic and religious groups and other subgroups.

Cultural Subgroups Within the Dominant Culture

The United States can be described as a beautiful mosaic of cultures. There are approximately 100 diverse ethnic groups living in the United States. Immigrants come to the United States from all over the world, bringing rich cultural patterns with them (Display 3-3 and Table 3-1). The fastest-growing ethnic group in the United States is Hispanic-American, with a growth rate of 12% annually. Hispanic-Americans represent 9% of the population currently and come from several countries of origin. African-Americans represent 12%, Asian-Americans 3%, and Native Americans 1% of the population. By the year 2050, it is projected that Hispanic-Americans will make up 21% of the U.S. population, African-Americans 15%, and Asian-Americans 10% (U.S. Bureau of Census, 1992). The percentage of European-Americans will decrease but will still be the majority. Display 3-4 lists factors indicating heritage consistency.

DISPLAY 3-3
Place of Birth of Foreign-Born Persons: 1990

Europe: 20%
Former Soviet Union: 2%
Asia: 25%
North America: 41%
South America: 5%
Africa: 2%
Oceana: 1%
Area Not Reported: 4%

(Source: Bureau of Census [1993]. 1990 Census of Population, Social and Economic Characteristics. Washington DC: U.S. Government Printing Office.)

TABLE 3-1. Top 10 Countries of Origin for Immigrants in Fiscal Year 1994

Country	Numbers
Mexico	6.2 million
Phillipines	1 million
Cuba	805,000
El Savador	718,000
Canada	679,000
Germany	625,000
China	565,000
Dominican Republic	556,000
South Korea	533,000
Vietnam	496,000

(*From:* United States Census Bureau Study, 8/28/1995; reported by the Associated Press, in *The Boston Globe,* v. 248, #60, August 29, 1995, p. 3.)

DISPLAY 3-4
Factors Indicating Heritage Consistency

1. Childhood development occurred in the person's country of origin or in an immigrant neighborhood in the United States of like ethnic group.
2. Extended family members encouraged participation in traditional religious or cultural activities.
3. Individual engages in frequent visits to country of origin or to the "old neighborhood" in the United States.
4. Family homes are within the ethnic community.
5. Individual participants in ethnic cultural events, such as religious festivals or national holidays.
6. Individual was raised in an extended family setting.
7. Individual maintains regular contact with the extended family.
8. Individual's name has not been Americanized.
9. Individual was educated in a parochial (nonpublic) school with a religious or ethnic philosophy similar to the family's background.
10. Individual engages in social activities primarily with others of the same ethnic background.
11. Individual has knowledge of the culture and language of origin.
12. Individual possesses elements of personal pride about heritage.

(*Spector R [1996].* Cultural Diversity in Health and Illness, *4th ed. Stamford, CT: Appleton and Lange.*

Cultural aggregates are further divided between elderly and youth cultures. These generational differences are magnified when immigrant families strive to adapt to and assimilate into the dominant American culture. Teenagers readily achieve this. Peer pressure and their sensitivity about being different from the dominant culture often cause teenagers to reject their traditional language and culture. At the same time, elderly family members find it difficult to learn new ways and languages readily. They cannot change so easily, and they persist with the old, familiar cultural ways. Conflicts occur because of differing allegiances.

Cultures are not defined only by ethnicity. There is also a generation gap in the dominant American culture; think of generational differences in music and dress preferences. We identify yuppie, gay, and street cultures. There are other divisions in all cultures, such as blue collar vs. white collar, rural vs. urban, and liberal vs. conservative.

Concepts as well as words have different meanings among different cultural groups. Some of these important concepts are suffering, health, healers, cause of illness, role of family, gift giving, caregivers, nourishing foods, family, religion, authority, appropriate sexual expression, time, personal space, death, and beliefs and practices about dying. (See Appendix A for customs about death and dying in various religious groups.)

Cultural Assessments

Making assumptions about a client's cultural background can be risky. Do not make assumptions on data such as race or appearance. For instance, some Filipinos closely resemble Hispanics or Asians. Migration and intermarriage make it difficult to identify ethnicity or race by appearance. Clients often have cultural heritages different than a glance at their face would lead you to believe. It is difficult to interpret a client's nonverbal communication unless you are familiar with his or her culture.

Making quick assumptions about people can also lead to stereotyping. Stereotypes are preconceived, oversimplified ideas, often with negative beliefs about a particular group. Even when stereotypes are positive, the results can be negative if individuality is ignored. The danger of stereotyping is that people are no longer considered as individuals.

Cultural assessments should be made by attentive listening and observation with a caring, respectful attitude (Display 3-5). Read about the culture and, more importantly, find reliable people within that group who will tell you about it. Often an assessment guide (Display 3-6) will help you remember the questions to ask in a formal or informal interview. Assessment guides can be simple or comprehensive, depending on their intended use. The cultural assessment includes the five most important topics for nurses to learn about their clients: health-care beliefs and practices; illness beliefs and practices; interpersonal relations; spiritual practices; and world view and social structures.

Until recently, spiritual needs and practices were neglected by the nursing and medical professions and relegated to the clergy. Now we recognize their relevance to health, healing, and nursing practice. Figure 3-1 illustrates the many influences affecting a person's personal health traditions, including ethnicity, culture, and religion. Table 3-2 lists the major religious affiliations in the United States as of 1994.

(text continues on p. 65)

DISPLAY 3-5
Strategies to Reduce Defensiveness and Resistance

1. State what you feel. Express empathy by reflecting feeling. "What you just said made me uncomfortable. Can we talk about it some more?" Reflecting your reactions attests to your integrity, honesty, and interest. There is no need to apologize for feelings.

2. Use humor, including humor that is self-directed. "Yes, I know I am late. I am sorry to keep you waiting. It seems I was born late, and I've been running to catch up ever since!"

3. Disclose selected, appropriate information to promote sharing and a sense of acceptance. "I know it's hard. My own baby never wanted me to do that to him either, but here's what I found worked for me . . ."

4. Acknowledge and describe briefly your own beliefs, behaviors, and responses in non-judgmental ways. "I personally have never believed in spanking children, but I know people have different ideas about raising them."

5. Get help from others; you do not have to do everything alone. "I don't know very much about your mother's values and beliefs. Could you tell me about them so that I can provide the kind of care she expects and will find appropriate?"

6. Accept responsibility for behavioral errors by acknowledging them and apologizing to reinforce positive expectations for the relationship. "I am sorry that I did not know today is a religious holiday for you. Will you tell me about it?"

7. Be flexible; it prevents frustration. Plans are necessary for meeting goals, but flexibility is needed to meet clients' needs and expectations realistically. "I was hoping you might be able to take him to see the doctor Monday, but will it be all right if I arrange it for Thursday?"

8. Show acceptance and understanding by clearly identifying and reflecting the client's concern or understanding of the problem. "I understand that you think rubbing horse liniment on your knee will help the arthritis, but I wonder if you would also like to try this other medication."

9. Assess coping response patterns (including your own) to problematic and stressful situations. Such assessment promotes recognition of resistant or defensive responses.

10. Ask questions. Different cultural groups expect questions to be asked in different ways (perhaps indirectly or after considerable small talk), but nurses need information. "What would you like me to do for you?"

11. Recommend interventions that are not likely to meet with resistance or defensiveness. "I understand that your ethnic foods are very important to you. Will you help me figure out which ones will fit into this diet that the doctor wants you to be on?"

12. Openly acknowledge discrepancies between your views and the client's. "I know you do not like to drive in the snow, but I am concerned about Sara missing her physical therapy sessions."

13. To let it be known you understand them, accurately reflect, clarify, and interpret the client's behaviors, concerns, or ideas. "I think I heard you say that Juan's illness is because of the evil eye. Would you tell me more about that?"

14. Reflect and adjust your voice, body position, and other aspects of nonverbal communication to synchronize with those of the client.

15. Get to know the client's informal system of social support. The client is part of a network and usually does not make decisions or act entirely without support from others. "Is there someone from your church who might stay with the children while you have that examination at the clinic?"

(Adapted from Pederson P [1988]. A Handbook for Developing Multicultural Awareness. *Alexandria, VA: American Association for Counseling and Development.)*

DISPLAY 3-6
Cultural Assessment Interview Guide

The following interview guide is one tool for data collection. The guide includes broad statements and open-ended questions to encourage clients to express themselves fully with descriptive responses. This is just a sampling of the type of questions that can be asked. It can be expanded and adapted to meet the needs of those using it. Those using the guide should be flexible: ask only the appropriate questions, and use a language and conversational level suitable to the client and the setting. Remember: in cultural assessment, the client teaches and the nurse learns.

HEALTH-CARE BELIEFS AND PRACTICES

1. I would like to learn what health means to you. Imagine yourself totally healthy. Tell me what it would be like for you. Tell me how you know when you are healthy. I am wondering how you believe people of your culture stay healthy.
2. Can you explain about the types of food you eat, how food is prepared, when your meal times are and with whom you share your meals?
3. Can you recall activities that were performed by your family to keep people healthy? What did your mother do to keep you from getting sick? How do you keep yourself from getting sick?

ILLNESS BELIEFS AND CUSTOMS

1. How do you describe "illness?"
2. Which of the following things do you believe causes illness: poor eating habits, incorrect food combinations, germs, God's punishment for sin, the "Evil Eye," other people's hexes or spells, witchcraft, changes in environment (ie, cold or hot weather), exposure to drafts, overwork, underwork, grief and loss, others?
3. Can you recall special folk beliefs and practices about illness? What home remedies did your mother use to treat illness? What home remedies do you use?

INTERPERSONAL RELATIONS

1. As you think about the ways that people in your culture communicate with each other, do you notice differences from the dominant culture—for example, the use of silence, how close to each other you stand, touching people, use of your body and hands?
2. I am wondering about family life. Could you identify and tell me about the members of your family? I would like to learn about women's duties, men's duties, and how the men and women relate to each other.
3. Tell me about your philosophy of raising children and disciplining them and their place in the family.

SPIRITUAL PRACTICES

1. Can you tell me about your religious and spiritual self? I would like to hear about your beliefs and practices.
2. As you think about your life experiences, could you share your feelings about life and death?

DISPLAY 3-6 (Continued)

3. Can you tell me about your beliefs and practices related to the death of a loved one—about the funeral, mourning customs, and your beliefs about souls, spirits, and the afterlife? When is it appropriate for men and women to express their feelings when a loved one dies?

WORLD VIEW AND OTHER SOCIAL STRUCTURES

1. I would like to learn about what is important in life to you.
2. I am interested in learning what languages are spoken in your home and the languages that you understand and speak.
3. Can you reflect on the kinds of jobs that members of your family have and how finances influence your way of life?
4. Can you reflect on what education means to you and your family? Please describe the kind of education you received and what education you hope your children will receive.

(Adapted from Rosenbaum [1991]. A Cultural Assessment Guide. Canadian Nurse 87:21–22.)

TABLE 3-2. Religious Affiliation in the United States, 1994

Religious Group	Percentage
Protestant	59.35
Baptist	20.8
Methodist	9.4
Lutheran	6.6
Presbyterian	4.75
Episcopal	2.2
No denomination given or nondenominational	15.6
Catholic	25.5
Jewish	2.0
None	9.2
Other–not Christian	3.9
Total	99.95

Reprinted by permission. Spector R [1996]. *Cultural Diversity in Health and Illness*, 4th ed. Stanford, CT: Appleton and Lange, pg. 73 (Based on data from Smith, T. W. [1994]. National Opinion Research Center [Chicago, IL: University of Chicago, 1994.])

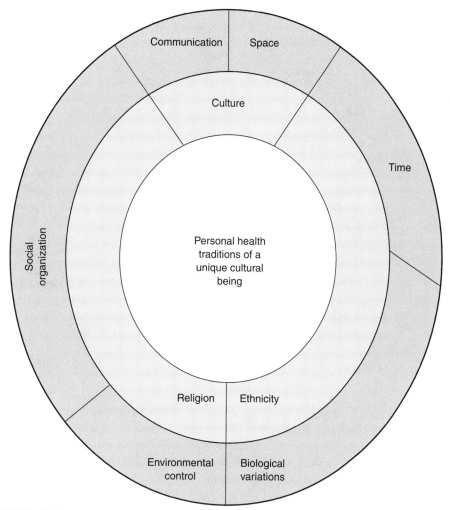

FIGURE 3-1
Many factors influence a person's health traditions. (Reprinted by permission. Spector R [1996]. *Cultural Diversity in Health and Illness,* 4th ed. Stamford, CT: Appleton and Lange.)

Spirituality and Religious Considerations

"The symbols, patterns and gestures, art forms and prayer and meditation commonly associated with religion often make it difficult to separate religious from cultural factors" (Spruhan, 1996). By ignoring clients' religious beliefs and practices and spiritual needs, we do them a great disservice. The mass media trivializes religious devotion, but polls indicate that nine of 10 Americans believe in God and the efficacy of prayer. At a 1997 conference sponsored by Harvard Medical School and the Mind/Body Institute, George

Gallup said,

> In the 6 decades my family has been involved with national Gallup polls, there has never been such an interest in spirituality as there is today, nor such hunger for God. Ninety percent of Americans say they believe in God and 9 out of 10 believe in an afterlife. Scientific discoveries are undergirding this.

Studies conducted at Duke University show how much Americans rely on religion to cope (Fig. 3-2). Other studies show a positive correlation between religious practice and physical health and well-being. Recent studies show that persons who attend church once or more a week only spend one third the amount of time in the hospital as those who never or rarely attend church. Important scientific studies are being conducted at several locations regarding the healing effects of prayer. One of the most famous experiments was conducted by Dr. R. C. Byrd among 393 patients in a coronary care unit in San Francisco. This study showed that a person's thoughts and prayers can influence another person's healing at a distance, without the persons meeting each other. Intercessory prayer was conducted on half of the 393 patients. This was a double-blind study; neither those who gathered the data nor the patients themselves knew who was receiving prayer. This study was well designed and corrected for the placebo effect in that the patients did not know if they were being prayed for. Those who received prayer healed much more quickly and had significantly fewer complications (Byrd, 1988).

Many nurses, especially holistic, parish, and hospice nurses, routinely pray for and with their clients, with their permission. Similar to the old religious tradition of ''laying on of hands,'' nurses have developed therapeutic touch and healing touch strategies in an attempt to decrease clients' pain and need for analgesia. ''Meditative in stance when they care for patients, practitioners believe that even if actual contact is not made, their healing energy field connects with patients,'' wrote Dr. Herbert Benson (1997), a professor at Harvard Medical School. Benson spent years studying all faith traditions and found they all have some mystical traditions of meditation, similar to what he dubbed ''the relaxation response.'' He found that the relaxation response is best elicited by using a meaningful phrase from one's faith tradition to focus one's thoughts. The relaxation response results in physiologic changes just the opposite of stressful fight-or-flight reactions. Blood pressure drops, as does muscle tension and metabolism.

To induce the relaxation response, select a focus word, brief prayer, or phrase rooted in your belief system. Sitting quietly, comfortably, and undisturbed, close your eyes, breathe slowly, and relax your muscles. Repeat the focus word as you exhale. When other thoughts intrude, assume a passive attitude, let them pass by, and return to the repetition. After 10 to 20 minutes, gently and gradually return to an active state by opening your eyes and sitting quietly for a few minutes. For maximal physical, mental, and spiritual benefits, practice this meditation once or twice daily.

Spirituality and religion are not exactly the same thing. Spirituality is the sensitivity and quest for the transcendent and is more generic. Religion is the practice of a particular faith tradition. The success of Alcoholics Anonymous is largely accredited to its spiritual basis of trusting in a higher power. One of this group's famous sayings is, ''Let go and let God.'' To summon the healing effect of the relaxation response, we need to surrender everyday worries and tensions. Faith in the Absolute is the most powerful road to healing

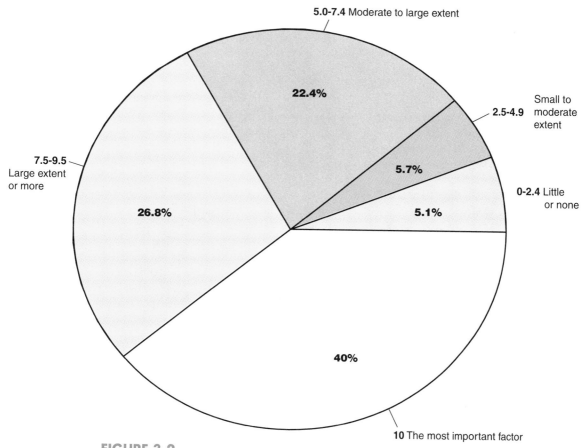

FIGURE 3-2
Self-rated religious coping (On a 0–10 scale, how much do you use religion to cope?) Responses by 298 consecutively admitted patients to Duke Hospital. (Reprinted with permission. Koenig HG [1997]. *Is Religion Good for Your Health?* Binghamton, NY: Haworth Press.)

because it deals with the whole person. Florence Nightingale, a deeply spiritual person, believed that humans have a remarkable self-healing capacity for adaptation and survival.

This is not in any way to negate the value of conventional medicine and surgery. However, much could be done to reduce health-care costs in this country if people regularly used stress-reduction and proven health and healing practices. Benson (1997) estimated that half of the stress-related office visits, or 37.5% of all visits, could be eliminated by placing greater emphasis on "mind–body health and remembered wellness." He used 1994 statistics to show that by reducing office visits by 37.5%, the cost savings would be $54.5 billion per year.

THE NURSE SPEAKS . . .
About an Ethical Dilemma

I am assigned to work at an HIV testing clinic. A fellow named Bob seemed to feel like talking one day, so I made extra time to sit down with him. He had come to the clinic three or four times in the past and seemed quite comfortable with me. His HIV tests were always negative.

Bob: "You know, one of these days this test is going to show I have AIDS. I've been sharing needles to shoot up. I try not to do it, but it keeps happening. Some of the other people could have AIDS—probably do, in fact."

Me: "You've been shooting drugs and sharing needles? How long have you been doing drugs?"

Bob: "Too long. I hate myself for it, but I just can't get off the stuff. It costs a fortune."

Me: "How do you manage the cost? You told me you couldn't find a job."

Bob: "How do you think? We rob houses. It's disgusting, actually. Most of the burglaries in this town are done to support a habit. We even have a system about who gets to do which neighborhood. I'm not proud of it."

My own problem was that my home had just been robbed about 10 days beforehand, and some very precious things I loved were stolen. I was still feeling personally violated and furious about the burglary. You can imagine the conflict I felt at that moment. I yearned to pick up the phone and call the police to report this guy. Then I remembered my nursing responsibility to maintain confidentiality. For a few moments I was so upset that I had to make an excuse and leave the room to regain my composure and think clearly. When I returned, I talked with Bob about the methadone maintenance program, reflecting his self-disgust with his current lifestyle and his fear of AIDS. The timing was right, and he agreed to a referral to the methadone clinic as well as a contract between the two of us. I agreed to continue to monitor his progress and lend support; Bob agreed to enter the methadone program, which would enable him to stop the robberies and stop sharing needles with other addicts.

This plan worked well for almost a year, at which point Bob moved back to his hometown and I lost track of him. At the time of his move, he had reduced his methadone dose so much and felt so much better about himself that I am optimistic he was able to get off drugs entirely with some supportive services in his hometown.

Jack
PUBLIC HEALTH NURSE

CLINICAL APPLICATION

A Critical Thinking Case Study About a Conflict of Values Due to Cultural Differences

You work as a nurse for the county department of health and receive a referral for an evaluation from the department of social services. A family on welfare has requested a 24-hour live-in personal care aide (PCA) financed by Medicaid due to an urgent situation. Mrs. R, a mother of nine children, delivered twins 6 days ago, developed thrombophlebitis, and has been ordered to stay on bed rest.

You notice that the family lives in a community of people who belong to a religious sect. In the past, you found the families of that community very demanding and persistent about receiving the care they desired; in fact, this led you to request a special in-service class for nurses at your agency about this group's beliefs and culture. You learned that this sect believes that these health and welfare services are awarded them by God, and the health-care providers are the mere vehicles of the gift.

When you arrive the house is full of people. Mrs. R is in bed with warm soaks on her left leg. Her mother and sister are present and all three are wearing scarves over their shaved heads. The twin babies have just been fed and look clean and comfortable. You estimate their weight at about 5 lb each. Seven other small children are playing actively in the house. Three of the children belong to the R family, the rest to Mrs. R's sister.

Mr. R is wearing a long black wool coat, the group's traditional garb for men. Mrs. R explains that it is their tradition that the men spend most of their time studying their sacred writings and praying. It is a hot day, and there is a strong, stale odor from the coat and other woolen clothing in the room. The air in the room is very stuffy, and the house is cluttered.

 and Think!

- Describe all the ways your personal value system is at odds with this situation.
- In what ways are your own values apt to prejudice you?
- How can you deal with your prejudices?

You assess the need for the requested PCA services. Mrs. R's mother explains that 24 hours of care are needed because the twins must be fed every 3 hours during the night and Mrs. R cannot get out of bed. She adds that she still has young children at home and heavy responsibilities, so she cannot be here all the time. The sister adds that she has 11 children and is in the same situation. All three women look worn and tired, and your heart goes out to them.

You explain that PCAs are not legally allowed to do treatments like the warm soaks on Mrs. R's leg. The mother hastily adds that she lives nearby and can come do them several times a day as ordered. When asked what they want the PCA to do,

Mrs. R says she wants her to clean and cook and care for the children, adding that she wants to feed and bathe the twins herself if someone can bring what is needed to her bed.

You assess Mrs. R physically and reinforce instructions about the warm soaks to her left leg. You examine the babies.

 and Think!

- Your decision is to deny the request for a 24-hour live-in PCA. Give your reasons for the denial.
- Are you influenced by the fact that Mr. R, who does not work, should be helping more with the household and the children he helped create?
- Do you think the mother and sister should be willing to help more?
- Do you think you understand this culture adequately to do your job? If not, how can you learn more?
- Are you making an objective, professional judgment in this situation?

Your professional responsibility is to assign the most appropriate and least costly level of care. To do this, you must take the client's culture into consideration and must not be biased by past experiences or your personal values. You report to the department of social services that personal care services are not needed or desired in this situation because Mrs. R wants to take care of herself and the twins. What is needed is a homemaker to cook and care for the house and the older children during the day. At night, Mr. R can place the twins and supplies on Mrs. R's bed and may even want to help feed them, because they are receiving bottles.

The family seems satisfied with the arrangement. You continue to call and visit every 2 weeks to assess the family and evaluate the situation.

Chapter SUMMARY

Legal, ethical, and cultural considerations are presented, with emphasis on applications for the community health nurse. Various strategies for data collection and nursing interventions are included under each category. The purposes of and inconsistencies in public health laws are described. Sources of public health laws are federal, state, and local ordinances emanating from all three branches of government: administrative, legislative, and judicial. The developmental process from the time legislation is proposed until it becomes law is discussed to show how nurses can have input into regulations. Legal responsibilities of community health nurses are described, along with common legal risks. A distinction is made between law and ethics.

Values are stressed as the building blocks of a personal or professional code of ethics. Values clarification strategies are noted. Ethical decisions and dilemmas are described, along with the most common conflicts of ethical principles. Culture is defined and statistics are provided about major ethnic groups in the United States, now and in the future. Cultural aggregates are described. Information on how to do a cultural assessment is given. Spirituality and religious practices support healing and illness prevention, according to experiments, and most Americans believe in God, the efficacy of prayer, and an afterlife. Nurses and doctors must be more sensitive to clients' spiritual needs.

A list of references and additional readings for this chapter appears at the end of Part 1.

4

The Family and the Community as the Client

Key Terms

aggregates
blended families
Centers for Disease Control and Prevention
clinical trials
community assessment
control group
descriptive study
double-blind study
dyads
dysfunctional families

endemic
epidemiology
experimental trials
family assessment
genogram
health planning
identified patient
incidence
mandated reportable disease
milestone chart
morbidity

mortality
multiproblem families
nuclear families
pandemic
prevalence
prospective studies
research survey
retrospective studies
triage
web of causation

Learning Objectives

1. Explain why and when the family is the client and the community is the client.

2. Identify four types of families.

3. Determine the implications for family life regarding new findings on early brain development.

4. Analyze the effect of divorce on adolescents.

5. Identify reasons for the declining rate of teenage pregnancies.

6. Explain why elderly people often prefer to live in retirement communities.

7. Differentiate between multiproblem and dysfunctional families.

8. List the strengths and weaknesses you see in your own family.

9. Identify the elements of a family.

10. Describe various methods of data collection.

11. Explain the complexities of health planning for a community.

12. Define the science of epidemiology.

13. Describe the various types of epidemiologic investigations.

14. **Explain the role of the Centers for Disease Control and Prevention.**

15. **Compare and contrast natural and man-made disasters.**

16. **Describe the role of the nurse during disasters.**

17. **Perform a community assessment.**

The Family as Client

The Family as a System

Family-centered nursing care was established by Florence Nightingale and continues to the present as one of the core practices of community health nursing. In the past, family care often focused on the needs of a person within the family context. Today we understand a family as a system or a unit of care, with the person as the context. An example of this type of family nursing occurs in home care when the community health nurse assesses a family's ability to care for a member at home, teaches the elderly woman about the care of her spouse, assesses her physical ability to provide care, and provides emotional support to her. At the same time, the nurse focuses on the adult children and their ability and motivation to help their parents and the problems they face in doing so. The actions of each of the members directly affects the family as a whole. Thus, the family as a unit or system is the client. The elderly male spouse may be the "identified patient," but the family system is really the client (Fig. 4-1). The nurse must be aware that families operate as a system.

Types of Families

The image of the traditional American family as portrayed in many popular television programs of the 1950s and 1960s is not realistic today. The nuclear family, with a father, mother, and children living together, is no longer the dominant pattern of family life in the United States. In fact, the pattern during the 1950s was the exception through U.S. history. Extended and multigenerational families were a pattern during the 19th century, mainly for economic reasons. Today the pattern has again changed. Among the middle class, most grandparents prefer to live on their own rather than with their children if they can afford to do so. It is also less common to see aunts and uncles and other extended family members boarding with one another, because more people can afford to live alone. Although this independence may seem more appealing for people in many respects, it also leads to greater isolation and loss of support systems, especially as people become elderly or widowed.

Children are an essential part of some people's definition of a family. However, more adult married couples, called dyad families, are choosing not to have children. By the year 2010, the Census Bureau estimates that three in five American families will have no children under 18 living at home. Dyads include elderly couples with adult children who live elsewhere. Childless couples and siblings living together are also dyads. Traditionally, cohabiting heterosexual or homosexual couples have not been legally considered families, although this is being challenged by gay and lesbian groups.

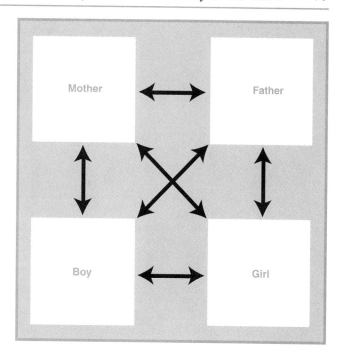

FIGURE 4-1
The family as a system.

Single-parent families are common in the United States and are rapidly increasing in number. However, a single parent usually must work to support the family, so many children are spending their early years in day-care centers of variable quality. Some of these children receive excellent parenting despite all the demands on a single parent's time and energy. Others, however, receive inadequate parental guidance and attention, with resultant adjustment and behavior problems. Recent findings regarding how a young child's brain develops have profound implications for parenting, early education, and policy (Nash, 1997). At Baylor College of Medicine, researchers found that babies who are not frequently touched or stimulated by play develop brains that are 20% to 30% smaller than normal. Stimulation by positive attention causes neural activity and growth that actually changes the structure of the brain, increasing learning capacity.

Blended families, in which divorced or widowed parents remarry, combining the children from previous marriages, are also increasing in number. These families face unique challenges as old loyalties are tested and new relationships are defined. Children of these unions spend an average of 6 years in single-parent families before the remarriage, compounding the adjustments required.

In 1996, the Substance Abuse and Mental Health Services Administration (SAMHSA) reported that adolescents living with two biologic or adoptive parents are significantly less likely to use illicit drugs, alcohol, or cigarettes than adolescents in other family structures (USDHHS, PHS, 1996a). SAMHSA's Office of Applied Studies surveyed 22,000

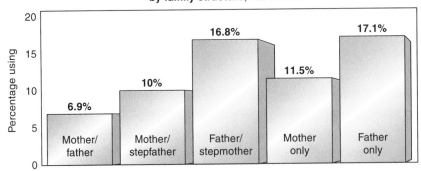

FIGURE 4-2
Study shows two-parent family lowers teen drug use. (Source: The Relationship Between Family Structure & Adolescent Substance Use. Office of Applied Studies, Substance Abuse and Mental Health Services Administration.)

respondents ages 12 to 17 in 1991, 1992, and 1993. The adolescents' gender, race, and ethnicity did not change the percentages at all. Adolescents living with both biologic or adoptive parents are 50% to 150% less likely to use and abuse chemicals (Fig. 4-2).

Many single women are raising families. Some are single women who never marry.

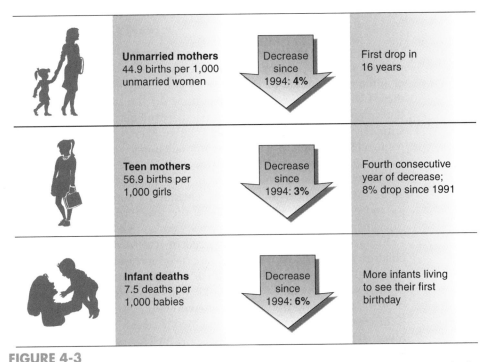

FIGURE 4-3
Birth rate trends. Fewer babies were born to unwed or teenage U.S. mothers in 1995, and infant mortality rates hit a record low. (Source: Centers for Disease Control and Prevention.)

The rates of unwed mothers and teenage mothers have been dropping (Fig. 4-3). In 1995, about 57 teenagers per 1,000 gave birth, compared with 63 per 1,000 in 1970. Teenagers give birth to 13% of the newborns in the United States, one of the highest rates in the industrial world.

Most single-parent families result from divorce, which ends 60% of American marriages. Divorce is usually very destructive to children, but sometimes it brings release from abusive, dysfunctional situations. Divorce contributes greatly to childhood

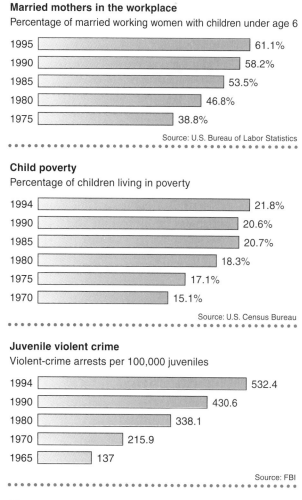

Married mothers in the workplace
Percentage of married working women with children under age 6

1995	61.1%
1990	58.2%
1985	53.5%
1980	46.8%
1975	38.8%

Source: U.S. Bureau of Labor Statistics

Child poverty
Percentage of children living in poverty

1994	21.8%
1990	20.6%
1985	20.7%
1980	18.3%
1975	17.1%
1970	15.1%

Source: U.S. Census Bureau

Juvenile violent crime
Violent-crime arrests per 100,000 juveniles

1994	532.4
1990	430.6
1980	338.1
1970	215.9
1965	137

Source: FBI

Most noncustodial fathers don't pay child support
Percentage of noncustodial fathers
who paid child support, 1989
62.5% – Paid nothing
25.5% – Paid full amount
12% – Paid partial amount

Source: U.S. Census Bureau

FIGURE 4-4
Vital statistics. These numbers may help you decide where you stand on the issues. (Source: USA Weekend, *Aug. 9–11, 1996.*)

poverty (Fig. 4-4). Children have replaced seniors as the poorest segment of the population. In 1996, the last year for which data were complete, 10 million children under age 18 had no health insurance coverage (Associated Press, 1997a). About 3 million children come from families eligible for Medicaid, so those children, in terms of medical coverage, are usually more fortunate unless block grants or welfare reform decrease their eligibility. Among the homeless, women with children are the fastest-growing group. Many fathers who do not have custody do not provide financially for their children (see Fig. 4-4).

Elderly Family Members

The entitlement programs of Medicare and Social Security are largely responsible for the improving economic status of the elderly population during the past 30 years. Elderly people are generally defined as those age 65 and over. Persons age 65 to 75 are usually the "well elderly." Most continue to lead active lives in their communities. Some people move to warmer climates after retirement, where they can play golf or walk during the winter. Health needs of the elderly are described in Chapter 11.

As elderly people reach their mid-70s, many choose to move into senior citizen housing complexes or retirement communities, if they can afford to do so. These communities offer various levels of care, depending on need. Independent living in apartments or small homes is available in most subsidized, community-sponsored senior citizen complexes. Some private communities also provide assisted living as the next level of care. Assisted living provides a small amount of nursing supervision and minimal assistance with bathing and dressing, but residents must be able to walk to the dining room for meals. Full care is available in a nursing facility when residents need 24-hour nursing assistance and supervision.

When these three levels of care are available on one campus, elderly people can remain near their friends even when their needs change; they avoid the readjustment of a major move. Many elderly people prefer these facilities because they provide as much independence as possible at each stage of old age. A major reason cited is that people dread becoming a burden on their children in their old age. As life expectancy increases, elderly people face the reality of years of chronic disease and physical limitations. However, members of some cultural and ethnic groups consider it wrong to "reject" their parents by allowing them to live alone.

Identified Patients Within the Family

Although health professionals consider the family as a whole to be the client, family members often identify one member as the patient—perhaps an elderly sick person, a physically or mentally disabled person, a dying person, a new mother and baby, or a person with a contagious disease. A child who is acting out anger and developing behavior problems at school is often a family's identified patient, but that child's behavior is usually a symptom of the problems of the real patient, the family. Everyone in a family is affected by what is happening to each family member. This is particularly obvious in the families of alcoholics, where the negative effects of alcoholism cause long-term problems in spouses and children.

Multiproblem Families and Dysfunctional Families

An example of a multiproblem family is shown in the Clinical Application in Chapter 1, in which a basically healthy family is confronted with many serious problems. Dysfunctional families usually result from unhealthy or inadequate communication and behavior patterns and poor definitions of family values. Alcoholism and other chemical dependencies create dysfunctional families because all family members are affected by the addiction. Families of persons with some personality disorders or other types of mental illness may become dysfunctional because of the "stably unstable" nature of some mental illnesses. See Chapter 10 for more about addictions and mental health problems.

Characteristics of Adequately Functioning Families

Some people ask, "Isn't every family somewhat dysfunctional?" In a sense, yes: no family is perfect, and every family is dysfunctional at times. However, families that function adequately have certain core characteristics and are said to be basically healthy. Healthy families:

- Provide a sense of security and support
- Promote good communication among members
- Are adaptable and perform roles flexibly
- Have values and a spiritual orientation
- Promote family unity, cooperation, and loyalty
- Promote pride and acceptance of one another
- Have good relationships in the wider community

Making a Family Assessment

A simple, quick way to assess a family is to identify its strengths and weaknesses. Many family assessment tools exist to help make a thorough family assessment (Displays 4-1 and 4-2). A genogram is a family assessment tool used to plot out genealogy for various purposes (Fig. 4-5). Genograms are particularly useful in identifying genetic diseases within a family.

The Community as Client

Communities Are Defined

The definition of community as client is demonstrated when nursing service is focused on the community as a whole. A community is a collection of people in a place who interact with one another and whose common interests and goals give them a sense of belonging. The defining characteristics of a community include a population within certain boundaries. Those boundaries are often geographic, such as a city, county, state, nation, or census tract. Much epidemiologic and statistical data about health are based on census tract information; this is especially useful for health planning. Libraries and health departments have census maps and data available. The U.S. Census Bureau gathers data about the national population every 10 years.

(text continues on p. 84)

DISPLAY 4-1
Open-Ended Family Assessment

Family Name

Family Constellation

Member names	Occupation	Educational background

Significant change in family life

Coping ability of family

Energy level

Decision-making process within the family

Parenting skills

Support systems of the family

Use of health care (include plans for emergencies)

Financial status

Other impressions

Signature of Nurse _____ Date _____

Categories of data collection for family health assessment

Assessment Categories	Family strengths and self-care abilities	Family stresses and problems	Family resources
1. Family demographics 2. Physical environment 3. Psychological and spiritual environment 4. Family structure/roles 5. Family functions 6. Family values and beliefs 7. Family communication patterns 8. Family decision-making patterns 9. Family problem-solving patterns 10. Family coping patterns 11. Family health behavior 12. Family social and cultural patterns			

(*Spradley BW, Allender JA [1996].* Community Health Nursing: Concepts and Practice. *Philadelphia: Lippincott-Raven.*)

DISPLAY 4-2
Family Assessment Tool

Family Name _____

Family Constellation

Member	Birth Date	Sex	Marital Status	Education	Occupation	Community Involvement

Financial Status _____

Using the following scale, score the family based on your professional observations and judgment:

0 = Never   3 = Frequently
1 = Seldom   4 = Most of the time
2 = Occasionally   N = Not observed

	score	date	score	date	score	date	score	date
Facilitative Interaction Among Members								
a. Is there frequent communication among all members?								
b. Do conflicts get resolved?								
c. Are relationships supportive?								
d. Are love and caring shown among all members?								
e. Do members work collaboratively?								
Comments_____								
Totals								

DISPLAY 4-2
Family Assessment Tool (continued)

	score	date	score	date	score	date	score	date

Enhancement of Individual Development
a. Does family respond appropriately to members' developmental needs?
b. Does it tolerate disagreement?
c. Does it accept members as they are?
d. Does it promote member autonomy?

Comments_____

Totals

Effective Structuring of Relationships
a. Is decision making allocated to appropriate members?
b. Do member roles meet family needs?
c. Is there flexible distribution of tasks?
d. Are controls appropriate for family stage of development?

Comments_____

Totals

Active Coping Effort
a. Is family aware when there is a need for change?
b. Is it receptive to new ideas?
c. Does it actively seek resources?
d. Does it make good use of resources?
e. Does it creatively solve problems?

Comments_____

Totals

Healthy Environment and Life-style
a. Is family life-style health promoting?
b. Are living conditions safe and hygienic?
c. Is emotional climate conductive to good health?
d. Do members practice good health measures?

Comments_____

Totals

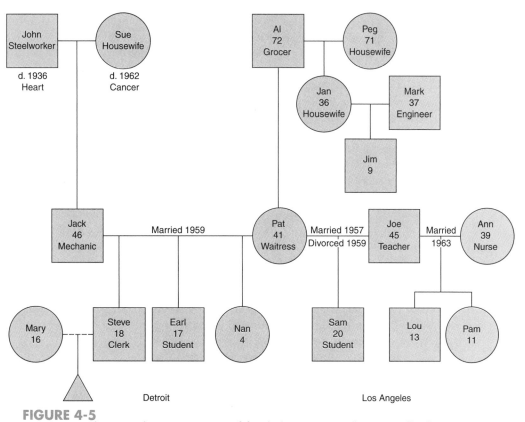

FIGURE 4-5
A genogram depicting three generations of family history. (Spradley BW, Allender JA [1996]. *Community Health Nursing: Concepts and Practice.* 4th ed. Philadelphia: Lippincott-Raven.)

Communities, Aggregates, and Groups

Many people do not define a community as a geographic location or place; instead, they speak of a community as a relationship—for example, the gay community, the elderly community, the business community, the black community, the religious community, or the homeless community. They say that community boundaries have to do only with the concerns people hold in common. In this context, the term *aggregate* is more precise. An aggregate is a group of people who share a common goal or interest and who are considered a unified whole. It is similar to the word *population*. A community is made up of many aggregates, and many of these aggregates extend beyond the geographic community. Persons who make up an aggregate seldom all meet one another, especially when the aggregate is large (ie, pregnant women). Thus, an aggregate differs from a group, whose members have face-to-face communication (ie, a support group). A school nurse provides service to an aggregate (schoolchildren) within a community (school district). Community health nurses serve aggregates and groups as well as communities.

Performing a Community Assessment

A community's needs can be assessed at various levels of complexity. A comprehensive assessment requires a great deal of work to gather and understand all the data relevant to the community's needs. Basic components of a community assessment are shown in Table 4-1. Some assessments rely on existing data and do not attempt comprehensive data collection. Problem-oriented assessments are commonly done, focusing on a single problem and studying the community in terms of that problem. An even simpler assessment is performed when only one aspect or dimension of the community is studied in reference to a problem.

The simplest type of community assessment is a survey. Descriptive epidemiologic studies might also be conducted regarding health problems. These are observational studies that describe what is naturally occurring regarding the health problems being studied. Data are organized and patterns are determined. Rates are studied, such as infant mortality rates. When the causes of a particular health problem are sought, an analytic study is conducted. Experimental studies are the most complex. These are epidemiologic investigations and will be covered later in this chapter.

In conducting a community assessment, information about aspects of the location or the geographic environment is gathered (Table 4-2). Aspects of the population and the social systems are observed (Table 4-3). All aspects of the health-care system are surveyed when community health nurses do a community assessment. Local telephone directories frequently list health and social welfare services; libraries are other excellent sources of information.

Health Planning—Implementation and Evaluation

Health planning for communities is much more complex than planning for individual clients because of the multiplicity of factors involved. Often community health planning becomes multidisciplinary, bringing into play the collaborative role of the nurse. Making

TABLE 4-1. Community Profile Inventory: Location Perspective

Location Variables	Community Health Implications	Community Assessment Questions	Information Sources
Boundary of community	Community boundaries serve as basis for measuring incidence of wellness and illness and for determining spread of disease.	Where is the community located? What is its boundary? Is it a part of a larger community? What smaller communities does it include?	Atlas State maps County maps City maps Telephone book City directory Public library
Location of health services	Use of health services depends on availability and accessibility.	Where are the major health institutions located? What necessary health institutions are outside the community? Where are they?	Telephone book Chamber of commerce State health department County or local health departments Maps Public library
Geographic features	Injury, death, and destruction may be caused by floods, earthquakes, volcanoes, tornadoes, or hurricanes. Recreational opportunities at lakes, seashore, mountains promote health and fitness.	What major landforms are in or near the community? What geographical features pose possible threats? What geographic features offer opportunities for healthful activities?	Atlas Chamber of commerce Maps State health department Public library
Climate	Extremes of heat and cold affect health and illness. Extremes of temperature and precipitation may tax community's coping ability.	What are the average temperature and precipitation? What are the extremes? What climatic features affect health and illness? Is the community prepared to cope with emergencies?	Weather atlas Chamber of commerce State health department Maps Local government Weather bureau Public library
Flora and fauna	Poisonous plants and disease-carrying animals can affect community health. Plants and animals offer resources as well as dangers.	What plants and animals pose possible threats to health?	State health department Poison control center Police department Emergency rooms Encyclopedia Public library
Human-made environment	All human influences on environment (housing, dams, farming, type of industry, chemical waste, air pollution, etc.) can influence levels of community wellness.	What are the major industries? How have air, land, and water been affected by humans? What is the quality of housing? Do highways allow access to health institutions?	Chamber of commerce Local government City directory State health department University research reports Public library

(Spradley BW, Allender JA [1996]. *Community Health Nursing: Concepts and Practice.* Philadelphia: Lippincott-Raven.)

TABLE 4-2. Community Profile Inventory: Population Perspective

Population Variables	Community Health Implications	Community Assessment Questions	Information Sources
Size	The number of people influences the number and size of health-care institutions. Size affects homogeneity of the population and its needs.	What is the population of the community? Is it an urban, suburban, or rural community?	State health department Census data Maps City or town officials Chamber of commerce
Density	Increased density may increase stress. High and low density often affect the availability of health services.	What is the density of the population per square mile?	Census data State health department
Composition	Composition of the population often determines types of health needs.	What is the age composition of the community? What is the sex composition of the community? What is the marital status of community members? What occupations are represented and in what percentages?	Census data State health department Chamber of commerce U.S. Department of Labor Statistics
Rate of growth or decline	Rapidly growing communities may place excessive demands on health services. Marked decline in population may signal a poorly functioning community.	How has population size changed over the past two decades? What are the health implications of this change?	Census data State health department
Cultural differences	Health needs vary among subcultural and ethnic populations. Use of health services varies with culture. Health practices and extent of knowledge are affected by culture.	What is the ethnic breakdown of population? What racial groups are represented? What subcultural populations exist in the community? Do any of the subcultural groups have unique health needs and practices? Are different ethnic and cultural groups included in health planning?	Census data State health department Social and cultural research reports Human rights commission City government Health planning boards
Social class	Class differences influence use of health services. Class composition influences cost of public health services.	What percentage of the population falls into each social class? What do class differences suggest for health needs and services?	State health department Census data Sociologic reports
Mobility	Mobility of the population affects continuity of care. Mobility affects availability of service to highly mobile population.	How frequently do members move into and out of the community? How frequently do members move within the community? Are there any specific populations, such as migrant workers, that are highly mobile? How does the pattern of mobility affect the health of the community? Is the community organized to meet the health needs of mobile groups?	State health department Census data Health agencies serving migrant workers Farm labor offices Program serving transients and the homeless

(Spradley BW, Allender JA [1996]. *Community Health Nursing: Concepts and Practice.* Philadelphia: Lippincott-Raven.)

TABLE 4-3. Community Profile Inventory: Social System Perspective

Social System Variables	Community Health Implications	Community Assessment Questions	Information Sources
Health system Family system Economic system Educational system Religious system Welfare system Political system Recreational system Legal system Communication system	Each system must fulfill its functions for a healthy community. Collaboration among the systems to identify goals and problems affects health of community. Undue influence of one system on another may lower the health of the community. Agreement on the means to achieve community goals affects community health. Communication among organizations in each system affects community health.	What are the functions of each major system? What are the major subsystems of each system? What are the major organizations in each subsystem? How well do the various organizations function? Are the subsystems in each major system in conflict? Is there adequate communication among the major systems? Is there agreement on community goals? Are there mechanisms for resolving conflict? Do any parts of the total system dominate the others? What community needs are not being met?	Chamber of commerce Telephone book City directory Organizational literature Officials in organizations Community self-study Community survey Local library Key informants

(Spradley BW, Allender JA [1996]. *Community Health Nursing: Concepts and Practice*. Philadelphia: Lippincott-Raven.)

the necessary changes requires excellent communication skills and possibly political involvement. Obviously, members of the community must be involved in the change process if plans are to be successfully implemented.

The phases of the health planning process resemble the phases of the nursing process. Evaluation of outcomes must be included when the plans are formulated.

An excellent tool for health planning is the Gantt milestone chart. This chart, developed by Henry Gantt almost 80 years ago, establishes milestones and identifies the needed tasks, the persons assigned to complete the tasks, and the time frame in which they are to be completed.

The national objectives for the year 2000, *Healthy People 2000*, contain excellent ideas for local health planning. Although there was considerable impetus for health planning nationally during the 1960s and 1970s with the health planning acts of 1966 and 1974, little was done during the 1980s. Since 1990, there has been great interest in health planning again with the implementation of the *Healthy People 2000* objectives. That project is described in Chapter 5.

The Science of Epidemiology

Epidemiologists systematically study conditions related to health and disease patterns. Investigators in this branch of science seek to answer how and why diseases occur and what causes them. The community or aggregate is the client. When there is an outbreak of an unknown disease, epidemiologic investigation becomes detective work. Historically, epidemiologists studied epidemics. They still do, although they also study major causes of death (mortality) and illness (morbidity). Acquired immunodeficiencey syndrome (AIDS), which is a pandemic, worldwide epidemic, is being surveyed and tracked constantly by epidemiologic agencies such as local and state health departments, the Centers for Disease Control and Prevention (CDC), and the World Health Organization. It was discovered that AIDS exists almost entirely as a heterosexual disease in Central Africa; in the United States, AIDS exists mainly among homosexual men. Now epidemiologists tell us that the incidence of AIDS is growing most rapidly in the United States among heterosexual minority women.

Only by studying the how and why and what of terrible diseases such as AIDS can we hope to control and cure them. This is why the science of epidemiology is so important and so relevant to community health nursing.

All nurses are taught the epidemiologic triangle regarding the relation of agent, host, and environment in contributing to disease: the agent must be present in sufficient numbers and pathogenicity, the host must be susceptible, and the environment must be conducive to an illness state. An increase in any of these factors has the potential of producing disease. Intervention strategies may focus on any one of these factors to break the chain of infection (Fig. 4-6). The complexity of modern life, with people living longer and developing several chronic diseases, results in multiple causes of illness, prompting epidemiologists to speak of a "web of causation" rather than the simple epidemiologic triangle.

Epidemiologic surveys are reported in rates and ratios rather than raw numbers so they can be more universally understood. The term *incidence* is used to report when diseases first occur within a population. The term *prevalence* is used to refer to the number of cases that exist, whether newly diagnosed or chronic. Data on morbidity and mortality are collected. Certain diseases require mandatory reporting to local and state health departments and the CDC (Display 4-3).

Types of Epidemiologic Investigations

Investigations of disease or health factors can be formal or informal. "The Nurse Speaks" in this chapter gives an example of an informal investigation by a community health nurse that actually occurred. Formal studies vary in their degree of sophistication. Epidemiologic investigations can study past data (retrospective studies) or future data (prospective studies).

Experimental trials are conducted to learn about cause-and-effect relations or to test hypotheses. An experimental or clinical trial requires that the investigator control or change certain factors. If a new treatment for a disease is being studied, there must be a control group of persons with the same disease who will not receive the new treatment. Most such studies are called "double-blind studies" because neither the clients nor the investigators know which clients are receiving the real treatment and which are receiving placebos until the study is completed.

Because some clients in experimental trials may experience increased illness or suffering, such studies would not be ethical unless the clients are fully informed of the risks. An infamous experimental study was conducted on African-American prisoners

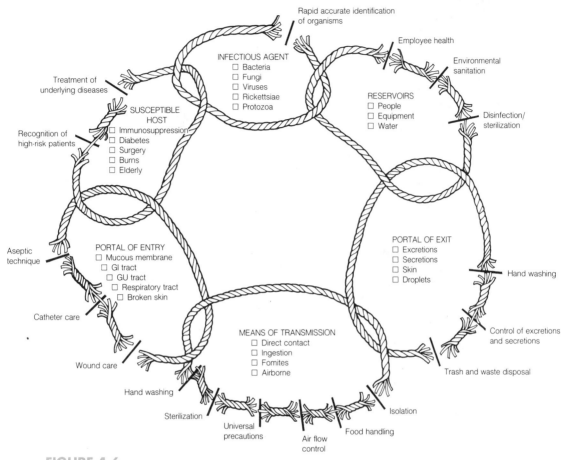

FIGURE 4-6
Health-care workers' interventions used to break the chain of infection transmission. (Smeltzer S, Bare B [1996]. *Brunner and Suddarth's Textbook of Medical-Surgical Nursing.* 8th ed. Philadelphia: Lippincott-Raven.)

with syphilis many years ago in Tuskegee, Alabama, without their knowledge or consent. The control group did not receive treatment for their disease and suffered greatly as a result. Today, strict guidelines for experimental studies ensure the rights of human subjects.

Most studies today are observational or descriptive in nature. Local and state health departments collect data about certain mandated reportable diseases within their area. This list is similar from state to state except for certain diseases that are endemic to a particular region (see Display 4-3). These data are also sent to the CDC, where they are surveyed and analyzed for patterns within the United States.

The Centers for Disease Control and Prevention

The primary source of information on communicable diseases within the United States is the CDC. It is one of the six agencies in the Public Health Service. The main CDC

Reportable Communicable Diseases

REPORT IMMEDIATELY BY TELEPHONE

Anthrax
Botulism (infant, foodborne, wound)
Cholera
Dengue
Diarrhea of the newborn (outbreaks)
Diphtheria
Food poisoning (when two or more cases or suspected cases of food-associated illness from separate households are suspected to have the same source)
Haemophilus influenzae, invasive disease
Hepatitis A

Measles (rubeola)
Meningococcal infections
Outbreaks or clusters of any kind
Plague
Poliomyelitis, paralytic
Rabies, human and animal
Relapsing fever
Syphilis (primary & secondary cases, and cases in pregnant women; also congenital cases)
Yellow fever

REPORT BY TELEPHONE OR MAIL WITHIN 1 WORKING DAY

Amebiasis
Campylobacteriosis
Conjunctivitis, acute infectious of the newborn (specify etiology)
Encephalitis: Viral, bacterial, fungal, parasitic (specify etiology)
Listeriosis
Malaria
Meningitis: Viral, bacterial, fungal, parasitic (specify etiology)
Pertussis (whooping cough)

Psittacosis
Q fever
Salmonellosis
Shigellosis
Streptococcal infections (outbreaks and cases in food handlers and dairy workers only)
Syphilis (all other cases)
Trichinosis
Typhoid fever (cases and carriers)

REPORT WITHIN 7 CALENDAR DAYS FROM THE TIME OF IDENTIFICATION

AIDS
Alzheimer's disease & related conditions
Brucellosis
Chancroid
Chlamydial infections
Coccidioidomycosis
Cryptosporidiosis
Cysticercosis
Disorders characterized by lapses of consciousness
Giardiasis
Gonococcal infections
Granuloma inguinale
Hepatitis B (cases and carrier, specify)
Hepatitis, delta (D)
Hepatitis, non-A, non-B (hepatitis C)
Legionellosis
Leprosy (Hansen's disease)

Leptospirosis
Lyme disease
Lymphogranuloma venereum
Mumps
Neoplasm, cancer
Nongonococcal urethritis (NGU)
Pelvic inflammatory disease (PID)
Reye syndrome
Rheumatic fever, acute
Rocky Mountain spotted fever
Rubella: Acute, congenital (German measles)
Tetanus
Toxic shock syndrome (TSS)
Tuberculosis
Tularemia
Typhus fever
Vibrio species

offices are in Atlanta, Georgia. Both the Public Health Service and the CDC were created by Congress to collect, coordinate, analyze, and share data on health and disease. *Morbidity and Mortality Weekly Report* is published by the CDC as a means of sharing this information. A yearly summary is also published. The CDC uses modern technology to track and monitor data related to health and disease and sends teams of epidemiologists to investigate and contain unusual outbreaks of disease. In recent years, its investigations have included an epidemic of cryptosporidiosis in Milwaukee, where the causative agent was found in the water supply. Unexplained, sudden acute fevers and rapid deaths among healthy young Native Americans in rural northern New Mexico were traced to field mice as the vectors in transmitting the Hansa virus. Legionellosis killed several men attending an American Legion convention at a Philadelphia hotel; the CDC found that legionellosis was transmitted by polluted air in the venting system of the hotel, and the disease was named for the convention where it was first identified.

Current Issues in Epidemiology

At the forefront of epidemiologic concern is HIV/AIDS because it is a fatal disease and has a very long incubation period, during which it is contagious. Its incidence and prevalence are rising rapidly. In the United States, an estimated 1 million or more persons are HIV-positive. In other parts of the world, outbreaks of virulent, rapidly fatal diseases such as Ebola fever are also alarming because there is so much international travel, providing opportunities for pathogens to migrate. New strains of drug-resistant microorganisms in the United States are another serious concern, as are environmental hazards. The cutbacks in funding for the CDC that began in the 1980s are deeply distressing because there is so much to be done to prevent infectious disease transmission.

Environmental Health of the Community as Client

The Nurse's Environmental Responsibility

Community nurses must work to protect the health and safety of the environment. They must be aware of threats to the environment, know to whom problems should be reported, and be cognizant of issues and efforts to maintain a healthy environment. In all workplaces, including clients' homes, nurses must be alert for environmental hazards. Nurses must work collaboratively with environmental sanitarians, other health professionals, and members of the community to reduce current hazards and prevent future ones. Client teaching regarding environmental hazards is a basic role of community health nurses. The client may be an individual, a family, a community, or an aggregate, and the teaching may be formal or informal. Nurses should advocate policies that support environmental health and safety and oppose forces that support a status quo of unhealthy practices.

Research is necessary to produce accurate data that lend credence to this advocacy role. The Nurses' Environmental Health Watch is an organization dedicated to educating nurses and the public about current issues in this field. The role of local health departments in safeguarding the environment is covered in Chapter 6.

Current Issues in Environmental Health and Safety (Display 4-4)

Air pollution is a major worldwide concern. Years ago, the fictional detective Sherlock Holmes commented on the terrible smog of London, caused by burning coal. Today cities such as Shanghai, Cairo, and Bangkok have that problem, with added pollutants from industry and automobile emissions. Areas of the former Soviet Union have horrible air pollution problems resulting from years of neglect of air quality. Cities such as Los Angeles and New York have air pollution problems because of heavy traffic and high buildings or mountains that inhibit air circulation. The use of lead-free gasoline and other efforts are lessening the problem. Buildings are home to chemical pollutants such as asbestos, lead, radon, and cigarette smoke. Asthma has produced increasing morbidity and mortality rates and is a major health problem. Air pollutants contribute to lung diseases such as emphysema and pneumoconiosis; an estimated 8% of Americans suffer from chronic lung problems (Moeller, 1992). Depletion of the ozone layer, which shields the earth from ultraviolet radiation, has ominous implications for the future. The marked increase in the incidence of melanoma, a virulent skin cancer, seems related to ozone depletion.

Another long-term result of air pollution is acid rain; the resultant greenhouse effect seems to be changing the earth's ecosystem and could ultimately result in loss of human life on earth. The results at Chernobyl, Hiroshima, and Nagasaki all point to possible global extermination if a large-scale nuclear explosion or accident occurs.

Water pollution, either biologic or chemical, presents another dangerous scenario. We take safe drinking water for granted in the United States and feel inconvenienced when we travel overseas and must boil and filter water and be immunized to protect ourselves from water pollutants. Cholera, typhoid, polio, bacterial dysentery, and hepatitis A are all transmitted by contaminated water and kill many Third World residents each year. The parasite *Giardia lamblia* infects the drinking water in St. Petersburg, Russia. A few years ago a major epidemic of hepatitis A occurred in Naples, Italy. Investigators could not pinpoint the cause until it was found that some ancient, broken pipes were channeling raw sewage into Naples Bay. Fishermen were harvesting mussels and oysters from those waters, and the seafood was often eaten raw. Hepatitis A virus, which is shed in human feces, had found its way into that seafood and then into the mouths of the persons who became infected. Seafood should not be eaten raw. Third World countries, particularly places with open sewers, are notorious for having biologically polluted water.

Most of the danger in the United States seems to result from chemical pollution. Much drinking water comes from underground aquifers, which are fed from groundwater filtering through the soil. Toxic substances can seep into aquifers from agricultural pesticides, oil spills, and dumping or burying hazardous wastes. Superfund legislation was passed to help fund the clean-up of industrial hazardous wastes that had been disposed of improperly. Bioremediation is the process of using special bacteria to break down hazardous waste materials and render them nonhazardous. Leukemia and other cancers, sterility, blindness, birth defects, and various acute and chronic illnesses have been linked to hazardous wastes.

Contaminated foods are also a threat. Microorganisms such as *Staphylococcus aureus*, *Salmonella enteritidis*, *Trichinosis spiralis*, and *Clostridium botulinum* can cause serious illness and death. Most people know to cook pork thoroughly, but

DISPLAY 4-4

National Health Objectives for Environmental Health-Related Problems by the Year 2000

1. Reduce asthma morbidity, measured by reduced asthma hospitalizations, to no greater than 160 per 100,000 population.
   Special target populations:
   Blacks and nonwhites
   Children

2. Reduce prevalence of serious mental retardation among school-aged children to no more than 2 per 1,000 children.

3. Reduce outbreaks of waterborne disease from infectious agents and chemical poisoning to no more than 11 per year.
   Special target populations:
   People served by public or investor-owned water systems

4. Reduce the prevalence of blood lead levels exceeding 15 ug/dL and 25 ug/dL among children aged 6 months through 5 years to no more than 500,000 and zero respectively.
   Special target population—Inner-city, low-income black children

5. Reduce human exposure to criteria air pollutants, measured by an increase to 85% or more in the proportion of people who live in counties where any Environmental Protection Agency standard for air quality has not been exceeded in the past 12 months.
   Target air pollutants
   Ozone, carbon monoxide, nitrogen dioxide, sulfur dioxide, particulates, lead

6. Increase the proportion of homes to 40% or more where owner or occupant radon testing shows minimal risk or has been modified to reduce health risk.
   Target populations at 50%:
   Homes with smokers and former smokers
   Homes with children

7. Reduce human exposure to toxic agents by confining total pounds of toxic agents released into the air, water, and soil each year. Goal is no more than:
   0.24 billion pounds of toxic agents on DHHS carcinogens list
   2.6 billion pounds of toxic agents on Agency for Toxic Substances and Disease Registry list for most toxic chemicals

8. Reduce human exposure to solid waste-related water, air, and soil contamination. This will be measured by a reduction in average pounds of municipal solid waste produced per person per day to no more than 3.6 pounds.

9. Increase the proportion of people to at least 85% who receive safe drinking water supplies measured by EPA standards.

10. Reduce potential risks to human health from surface water. This will be measured by a decrease in the proportion of surface waters (lakes, streams, etc.) to no more than 15% that do not support beneficial uses, such as fishing and swimming.

11. Provide testing for lead-based paint in at least 50% of homes built before 1950.

12. Expand the number of states to at least 35 where 75% of local jurisdictions have adopted construction standards and techniques to minimize elevated indoor radon levels.

13. Increase the number of states to at least 30 that require disclosure of lead-based paint and radon concentrations to prospective buyers of buildings for sale.

14. Eliminate significant health risks from hazardous waste sites on the EPA's National Priority List. This will be measured by performing site clean-ups sufficient to eliminate specified health threats.

15. Establish programs for recyclable materials and household hazardous waste in at least 75% of counties.

DISPLAY 4-4
National Health Objectives for Environmental Health-Related Problems by the Year 2000 (continued)

(continued)

16. Establish and monitor plans to define and track sentinel environmental diseases in at least 35 states. (These diseases include lead poisoning, other heavy metal poisoning, pesticide poisoning, carbon monoxide poisoning, heatstroke, hypothermia, acute chemical poisoning, methemoglobinemia, and respiratory diseases due to environmental factors.)

(Source: U.S. Department of Health and Human Services. (1991). Healthy People 2000: National health promotion and disease prevention objectives. *Washington, DC: Government Printing Office.)*

many people eat rare beef; it should be cooked until well done. Hamburger meat is particularly hazardous. An estimated one third of all poultry is contaminated with salmonella during processing and shipping (Blumenthal, 1994). Separate cutting boards and implements should be used when preparing poultry for cooking, and hands should be washed thoroughly. Food contamination can also occur with insects, mice and rat feces, dirt, and hairs, fungi, and pesticides. Food handlers and restaurant employees should wash their hands thoroughly and frequently, particularly after using the toilet.

Some food additives have been found to be toxic. Red dye #2 was found to be carcinogenic and is no longer used. The long-term effects of flavor enhancers, preservatives, and synthetic products such as aspartame and Olestra are still unknown.

Vectors and the disposal of garbage are a big problem in the United States. Much of our garbage, such as disposable diapers, is not biodegradable. Disposable diapers are estimated to last up to five centuries, and about 18 million diapers are disposed of each year, usually with feces intact. This dumps a great deal of raw sewage into landfills, attracts vectors such as rats and flies, and helps spread disease. Burning of refuse is no longer allowed because of air pollution problems. Sanitary landfills are replacing municipal dumps because they are safer. The process of daily covering and sealing of garbage has reduced the risks from vectors such as rodents and insects.

However, developing countries still have a high prevalence of vector-borne diseases. Malaria, the most common disease worldwide, is transmitted by the *Anopheles* mosquito and infects an estimated 200 million people annually. A relatively new and serious condition, Lyme disease, is transmitted by deer ticks. It has already reached epidemic proportions in some areas of the northern states, extending west from the Atlantic coast through the Midwest thus far.

Regulatory governmental agencies exist to help protect the environment. The Environmental Protection Agency was given considerable authority over environment matters in 1971. Within the Public Health Service, the Food and Drug Administration was established in 1968, the Occupational Safety and Health Administration in 1970. The former monitors food safety and tests new medications for approval and release. The latter sets policy to ensure safe and healthy workplaces.

Environmental Disasters: Natural and Man-Made

Hurricanes Hugo and Andrew, the California earthquakes, and the Midwestern floods and tornadoes are examples of recent natural disasters in the United States. The Oklahoma City and World Trade Center bombings are examples of man-made disasters. The impact of the latter seems more difficult to bear, but all major disasters have an enormous, prolonged impact on communities. The incidence of post-traumatic stress disorder increases in communities after a disaster occurs. The physical and financial hardships are immense.

Nursing in Disasters

Nurses play a major role during disasters and prepare for that role by participating in disaster planning, education, and prevention drills. In many cases, natural disasters are prone to recur—for example, tornadoes in Kansas and hurricanes in the Gulf region. Some disasters develop slowly, allowing time for warning and preparation. This was true with the floods in the Midwest and helped reduce the loss of life.

The American Nurses Association has been working with other organizations to develop a national disaster preparedness plan for nurses (Turner, 1993). According to the American Red Cross, there is a need for more specialty-prepared nurses to participate in this effort. The Red Cross Disaster Services regulations mandate that at least one registered nurse must be present at all times while emergency aid stations are operating. Disaster victims' needs are enormous and range from shelter, water, and food to psychological counseling and medical care. Physicians are needed at hospitals to provide medical treatment.

Nurses often wonder if they can assist in a disaster in states other than where they are licensed. A federal mandate protects nurses working with the American Red Cross anywhere during a disaster. For more information about the volunteer needs of the American Red Cross, see Chapter 7.

Triage is one of the most emotionally taxing tasks of the nurse during a disaster. The Red Cross uses a color-coding system to prioritize victims for care. First-priority victims with life-threatening injuries are coded red. Second-priority victims, those who are not yet in shock or hypoxic but have that potential, are coded yellow. Third-priority victims, those with minimal injuries who can wait several hours for treatment, are coded green. Dead victims or those who are hopelessly injured are coded black. It is heart-rending to leave a dying victim alone if personnel are scarce. The nurse must think in terms of the chance of survival for the greatest number of victims and use personnel, equipment, and medications where they can do the most good.

THE NURSE SPEAKS . . .
About an Informal Epidemiologic Investigation

work in a community health center in a rundown inner-city neighborhood. I remember a situation that happened a couple of years ago.

It was about 5 o'clock on a winter Wednesday evening when I noticed a flashy-dressed young man flirting with the clinic's clerk in the reception room. Because of the flamboyant way he was dressed, I remembered seeing him at the clinic the previous week and once or twice before. He was not a client himself but brought his friends in for treatment. They each had vague complaints such as fatigue, anorexia, or upper respiratory infections and complained of having the flu. The woman he brought that particular evening had a bad cold and also told the doctor she thought she was coming down with the flu. She was dressing after the examination when I first noticed her friend out in the visiting room.

Suddenly the thought hit me that her diagnosis might be hepatitis. I went to talk to her so that I could look at the sclera of her eyes. They were a dark, creamy color. It was difficult to see whether that was her normal sclera color because her skin was dark also. I asked her about her eye color, but she said she hadn't noticed. She repeated what she had said earlier about feeling "blah" for the past few weeks and added that the flu seemed to be "going around" because some of her friends were feeling the same way. I asked if the fellow in the reception room was her boyfriend, and she answered, "Sort of." I asked if they had sex together, and she answered, "Sometimes." I asked if he had been feeling "blah" also and she answered, "No, he feels just fine." While she finished dressing, I spoke with the doctor privately.

The doctor agreed that testing for hepatitis was appropriate when I explained my suspicions that the man who brought her in might be a hepatitis B virus carrier. I was asked to try to persuade the man to be tested also. He refused, saying, "We ain't got AIDS, if that's what you're wondering about. We've been tested recently at the health department. I feel fine and I definitely ain't going to let anybody stick me for a blood test." Neither the doctor nor I could persuade him. We reminded them to be sure to use condoms. We made sure we had his name and address on the young woman's chart, and we made an appointment for the young woman to return when the results of her tests were known.

Sure enough, she had hepatitis B virus in her blood. Fortunately, the same man brought her in again, and this time he was willing to listen and to be tested. We explained that some people have hepatitis B virus without having any symptoms but can still transmit it to others in semen and in blood. We asked about his sexual relationships with other women, especially the other women he drove to the clinic earlier. He agreed that they should be tested and added, "I don't like rubbers and don't use rubbers when I'm with women unless I don't know them." He brought in additional women to be tested. In all, there were seven women positive for hepatitis B virus, as was the carrier, himself!

Chronic persistent hepatitis is an asymptomatic carrier state with HBsAG in the serum. Carriers provide a major source of the virus for infecting others. Complications such as chronic hepatitis and postnecrotic cirrhosis can occur, although generally hepatitis B is benign to the carrier. Given this man's very active sex life, his casual use of condoms, his elevated serum AST and ALT levels, indicative of chronic hepatitis, and the slight possibility of postnecrotic cirrhosis, we decided to treat him with alpha-interferon. Some of his recent negative sexual contacts were also given passive immunity with HBIg serum, which provides about 2 months of passive immunity against the disease.

Everyone who was infected was instructed about the importance of avoiding alcohol and hepatotoxic medications such as Tylenol for several months. Bed rest with minimal ambulation was recommended to the women to allow their livers to rest and heal. I taught them to eat a high-calorie, high-protein, low-fat diet after finding out what foods they liked to eat. Some of the women became jaundiced and complained of pruritus. They were advised to use an oil-based lotion instead of soap and to avoid tight clothing and hot baths. Most importantly, they were told to avoid sex or at least to be sure that condoms were always used, or else they would continue to spread the disease. Although they denied it, we had a strong suspicion that some of the women might be prostitutes working for the man who was the HBV carrier.

An amusing thing happened several months later, when we launched a big hepatitis prevention campaign in the community and encouraged vaccination against hepatitis B. The former hepatitis B virus carrier and all his girlfriends came to the clinic for the vaccine, greeting us like old friends. We explained again that they already had protective hepatitis antibodies from their disease and didn't need to be immunized. They seemed disappointed! Then they assured us that they knew lots of other people and would be sure to spread the news to come to our clinic for the vaccine.

Ethel
PUBLIC HEALTH CLINIC NURSE

CLINICAL APPLICATION

A Critical Thinking Case Study About Preventing Child Abuse

You decide to make a home visit to Sherry because of a comment she made during the well-child clinic when her three children were getting their check-ups. She said, "I hope nobody ever sees marks from beatings on their bodies. I was beat up as a kid and I don't want that to happen to them."

 and Think!

- What is significant about that remark?
- Why do you think it warrants a home visit?

The home is a tiny cottage in an old dilapidated bungalow colony behind a bar. As you approach, you see the children playing in the middle of a 12-foot-round circle of lush green grass near the bar. The rest of the ground has dirt and scanty grass. You detect a swamplike odor and observe the round area carefully while saying hello to the children.

 and Think!

- What do you suspect may be the cause of the round, lush green area?
- Should you do anything about it? If so, what?

Sherry is inside watching soap operas. The tiny room is neat, clean, and sparsely furnished. Sherry asks why you are here and seems on edge. You say that you like to make home visits to clinic families to have more time to talk in a relaxed way and to answer any questions she might have.

"I ain't got no questions," she says sullenly, turning back to the TV.

 and Think!

- How can you engage her in a nonthreatening way?
- What can you say to make her less defensive?
- Why is she so hostile?

You apologize for interrupting her TV show and excuse yourself to go see the children, telling her to call you when the show is over. This will give her time to gather her composure and feel more calm. Also, she may be sincerely angry by the TV interruption.

About 20 minutes later, she comes outside smiling and thanks you for waiting. She invites you in and you sit together on the old couch. You mention how much Robbie has been growing and that Cindy's hair is turning darker.

"What did you come to talk about?" she asks directly. You explain that you would like to hear more about what she said about being beaten as a child. She describes a father who became nasty when drunk and beat her, but never on the face. One day during a school physical exam, the school nurse noticed her bruises and went to see her parents. After that, the beatings stopped but she could never relax, always fearing when it might happen next. Her father constantly threatened and verbally abused her. She added, "Fortunately, he never done nothing weird, like sex or nothing. It was just his bad temper and all the fear. And then one day he just walked out on us."

 and Think!

- What should you say now?
- Should you bring up her comment about her own children?
- Why do you suppose she said what she did?
- Will you lose her trust if you comment about their possible risk of being abused?

"It must have been so hard for you as a child. (Pause) You seem very concerned about your own children and don't want them abused. Are you concerned about someone beating them? Your husband? (Long pause) Or have you heard it said that people who were abused as children often end up abusing their own children?" you ask.

"That's what I'm scared about the most. Sometimes when the weather is bad and we're all cooped up in here for days, I almost go crazy with the kids' noise. I want to scream and let them have it! (Silence) Dave's OK. It's not him. He don't even drink. We don't have much, but he works hard paving driveways. In the winter he does snow plowing. It's not him. It's me I'm scared about. Sometimes I think I've got my old man's temper. I'm so scared I might lose control. I really love these kids. I don't know why they can get on my nerves so much.''

 and Think!

- How should you respond?
- What can you do to help this family?
- Who is the client in this situation?

You reflect back her feelings of love for her children and her fear that she will lose control and beat them. This is the best way to express empathy and to say you understand what she has been saying. You suggest that you two make a contract. She will call you when she finds her anger mounting and fears loss of control. You will come support her and help her regain control. You also suggest that she try to discuss her fear with her husband, Dave. This is something she has always felt ashamed to do. You tell her you will revisit her in a month unless she needs you sooner.

 and Think!

- What follow-up is needed after this visit, and what additional information do you need to help this family?

You report the malfunctioning septic tank to the health department's environmental health office for follow-up, reminding them not to implicate Sherry or her children when they visit the bar and tell the owner the septic tank needs attention.

See if there are any nursery schools or day-care centers in that area that offer scholarships for needy children. Even 2 days a week would give Sherry valuable respite.

Listen actively and use broad opening questions on future visits to allow Sherry to express any priorities that may need follow-up. Remain faithful to the contract; respond promptly if she calls for your support. When you are not working, make certain a backup nurse is available to come in your place.

Chapter SUMMARY

Community health nurses regard the family as the client because they work with family units as a system. The nuclear family is not the dominant pattern in the United States. Dyads, single-parent families, and blended families are increasing in number, while multigenerational and extended families are decreasing in number. More and more elderly people choose to move into retirement communities. Characteristics of multiproblem, dysfunctional, and healthy families are described. Tools for family and community assessments are included.

In community health nursing, the community as a whole is the client. Communities, aggregates, and groups are differentiated. Methods of data collection include surveys and epidemiologic, observational, analytic, and experimental studies. Health planning is multidisciplinary and based on outcome measurements. *Healthy People 2000* established national goals for the year 2000 and involves local communities in achieving these goals.

Epidemiologists regard the community or the aggregate as the client and seek to answer how and why diseases occur and what causes them. The Centers for Disease Control and Prevention plays a major investigative role, as do local and state health departments.

The community is the client in environmental health issues and disasters. Major issues of the former include air and water pollution, contamination of food substances, and vector and garbage control. Regulatory governmental agencies are described. The work of the American Red Cross and the role of nurses during disasters is vitally important. Nurses are assigned to emergency aid stations and perform the difficult duty of triage during natural and man-made disasters. Nurses who work as Red Cross volunteers can assist in a disaster in states other than where they are licensed.

A list of references and additional readings for this chapter appears at the end of Part 1.

References and Additional Readings

Aaron H (1994). Health spending analysis: Thinking straight about medical costs. *Health Affairs* 13(5):7–13.

Adams C, et al (1995). Home health quality outcomes: Fee for service versus health maintenance organization enrollees. *JONA* 25:39–45.

American Academy of Nursing (1993). *Managed Care and National Health Care: Nurses Can Make it Work*. American Academy of Nursing.

American Nurses Association (1985). *Code for Nurses With Interpretive Statements*. Kansas City, MO: ANA.

American Nurses Association (1991). *Nursing's Agenda for Health Care Reform*. Washington DC: ANA.

Anderson E, McFarlane J (1996). *Community As Partner*. Philadelphia: Lippincott-Raven.

Andrews M, Boyle J (1995). *Transcultural Concepts in Nursing Care*, 2d ed. Philadelphia: JB Lippincott.

Associated Press (May 20, 1996). Infectious disease still a killer. *Rockland Journal-News.* Nyak, NY.

Associated Press (June 4, 1997). Tobacco state officials meet. *Hendersonville Times-News.*

Associated Press (June 4, 1997a). Medical savings accounts proposed. *Hendersonville Times-News.*

Bandman E, Bandman B (1995). *Nursing Ethics Through the Lifespan*, 3d ed. Stamford, CT: Appleton & Lange.

Begley S (1997). America 2000: Uncovering Secrets Big and Small. *Newsweek*, Jan. 27, 1997, pp. 63–73.

Benenson AS (1995). *Control of Communicable Diseases*, 16th ed. Washington DC: American Public Health Association.

Benner P, Tanner C, Chesla C (1995). *Expertise in Nursing Practice: Caring, Clinical Judgement, and Ethics.* New York: Springer.

Benson H (1997). *Timeless Healing: The Power and Biology of Belief.* New York: Simon & Schuster.

Benson M (March 19, 1997). United front plans attack to restrict HMOs' power. *Wall Street Journal.*

Blumenthal D, Ruttenber J (1994). *Introduction to Environmental Health,* 2nd ed. New York: Springer.

Boyle P (1997). *Getting Doctors to Listen—Ethics and Outcome Data in Context.* Baltimore, MD: Georgetown University Press.

Boyle (1995). *Transcultural Concepts in Nursing Care.* Philadelphia: JB Lippincott.

Braun I (1996). Varicella zoster virus: Trends and treatment. *MCN* 21(4):187–190.

Breslow L (1996). Public health and managed care: A California perspective. *Health Affairs* 15(1):92.

Brider P (1996). Portable health coverage at last; hospitals brace for welfare fallout. *AJN* 96(9):68–72.

Brider P (1996). Merging medical centers deny plans for layoffs. *AJN* 96(9):67.

Brook PS (1995). Legal context for community health nursing In Smith CS, Maurer F. *Community Health Nursing.* Philadelphia: WB Saunders.

Buhler-Winkerson K (1994). Bringing care to the people: Lillian Wald's legacy to public health nursing. *AJN* 83:1778–1786.

Burggrabe J, Miller K. (1991). *Developing a Healthy Lifestyle*. San Jose, CA: Resource Publications.

Burrell L (1997). *Adult Nursing in Hospital and Community Settings*. Stamford, CT: Appleton & Lange.

Butler R (1997). Living longer and loving it. *Secure Retirement* 6(1):12–18.

Callahan J et al (1995). Mental health/substance abuse treatment in managed care: The Massachusetts Medicaid experience. *Health Affairs* 14:173–184.

Cavendish R (1996). Traditional values: Are they in fact devalued? Society says it wants full-time mothers. *MCN* 21(4):203–204.

Centers for Disease Control & Prevention (1996). Infant Mortality—United States, 1993. *MMWR* 45(10):211.

Centers for Disease Control & Prevention (1996). Tuberculosis Morbidity—United States 1996. *MMWR* 46(30):695.

Chenevert M (1997). *The Pro Nurse Handbook.* St. Louis: Mosby-Yearbook.

Christiansen K (1996). Change and our home care paradigms. *Home Healthcare Nurse*, 14(2):144.

Churchill L (1997). Market meditopia: A glimpse at American health care in 2005. *Hastings Center Report* 27(1):5-6.

Clemen-Stone S et al (1995). *Comprehensive Community Health Care*, 4th ed. St. Louis: Mosby-Year Book.

Clinical Highlights (1996). The U.S. posts its lowest-ever infant mortality rate. *RN* 59(7):14.

Congressional Budget Office (1995). *The Effects of Managed Care and Managed Competition.* Washington DC: Congressional Budget Office.

Considine C (1996). Measurement of outcomes: What does it really mean? *Home Healthcare Nurse* 14(6):417-418.

Consumers Union (1995). Mental health insurance: Who pays? How much? *Consumers Report* 60(11):735-736.

Consumers Union (1996). Standing up for children. *Consumers Report* 61(6):9.

Cunningham R (1995). Medicare HMO's advocates fend off critics right and left. *Healthcare Leadership Review* 14(6).

Davis C et al (1997). Leadership for expanding nursing influence on health policy. In Spradley BW, Allender JA, eds. *Readings in Community Health Nursing.* Philadelphia: JB Lippincott.

De la Cruz F (1994). Clinical Decision Making Styles of Home Healthcare Nurses, *Image J Nurs Scholarship,* 26,222-226.

DiMeo E (1991). Rx for spiritual distress. *RN* March 1991:22-25.

Doheny M, Cook C, Stopper M (1997). *The Discipline of Nursing.* Stamford, CT: Appleton & Lange.

Donnelly E (1993). Health promotion, families, and the diagnostic process. In Wegner, Alexander, eds. *Readings in Family Nursing.* Philadelphia: JB Lippincott.

Doyle R et al (1994). *Healthcare Management Guidelines, Vol. 4: Home Care and Case Management.* Radnor, PA: Milliman & Robertson.

Dubos K, Rizzolo M (1994). Cruising the information superhighway. *AJN* 94(12):58-60.

Dunkle R (1996). Parish nurses help patients, body and soul. *RN* 59(5):55-57.

Dunlay J (1996). Making the cultural connection. *Health Technology* 3(4):9-12.

Editors (1996). Nursing the Net. *Nursing '96* 26(11):18.

Editors (1997). Home care. *The Johns Hopkins Medical Letter: Health After 50* 9(2):3.

Edward M (1995). *The Internet for Nurses and Allied Health Professionals.* New York: Springer.

Eisenberg DM et al (1993). Unconventional medicine in the United States. *N Engl J Med* 328(4):246.

Feingold E (1994). Health care reform—more than cost containment and universal access. *Am J Publ Health* 84(5):727-728.

Ferguson T (1996). *Health Online.* Reading, MA: Addison-Wesley.

Freudenheim M (Feb. 2, 1997). Knocking down gatekeepers' doors. *NY Times News Service.*

Friedemann M (1993). The concept of family nursing. In Wegner, Alexander, eds. *Readings In Family Nursing.* Philadelphia: JB Lippincott.

General Accounting Office. (1993). *Long-Term Care Case Management: State Experiences and Implications for Federal Policy.* Washington DC: Human Services Division, General Accounting Office.

General Accounting Office (1994). *Health Care Reforms: Potential Difficulties in Determining Eligibility for Low-Income People.* Gaithersburg, MD: General Accounting Office.

Gerberdine, JL (1996). Open trial of zidovudine, lamivudine and indinavir as postexposure prophylaxis in health care workers with occupational exposure to human immunodeficiency virus (HIV). *Epi-Center.* San Francisco: UCSF.

Giger (1994). *Transcultural Nursing.* St. Louis: Mosby.

Gingrich B, Ondech D (1995). *Clinical Pathways for the Multidisciplinary Home Care Team.* Gaithersburg, MD: Aspen.

Gloss E (1995). Community nursing yesterday, today and tomorrow. *J NY State Nurses Assoc* March, pp. 40-41.

Gorman M (1996). Culture clash: Working with a difficult patient. *AJN* 96(11):58.

Gorrie TM, McKinney ES, Murray S (1994). *Maternal-Newborn Nursing.* Philadelphia: WB Saunders.

Greenwald J (1997). Where jobs are superhot: 15 of the hottest fields. *Time* 149(3):54-63.

Greifzu S. (1996). Grieving families need your help. *RN* 59(9):22-28.

Grimes D, Grimes R (1997). Tuberculosis: What nurses need to know to help control the epidemic. In Spradley BW, Allender JA, eds. *Readings in Com-*

munity Health Nursing. Philadelphia: JB Lippincott.

Gross D (1996). What is a "good" parent? *MCN* 21(4):178-182.

Grossman D (1994). Enhancing your cultural competence. *AJN*:58-61.

Grossman D (1996). Cultural dimensions in home health nursing. *AJN* 18(7):33—-36.

Guido GW (1995). Legal and ethical issues. In Yoder-Wise P. *Leading and Managing In Nursing*. St. Louis: Mosby.

Haddad A (1990). *Ethical and Legal Issues in Home Healthcare*. Stamford, CT: Appleton & Lange.

Haddad A (1996). Ethics in action. *RN* 59(9):17-20.

Haddad A (1997). Ethics in action. *RN* 60(3):17-20.

Hall-Long B (1997). Nursing's past, present, and future. In Spradley BW, Allender JA, eds. *Readings in Community Health Nursing*. Philadelphia: Lippincott-Raven.

Halloran M (1982). Rational ethical judgements using a decision making tool. *Heart Lung* 11(6):566-570.

Hanson M, Callahan D (1995). *Life Choices—A Hastings Center Introduction to Bioethics*. Baltimore: Georgetown University Press.

Hanson (1995). *Family Health Care Nursing*. Philadelphia: FA Davis.

Harper M (1996). Caring for the special needs of aging minorities. *Health Technology* 3(4):17-23.

Harris M (1996). Medicare managed care. *Home Healthcare Nurse* 14(3):185-187.

Hayes B (1994). The new paradigm. *Public Health Nursing* 11(2):.

Health Insurance Association of America (1996). *Source Book of Health Insurance Data*. Washington DC: Health Insurance Institute of America.

Hicks LL et al (1993). *Role of the Nurse in Managed Care*. Washington, DC: American Nurses Publishing.

Hodgin L (1994). The wave of the future. *Continuing Care* 13(4):43-44.

Home Health Care Revenue Report (1995). *Preparing for Capitation in Home Health Care*. Gaithersburg, MD: Aspen.

Howe RS (1994). *Case Management for Healthcare Professionals*. Chicago: Precept Press.

Huch M (1995). Nursing and the next millennium. *Nursing Science Quarterly* 8:1.

Hunt (1997). *Nursing in the Community*. Philadelphia: Lippincott-Raven.

Hunt AR (May 8, 1997). Politics and people. *Wall Street Journal*.

Iglehart J (1994a). Changing course in turbulent times. *Health Affairs* 13(5):65-77.

Institute for Natural Resources. (1996). *The Internet: A Guide for Health Professionals*. Berkeley, CA: Institute for Natural Resources.

Irvine J (1995). *Sexuality Education Across Cultures: Working With Differences*. San Francisco: Jossey-Bass.

Joel L (1996). More than rearranging the deck chairs. *AJN* 96(8):7.

Kachoyeanos M (1996). Evaluating Research for Use in Clinical Practice. *MCN* 22(5):223-224.

Kavanagh K (1995). Values clarification for change and empowerment. In Smith C, Maurer F. *Community Health Nursing*. Philadelphia: WB Saunders.

Kavanagh K, Kennedy P (1992). *Promoting Cultural Diversity: Strategies for Health Care Professionals*. Newbury Park, CA: Sage.

Kelly LY, Joel LA (1995). *Dimensions of Professional Nursing*, 7th ed. New York: McGraw-Hill.

Kelly M (1995). Community health nursing in international disasters. *Home Healthcare Nurse* 13(4):75-76.

Kenyon V et al (1990). Clinical competencies for community health nursing. *Public Health Nursing* 7(1):33-39.

King G (1994). Health care reform and the Medicare program. *Health Affairs* 13(5):39-43.

Knowles (1980). *The Modern Practice of Adult Education*, 2d ed. Chicago: Follett.

Koenig H (1997). *Is Religion Good for Your Health?* Binghamton, NY: Haworth Press.

Koenig H (1997). Use of religion by patients with severe medical illness. *Mind/Body Medicine* 2(1):31-36.

Kongstvedt P (1997). *The Managed Health Care Handbook*. Frederick, MD: Aspen.

Kristjanson L, Chalmers K (1993). Preventive work with families: Issues facing public health nurses. In Wegner, Alexander, eds. *Readings in Family Nursing*. Philadelphia: JB Lippincott.

Lapp C et al (1993). Family-based practice: Discussion of a tool merging assessment with intervention. In Wegner, Alexander, eds. *Readings in Family Nursing*. Philadelphia: JB Lippincott.

Larson D, Milano M (1997). Making the case for spiritual interventions in clinical practice. *Journal of Clinical Behavioral Medicine* 2(1):20-30.

Lawrence D, Schaeffer L (1996). Debating nonprofit versus for-profit status for health plans. *Health Affairs* 15(1):237-238.

Leininger M (1995). *Transcultural Nursing Concepts,*

Theories, Research, and Practice. New York: McGraw-Hill.

Lewis P (1996). A review of prayer within the role of the holistic nurse. *J Holistic Nursing* 14(4):308–315.

Luft H (1996). Modifying managed competition to address cost and quality. *Health Affairs* 15(1):23–38.

Macrae J (1995). Nightingale's spiritual philosophy and its significance for modern nursing. *Image* 27: 8–10.

Mann T, Ornstein N (1995). *Intensive Care: How Washington Shapes Health Policy.* Washington: The Brookings Institution.

Maraldo P (1990). The nineties: A decade in search of meaning. *Nursing and Health Care* 11(1):11–14.

Marrelli TM (1994). *Handbook of Home Health Standards,* 2d ed. St. Louis: Mosby-Year Book.

Matthews D (1997). Religion and spirituality in primary care. *Mind/Body Medicine* 2(1):9–19.

Matthews D, Larson D (1997). Faith and medicine: Reconciling the twin traditions of healing. *Mind/Body Medicine* 2(1):3–6.

McAlindon M (1995). Managing information and technology. *Leading and Managing in Nursing.* St. Louis: Mosby-Year Book.

McCrystal P (1995). What kind of prescription? Do contraceptive drugs prevent life or destroy it? *Celebrate Life*, December, p. 23.

McGregor L (1996). Short, shorter, shortest: Continuing to improve the hospital stay for mothers and newborns. *MCN* 21(5):191–201.

McKinnon (1997). *Community Nursing Practice: Case Study.* Philadelphia: Lippincott-Raven.

McKnight J, Van Dover L (1994). Community as client: A challenge for nursing education. *J Public Health* 11(1):12–16.

Mechanic D (1994). *Inescapable Decisions: The Imperatives of Health Reform.* New Brunswick, NJ: Transaction Publishers.

Metler M, Kemper D (1996). *Healthwise for Life.* Boise, ID: Healthwise.

Miller M (1997). The nurse as change agent. In Spradley BW, Allender JA, eds. *Readings in Community Health Nursing.* Philadelphia: JB Lippincott.

Moeller, DW (1992). *Environmental Health.* Cambridge, MA: Harvard University Press.

Monteiro L (1997). Florence Nightingale on public health nursing. In Spradley BW, Allender JA, eds. *Readings in Community Health Nursing.* Philadelphia: JB Lippincott.

Morgan K, McClain S (1995). *Core Curriculum for Home Health Care Nursing.* Gaithersburg, MD: Aspen.

Moskowitz E, Jennings B (1996). *Coerced Contraception? Moral and Policy Changes of Long-Acting Birth Control.* Baltimore: Georgetown University Press.

Multistate Regulation Task Force (1996). Communique. *National Council of State Boards of Nursing*, December.

Nader P (1990). The concept of comprehensiveness in design and implementation. *J School Health* 60(4):133–138.

Nash, JM (1997). Fertile minds. *Time* 149(5):48–56.

National Association for Home Care (1994). *Basic Statistics About Home Care.* National Association for Home Care.

Navarro U (1989). Why some countries have national health insurance, others have national health services and the United States has neither. *International J Health* 19(3):383–404.

Nightingale F (1880). Introduction to the history of nursing in the home of the poor. In Rathbone W. *History and Progress of District Nursing of London.* London: McMillan & Co.

Nightingale F (1884). *Health and Local Government.* Aylesbury: Poulton & Co.

Nightingale F (1969). *Notes on Nursing.* New York: Dover Publications (originally published in 1860).

Nightingale F (1994). *Suggestions for Thought: Selections and Commentaries* (Calabria M, Macrae J, eds). Philadelphia: University of Pennsylvania Press.

Otto D, Valadez A (1995). Cultural diversity in healthcare. In Yoder Wise P. *Leading and Managing in Nursing.* St. Louis: Mosby.

Pare D (1995). Of families and other cultures: The shifting paradigm of family therapy. *Family Process* 34(1):1–19.

Parry JK, Ryan AS (1995). *A Cross-Cultural Look At Death, Dying, and Religion.* Chicago: Nelson-Hall.

Pearson MI et al (1992). Nosocomial transmission of multidrug-resistant *Mycobacterium* tuberculosis. *Ann Intern Med* 117:191–196.

Pedersen P (1988). *Handbook for Developing Multicultural Awareness.* Alexandria, VA: American Association for Counseling and Development.

Pincus H (1997). Commentary: Spirituality, religion, and health, expanding and using the knowledge base. *J Clinical Behavioral Medicine* 2(1):49.

Plumb J et al (1996). A collaborative community approach to homeless care. In Perkel R, Wender R, eds. *Primary Care Models of Ambulatory Care.* Philadelphia: WB Saunders.

Polit-O'Hara D, Hungler P (1995). *Nursing Research: Principles and Methods,* 5th ed. Philadelphia: JB Lippincott.

Post S (1997). Ethical aspects of religion in health care. *J Clinical Behavioral Medicine* 2(1):44-48.

President's Health Security Plan (1993). New York: Random House.

Public Health Foundation (1991). *Public Health Chartbook.* Washington DC: Public Health Foundation.

Rector C (1997). Innovative practice models in community health nursing. In Spradley BW, Allender JA, eds. *Readings in Community Health Nursing.* Philadelphia: JB Lippincott.

Rhodes A (1996). Immunity for reporting child abuse. *MCN* 21(4):169.

Roemer MI (1991). *National Health Care Systems of the World.* New York: Oxford University Press.

Romaine D (1995). Case management challenges, present and future. *Continuing Care* 14(1):24-31

Rosella J (1994). The need for multicultural diversity among health professionals. *Nurs Health Care* 15:242-246.

Rosenbaum J (1991). A cultural assessment guide. *Canadian Nurse* 87:21-22.

Ross B, Cobb K (1990). *Family Nursing: A Nursing Process Approach.* Redwood City, CA: Addison-Wesley Nursing.

Rother J (1997). Making sense of managed care. *Modern Maturity* 40(2):82-84.

Rubenfeld G, Scheffer B (1995). *Critical Thinking in Nursing: An Interactive Approach.* Philadelphia: JB Lippincott.

Rubin L (1994). *Families on the Faultline: America's Working Class Speaks About the Family, The Economy, Race and Ethnicity.* New York: Harper-Collins.

Schauffler H, Rodriguez T (1996). Exercising purchasing power for preventive care. *Health Affairs* 15(1):73-85.

Schuster S (1995). My patient, my friend: A community health nursing experience. *Home Health Care Nurse* 13:70-72.

Scott R (1996). The most important health factor your doctor isn't asking about. *Spirituality & Health* Fall 1996, pp. 26-27.

Shea M (1996). When a patient refuses treatment. *RN* 59(7):51-54.

Sheils J (1996). Why medical savings accounts increase costs. *Health Affairs* 15(1):241.

Shortell S et al (1994). The new world of managed care: Creating organized delivery systems. *Health Affairs* 13(5):46-64.

Shugars D, Bader J, eds. (1991). *Healthy America: Practitioners for 2005, An Agenda for Action for U.S. Professional Schools.* Durham, NC: Pew Health Professions Commission.

Smeltzer S, Bare B (1996). *Brunner and Suddarth's Textbook of Medical-Surgical Nursing,* 8th ed. Philadelphia: JB Lippincott.

Smith J (1997). Can you handle home care? *RN* 60(3):51-55.

Snyder R (1995). Ethical decisions: Home healthcare providers and patients who choose to die. *Home Health Care Nurse* 13(5):75-78.

Solomon J (1995). Retirement living equals jobs for nursing. *RN* 58:52.

Sowell R, Meadows T (1994). An integrated case management model: Developing standards, evaluation and outcome criteria. *Nurs Admin Q* 18(2):52-64.

Spector R (1996). *Cultural Diversity in Health & Illness,* 4th ed. Stamford, CT: Appleton & Lange.

Spradley BW, Allender JA (1996). *Community Health Nursing: Concepts and Practice,* 4th ed. Philadelphia: Lippincott-Raven.

Spradley BW, Allender JA (1997). *Readings in Community Health Nursing.* Philadelphia: Lippincott-Raven.

Spragins E (June 24, 1996). Does your HMO stack up? *Newsweek,* pp. 56-63.

Spruhan J (1996). Beyond traditional nursing care: Cultural awareness and successful home healthcare nursing. *Home Healthcare Nurse* 14:445-449.

Stackhouse J (1994). Death, dying, bereavement and spiritual distress. In Monahan F, Neighbors M, eds. *Nursing Care of Adults,* 2d ed. Philadelphia: WB Saunders.

Stackhouse J (1997). Facilitative verbal responses. In Leasia S, Monahan F, eds. *A Practical Guide for Health Assessment.* Philadelphia: WB Saunders.

Stanhope M, Knollmueller R (1996). *Handbook of Community and Home Health Nursing.* St. Louis: Mosby.

Stark J (1995). Critical thinking, taking the road less traveled. *Nursing '95* November, pp. 53-55.

Stolberg S (March 2, 1996). Report sees vastly different U.S. household in 15 years. *Los Angeles Times.*

Stolte KM (1996). *Wellness Nursing Diagnosis for Health Promotion.* Philadelphia: Lippincott-Raven.

Strasser J (1995). The cultural context for community health nursing. In Smith C, Maurer F, eds. *Community Health Nursing.* Philadelphia: WB Saunders.

Survey Reactions (1996). A grim prognosis for health care? *AJN* 96(11):40–44.

Tagliareni E, Murray J (1995). Community-based experiences in the associate degree nursing curriculum. *J Nursing Education* March.

Talbot L, Curtis L (1996). The challenge of assessing skin indicators in people of color. *Home Healthcare Nurse* 14(3):168–173.

Tammelleo A (1993). Legally speaking: Staying out of trouble on the telephone. *RN* October.

Thomasma D et al (1996). The ethics of caring for conjoined twins. *Hastings Center Report* 26(4): 4–12.

Tomaiuolo NG (1996). Accessing nursing resources on the Internet. *Computers in Nursing* 13(4): 159–164.

Tripp-Reimer T, Alfifi L (1989). Crosscultural perspective on patient teaching. *Nursing Clinics of North America* 24:613–619.

Turner UA (1993). ANA, Red Cross cite need for more RNs to be trained for disaster relief. *The American Nurse* September, p. 3.

U.S. Dept. of Commerce, Bureau of Census (1995). *Population Projection for the States: 1993–2020.* Current Population Report, Series P25-111.

U.S. Dept. of Health & Human Services (1994). *Registered Nurse Population.* Health Resources.

U.S. Dept. of Health & Human Services, Public Health Service (1996a). Study shows two-parent family lowers teen drug use. *SAMHSA Newsletter* IV(4): 25–26.

U.S. Dept. of Health & Human Services, Public Health Service, Centers for Disease Control & Prevention (1996). *Health United States 1996.* Washington DC: U.S. Govt. Printing Office.

Vahldieck R et al (1993). A framework for planning public health nursing services for families. In Wegner, Alexander, eds. *Readings in Family Nursing.* Philadelphia: JB Lippincott.

Vezeau T (1996). Cost care by task/define nursing by knowledge. *MCN* 21(5):253–254.

Whall A (1993). The family as the unit of care in nursing: A historical review. In Wegner, Alexander, eds. *Readings in Family Nursing.* Philadelphia: JB Lippincott.

Williams C (1992). Public health nursing: Does it have a future? In Aiken IA, Fagan C, eds. *Charting Nursing's Future: Agenda for the 1990s.* Philadelphia: JB Lippincott.

Williams C (1997). Community health nursing—what is it? In Spradley BW, Allender JA, eds. *Readings in Community Health Nursing,* 5th ed. Philadelphia: JB Lippincott.

Wills E (1996). Nurse-client alliance: A pattern of home health caring. *Home Healthcare Nurse* 14(6): 455–459.

Wilson HD (1993). Family caregiving for a relative with Alzheimer's dementia: Coping with negative choices. In Wegner, Alexander, eds. *Readings in Family Nursing.* Philadelphia: JB Lippincott.

Woodham-Smith C (1951). *Florence Nightingale.* New York: McGraw-Hill.

Wright L, Leahey M (1994). *Nurses and Families: A Guide to Family Assessment and Intervention.* Philadelphia: FA Davis.

Wurtz R et al (1996). A new class of close contacts: Home health care workers and occupational exposure to tuberculosis. *Home Health Care Management and Practice* 8(2):28–31.

Yoder Wise P (1995). *Leading and Managing in Nursing.* St. Louis: Mosby.

Zerwekh J (1993). Going to the people: Public health nursing today and tomorrow. *Am J Public Health* 83:1676–1678.

Part 2

Nursing Practice in Wellness Care

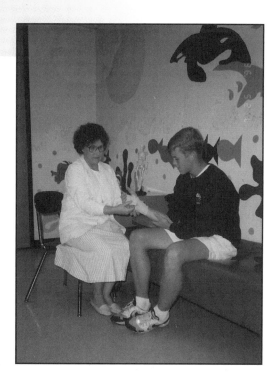

A school nurse.

5

Wellness Goals and Activities

Key Terms

affective learning

case finding

cognitive learning

empowerment

health fairs

health risk appraisal

Healthy People 2000

learning readiness

locus of control

measurable outcomes

multiphasic screening

noncompliance

nurse–client contracts

personal lifestyle choices

psychomotor learning

screening

self-efficacy

spirituality

teaching–learning process

World Health Organization

Learning Objectives

1. Define health.
2. List at least 15 steps to total wellness.
3. Perform a stress reduction exercise.
4. Identify at least 10 hassles and 10 uplifts in your daily life.
5. Explain the health value of promoting a sense of self-efficacy or internal locus of control.
6. Describe the *Healthy People 2000 process.*
7. List 20 of the 47 sentinel objectives of *Healthy People 2000.*
8. Identify at least 10 benefits of physical activity for older persons.
9. Compare your weight with the recommended weight range for your height.
10. Describe how to conduct a successful health fair.
11. Perform a health risk appraisal on yourself and a friend or a family member.
12. Use the classification and recommendations chart of the Joint National Committee on Detection, Evaluation, and Treatment of High Blood Pressure to conduct a hypertension screening program.
13. Identify, by percent, the factors that contribute to our health, based on National Institute of Health statistics.
14. Identify the highest risk factors in American life.
15. Explain in detail the steps of the teaching–learning process.
16. Develop a client–nurse contract.
17. Explain the value of holistic assessments.

Definition of Health or Wellness

In 1974, the World Health Organization (WHO) proposed a holistic definition of health: "Health is a state of complete physical, mental and social well-being and not merely the absence of disease and infirmity." We have realized during the past 25 years that health care must be holistic, and nurses have helped promote that recognition. The old medical model of health care as the treatment of illness has been replaced by a more positive approach of promoting wellness. The health-care system is now placing a priority on wellness care—that is, activities that promote health and help prevent disease.

Nurses are wonderfully equipped to provide wellness care. Community health nurses are concerned with family, community, societal, and environmental wellness as well as individual wellness.

Most of the factors that determine wellness are related to lifestyle choices (Fig. 5-1). We are holistic beings, but for the sake of clarity we will discuss the various factors of wellness separately: social, mental, emotional, spiritual, and physical (modified from Health EDCO., 1995).

Social
Create and cultivate close relationships.
Learn to interact well with others.
Act assertively, not passively nor aggressively.

Mental
Recognize special needs for love and stimulation.
View life's challenges as growth opportunities.
Practice time and stress management.

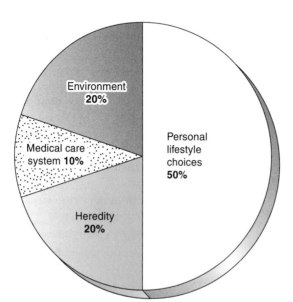

FIGURE 5-1
Factors contributing to health. (Based on 1996 figures from the National Center for Health Statistics, Centers for Disease Control, and National Institutes for Health.)

Seek and follow sound medical advice, and be informed.

Learn to become a good communicator.

Develop problem-solving strategies.

Emotional

Know and understand your feelings.

Engage in humor, fun, and celebration.

Express emotions appropriately to others.

Promote a positive outlook on life.

Promote a sense of well-being, even in adversity.

Spiritual

Find a meaningful purpose in life.

Seek harmony with yourself, others, and God.

Experience beauty in music, nature, and art.

Determine your personal values and act accordingly.

Practice forgiveness.

Do things for others.

Engage in prayer.

Physical

Exercise regularly and be physically active.

Avoid destructive habits (eg, smoking, drug and alcohol abuse).

Prevent illness and harm.

Use seat belts.

Keep immunizations up to date.

Practice regular, thorough handwashing.

Use protective measures against sexually transmitted diseases and HIV.

Do not drink while driving.

Avoid hazardous activities.

Rest adequately and get plenty of sleep.

Eat a nutritious diet with plenty of whole grains, fruits, and vegetables. Limit fats and sugars.

Maintain total cholesterol less than 200.

Maintain blood pressure less than 130/85.

Maintain a resting pulse rate less than 80.

Maintain body fat of 23% to 30% (women) or 16% to 25% (men).

Figure 5-2 illustrates a "protective bubble" of positive health behaviors in which to live our lives. Wellness behaviors require self-responsibility and self-discipline.

Empowerment to Change

People have more incentive to change unhealthy habits and take responsibility if they believe that control is possible and their actions will be effective. To realize their aims, people try in various degrees to exercise control over their lives. Those who believe in their personal capacity to cope with life are said to have perceived self-efficacy or

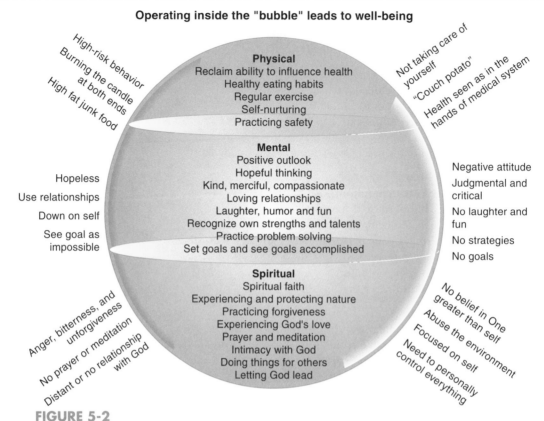

FIGURE 5-2
Health model for well-being of body, mind, and spirit. (Reprinted with permission. Adair M, Adair JB [1995]. Nashville, TN: Mountainbrook Foundation.)

an internal locus of control. Perceived low self-efficacy or external locus of control causes people to feel helpless, buffeted by external forces, and powerless to change things. This leads to lack of motivation and apathy about trying to improve their status or become responsible about their health needs.

Perceived self-efficacy regulates human functioning in four major ways, according to Dr. Albert Bandura, a professor of social science in psychology at Stanford University (1997).

1. Cognitive: High self-efficacy leads to sound, positive thinking, high aspirations, long-term goal setting, and a strong commitment to meeting those goals.
2. Motivational: High self-efficacy leads to forming beliefs about what one can do, setting goals, expending effort toward those goals, and persevering and demonstrating resiliency in the face of setbacks and failures. In contrast, people with low self-efficacy avoid difficult tasks and have low aspirations and a weak commitment to their goals.
3. Affect: Those who believe they can manage threats are less distressed by them; those with low self-efficacy magnify the risks. People with high self-efficacy can

tolerate and manage stress better by relaxation methods, diversion, and seeking help from their support group.

4. Depression: Perceived low self-efficacy can lead directly to depression because of the defeat of one's hopes. This, in turn, further lowers the sense of self-efficacy, creating more depression, and a vicious cycle results. These people also have a sense of social inefficacy, which means they do not have the social support that helps make chronic stress easier to bear.

Methods to improve self-efficacy have been called "internality training" because they improve the user's sense of internal locus of control and self-empowerment. The "internality" process is worth the considerable effort it takes, and nurses can help clients by doing the following:

1. Communicate a genuine, caring, therapeutic attitude.
2. Provide experiences of success or mastery in overcoming obstacles. Gradually increase the level of difficulties to be overcome. Avoid situations that are likely to cause failure, but increase the challenges with time and experience.
3. Provide contact with positive role models who have persevered and succeeded through similar circumstances.
4. Demonstrate genuine respect for the client and his or her ability to move forward. Build on recognized strengths.
5. Help the client recognize and structure the environment to reduce or eliminate unnecessary stress.
6. Teach the client to recognize physical fatigue, pain, anxiety, and tension for what it is and deal with it by using stress reduction strategies. Persons with perceived low self-efficacy tend to misperceive fatigue or tension as another indicator of failure.

Figure 5-3, Display 5-1, and Table 15-1 in Chapter 15 show examples of stress assessment and reduction techniques to use with clients.

Healthy People 2000 *National Goals*

Achieving good health requires a foundation of mental, emotional, spiritual, social, and physical elements. With a vision of achieving health from a multidimensional perspective, the *Healthy People 2000* national goals were established in 1990. Participants in the consortium came from across the country and represented more than 300 organizations, all the health professions, and every level of government. National goals were established, and many states developed objectives targeted to their specific populations. The process began in 1979 when the U.S. Public Health Service (PHS) published *Healthy People: The Surgeon General's Report on Health Promotion and Disease Prevention*. This document and other PHS publications established national health objectives with measurable outcomes for the next decade. The *Healthy People 2000* objectives grew out of that initial effort.

If the multidimensional goals and objectives of *Healthy People 2000* are to be achieved, all segments of American society must be aware of them and work toward

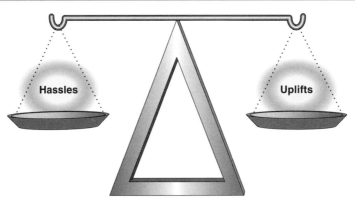

FIGURE 5-3
Balancing everyday stress: Hassles and uplifts
An overload of minor aggravations ("hassles") can cause major symptoms of stress. Good coping skills can help avoid these harmful effects. In addition, you can offset the hassles with small pleasures ("uplifts"). Be sure to build enough uplifts into your everyday life to balance the inevitable hassles that come your way. These examples will help you identify the hassles and uplifts that apply to you:

Hassles	**Uplifts**
Difficult people	Music
Misplacing things	Hugs and kisses
Waiting in line	Humor
Minor physical problems	Nature
Concerns about weight	Hobbies
Traffic jams	Relaxing
Problems with children	Prayer
Breaking a shoelace	Completing a task
Telephone sales calls	Daydreaming
Filling out forms	Entertainment (TV, movies, etc.)
Problems on the job	Sharing something
Too many interruptions	Friends

_____ _____
_____ _____

Richard S. Lazarus, Allen D. Kanner, et al (1981). Comparisons of two modes of stress measurements: Daily hassles and uplifts versus major life events. J. of Behavioral Medicine. University of California, Berkeley.

them. These goals go far beyond the health-care system itself, dealing with how people lead their daily lives. The three major goals are to

1. Increase the span of healthy life
2. Reduce health disparities among Americans
3. Provide preventive services for all Americans

A midcourse review performed in 1995 found that much progress had been achieved in many areas, but no progress had been made in some areas and a few areas had actually gotten worse (Table 5-1). Based on these data, additional objectives were added, many of which target specific groups.

(text continues on p. 120)

DISPLAY 5-1
Are You Vulnerable to Stress?

To find out, complete this check-up (based on research by Miller and Smith at Boston University Medical Center). By each question, write the score which most applies to you.

1 = almost always
2 = often
3 = sometimes
4 = hardly ever
5 = never

_____ **1.** I eat at least one full, balanced meal daily.
_____ **2.** I get enough sleep at least four nights per week.
_____ **3.** I give and get affection regularly.
_____ **4.** I have at least one close friend or relative who lives within 50 miles.
_____ **5.** I get vigorous exercise at least three times a week.
_____ **6.** I smoke less than half a pack of cigarettes daily.
_____ **7.** I consume fewer than five alcoholic drinks a week.
_____ **8.** I am within 10 pounds of my appropriate weight.
_____ **9.** I have enough money to meet basic expenses.
_____ **10.** I get strength from my religious faith.
_____ **11.** I have regular social activities.
_____ **12.** I have several friends and a larger number of acquaintances.
_____ **13.** I talk openly and frankly with one or a few close friends about personal matters.
_____ **14.** I am in good health or manage any chronic health problem well.
_____ **15.** I can express anger, joy, and other feelings freely.
_____ **16.** I have work to do which is satisfying and meaningful.
_____ **17.** I do something at least once a week for fun or recreation.
_____ **18.** I have enough time for important activities, work, and recreation.
_____ **19.** I take stimulants or tranquilizers only when prescribed by a doctor.
_____ **20.** I take some time out for myself every day.

_____ = **TOTAL**

___−20___ (now subtract 20 from the total)

_____ My final score

What my final score means:

(1–29)   I'm fairly stress-hardy at this point in life.
(30–49)   I'm somewhat vulnerable to stress.
(50–75)   I'm definitely vulnerable and can benefit from developing my ability to handle stress constructively.
(over 75)   I'm quite vulnerable to the effects of stress, and need to have adequate coping strategies and plans to avoid unwanted stress-related problems.

(Source: Burggrabe J. Miller, K. [1991]. Developing a Healthy Lifestyle. *San Jose, CA: Resource Publications.)*

TABLE 5-1. Progress on Forty Seven Sentinel Objectives

Objective	% Change Targeted	Baseline[a]	Update[g]	Year 2000 Targets	Right Direction	Wrong Direction	No Change	No Data
Health Promotion								
1. Physical activity								
• More people exercising regularly	+36%	22%[c]	24%[i]	30%	X			
• Fewer people never exercising	−38%	24%[c]	24%[i]	15%			X	
2. Nutrition								
• Fewer people overweight	−23%	26%[b]	34%[h]	20%		X		
• Lower-fat diets	−17%	36%[b]	34%[h]	30%	X			
3. Tobacco								
• Fewer people smoking cigarettes	−48%	29%	25%	15%	X			
• Fewer youth beginning to smoke	−50%	30%	27%	15%	X			
4. Alcohol and other drugs								
• Fewer alcohol-related automobile deaths (per 100,000)	−13%	9.8%	6.8	8.5	X			
• Less alcohol use among youth aged 12–17 years	−50%	25.2%[a]	18.0%	12.6%	X			
• Less marijuana use among youth aged 12–17 years	−50%	6.4%[e]	4.9%	3.2%	X			
5. Family planning								
• Fewer teen pregnancies (per 1,000)	−30%	71.1[c,f]	74.3[i,r]	50[r]		X		
• Fewer unintended pregnancies	−46%	56%[e]	NA	30%				X
6. Mental health and mental disorders								
• Fewer suicides (per 100,000)	−10%	11.7	11.2	10.5	X			
• Fewer people reporting stress-related problems	−21%	44.2%[c]	39.2%	35%	X			
7. Violent and abusive behavior								
• Fewer homicides (per 100,000)	−15%	8.5	10.3[k]	7.2		X		
• Fewer assault injuries (per 100,000)	−10%	9.7[d]	9.9[k]	8.7		X		

Objective								
8. Educational and community-based programs								
• More schools with comprehensive school health education	NA	NA	NA		75%			X
• More workplaces with health promotion programs	+31%	NA	65%c	81%k	85%	X		
Health Protection								
9. Unintentional injuries								
• Fewer unintentional injury deaths (per 100,000)	−16%		34.7	29.6	29.3	X		
• More people using automobile safety restraints	+102%		42%	67%l	85%	X		
10. Occupational safety and health								
• Fewer work-related deaths (per 100,000)	−33%		6m	5	4	X		
• Fewer work-related injuries (per 100,000)	−22%		7.7m	7.9	6.0		X	
11. Environmental health								
• No children with blood lead 25 µg/dl	−100%		234,000n	93,000h	0	X		
• More people with clear air in their communities	+71%		49.7%e	76.5%	85%	X		
• More people in radon-tested houses	+700%		5%f	11.4%	40%	X		
12. Food and drug safety								
• Fewer *Salmonella* outbreaks	−68%		77f	63	25	X		
13. Oral health								
• Fewer children with dental caries	−34%		54%	52%	35%	X		
• Fewer older people without teeth	−44%		36%d	30%	20%	X		
Preventive Services								
14. Maternal and infant health								
• Fewer newborns with low weight	−28%		6.9%	7.1%k	5%			X
• More mothers with first-trimester care	+18%		76.0%	77.7%k	90%	X		

(continues)

TABLE 5-1. (Continued)

Objective	% Change Targeted	Baseline[a]	Update[g]	Year 2000 Targets	Right Direction	Wrong Direction	No Change	No Data
15. Heart disease and stroke								
• Fewer coronary heart disease deaths (per 100,000)	−26%	135	114[k]	100	X			
• Fewer stroke deaths (per 100,000)	−34%	30.4	26.4	20.0	X			
• Better control of high blood pressure	+355%	11%[b]	21%[h]	50%	X			
• Lower cholesterol levels	−6%	213 mg/dl[b]	205 mg/dl[h]	200 mg%	X			
16. Cancer								
• Decreased cancer deaths (per 100,000)	−3%	134	133	130	X			
• Increased screening for breast cancer (age > 50)	+140%	25%	55%	60%	X			
• Increased screening for cervical cancer (age > 18)	+8%	88%	95%	95%	X			
• Increased fecal occult blood testing (age > 50)	+85%	27%	30%[k]	50%	X			
17. Diabetes and chronic disabling conditions								
• Fewer people disabled by chronic conditions	−15%	9.4%	10.6%	8%		X		
• Fewer diabetes-related deaths (per 100,000)	−11%	38[d]	38[k]	34			X	

Objective					Status			
18. HIV infection								
• Slower increase in HIV infection (per 100,000)	0%	400[f]	NA	400				X
19. Sexually transmitted diseases								
• Fewer gonorrhea infections (per 100,000)	−25%	300[f]	172	225	X			
• Fewer syphillis infections (per 100,000)	−45%	18.1[f]	10.4	10.0	X			
20. Immunization and infectious diseases								
• No measles cases	−100%	3058[e,q]	312[q]	0	X			
• Fewer pneumonia and influenza deaths (per 100,000)	−63%	19.9[o]	23.1[p]	7.3		X		
• Higher immunization levels (ages 19–35 months)	+53%	54–64%	67%	90%	X			
21. Clinical preventive services								
• No financial barrier to recommended preventive services	−100%	16%[f]	17%	0		X		
Surveillance and Data Systems								
22. Surveillance and data systems								
• Common and comparable health status indicators in use across States	0 States	48 States	40 States		X			
Total					33	9	2	3

[a] 1987 unless otherwise noted
[b] 1976–80
[c] 1985
[d] 1986
[e] 1988

[f] 1989
[g] 1993 unless otherwise noted
[h] 1988–91
[i] 1990
[j] 1991

[k] 1992
[l] 1994
[m] 1983–1987
[n] 1984

[o] 1979–80 through 1986–87 influenza seasons
[p] 1987–88 through 1989–90 influenza seasons
[q] Data are expressed as measles cases
[r] Rate per 1,000

(USD HHS [1996]. *Healthy People 2000, Midcourse Review and 1995 Revisions*, Washington DC: U.S. Govt. Printing Office.)

Health Promotion and Disease Prevention Activities

Exercise and Obesity

There is good evidence that exercise reduces the risk of many diseases and promotes physical, mental, and emotional wellness. Exercise is particularly important in maintaining independent healthy living as people grow older or develop chronic diseases (Display 5-2). Regular exercise is the best way to maintain daily functioning and independent living.

However, many Americans never exercise. One reason is the increasing amount of time we spend in front of the television and the computer. Consequently, obesity in America is increasing: about 58 million Americans are obese (120% or more of ideal weight). Table 5-2 lists recommended weight ranges. Each year, 300,000 people die from obesity-related complications. Obesity is the second leading cause of preventable death in the United States, exceeded only by cigarette smoking. One in five teenagers and one in three adults in America are overweight. Children need to spend more time being physically active. Obesity is a particular concern for certain racial and ethnic populations, such as Hispanics, African-Americans, and Native Americans. One of the goals in the 1995 revision of *Healthy People 2000* is to stress the adoption of appropriate weight-loss practices, with exercise and dietary changes, for these and other target groups.

The popular diet drug dexfluramine (Redux), released in 1996, has received a great deal of attention in the popular media. That is not surprising, because at any given moment, up to 50% of American women and 25% of men say they are trying to diet (*Johns Hopkins Medical Letter*, March 1997). However, Redux (or its predecessor "fen-phen," a combination of fenfluramine and phentermine), is not the answer for most

---

DISPLAY 5-2
Effects of Exercise

- Helps prevent or control chronic health conditions, such as arthritis
- Helps prevent certain cancers, such as colon and possibly breast cancer
- Prevents bone loss that leads to conditions such as osteoporosis
- Relieves stress and tension
- Improves mental outlook by easing depression, loneliness, anxiety
- Mitigates symptoms of menopause
- Increases energy
- Improves circulation
- Helps maintain weight or prevent obesity
- Acts as a natural laxative
- Maintains and builds muscle tissue
- Serves as a social outlet

(Adapted from AARP. [1996] Physical activity—It's never too late! Perspectives in Health Promotion and Aging, *vol. 2. November, pp. 1–5.)*

TABLE 5-2. Healthy Weight Range

Height (Inches)	Range (lbs)
58	91–119
60	97–127
62	103–136
64	111–146
66	118–156
68	125–165
70	133–175
72	140–185
74	148–195
76	156–205

(Source: National Institute of Health.)

overweight Americans. Appetite suppressants do not help everyone and should be used only after increased exercise and dietary measures have failed to produce results. These drugs are more apt to help those whose appetite is triggered truly by hunger, not by habit or stress. Redux is not safe for long-term maintenance. In addition to the side effects of insomnia, gastrointestinal disturbances, increased blood pressure, pulmonary hypertension, and cardiac damage can occur. This can become a fatal condition characterized by increased blood pressure in the arteries that supply the lungs. For these reasons, Redux was removed from the market in 1997.

Health Screening

Health screening is the term used when dealing with groups or aggregates. With increased awareness of the value of prevention, the use of health screening and referral has expanded in the United States. Free screening programs have existed for some time, with good results. Health fairs, which include screening programs, are increasingly popular; Displays 5-3 and 5-4 list strategies for planning and conducting a successful health fair.

Multiphasic screening is a battery of tests done at one time to detect several health problems. For example, multiphasic screening by a school nurse may include hearing, vision, height and weight, PPD skin testing, hematocrit or hemoglobin, urinalysis, and dental examination.

Hypertension screening is regularly performed by many community groups and health-care agencies (Table 5-3). A *Healthy People 2000* objective is to increase the control of hypertension in at least 50% of the people who have hypertension. Hypertension screening has already helped identify this "silent killer" in many asymptomatic people. The dramatic reduction over the past 25 years in the number of deaths caused by secondary conditions of high blood pressure (heart disease and stroke) owes much to these screening programs. *(text continues on p. 123)*

DISPLAY 5-3
Health Fairs

Background
Well suited to moderate to large groups, the health fair can be scheduled on its own or as part of a larger event. To emphasize the link of health and wholeness focus activities on choices and behaviors that are under personal or organizational control.

Strategies for a Successful Health Fair
Have Fun
Set a tone of enjoyment and fellowship: details such as bright colors, music, balloons, and clowns help develop enthusiasm for adopting healthy lifestyles.

Be Active
People learn and understand best when they are actively involved: "hands-on" experiences are memorable and meaningful.

Use Humor
Humor helps ideas gain acceptance and spices up necessary information; use a light approach when possible (such as "Go to Health" as a theme).

Use Variety
Balance activities that may arouse anxiety (such as measuring blood pressure) with those that are fun and feel good.

Volunteers
Recruit a few medical professionals to serve as volunteers for check-up activities and to answer health-related questions or refer participants to additional help.

Get Resources
Solicit "freebie" health promotion information and give-away items from community organizations (for instance, the Heart Association, Dairy Council, or Lung Association).

Get Help
Ask local junior colleges or high schools to participate with health promotion displays, "learning labs," or other successful health education techniques.

Health Fair: How to Proceed
GOALS: Decide what you want the health fair to accomplish. Arouse interest, motivate people's desire for better health, promote upcoming healthy lifestyle activities.

LEADERSHIP: Select a project coordinator, and divide specific responsibilities among others in the planning group—publicity, volunteers, displays, activities, food, etc.; or each member of the group may prefer to arrange and supervise one area of lifestyle choice—nutrition, stress, fitness, etc.

ORGANIZATION: Choose a date, place, and theme for the fair.

CONTENT: Brainstorm a list of possible activities and options for learning about healthful living. For each area of lifestyle choice, provide a background, one or more actions and one or more give-away options.

Nutrition
BACKGROUND: a display or posters of the nutrition triangle of basic food groups showing recommendations for the number of servings appropriate for each day.

ACTION: participants spoon onto one side of a balance scale their estimate of a "serving" of food (such as cottage cheese), then check themselves by adding the specified weight on the other side.

GIVE-AWAYS: "mystery treats"—small bites of healthy goodies such as bran muffins, raisin clusters, trail mix, or fruit leather.

Fitness
BACKGROUND: posters or photos showing people enjoying the benefits of fitness, such as lowered stress level, controlled weight, improved energy and mood.

ACTION: participants calculate their own "heart training rate" for aerobic exercise benefits.

GIVE-AWAYS: activity charts, sweatbands.

Stress Management
BACKGROUND: posters showing or listing the "hassles and uplifts" of everyday life.

DISPLAY 5-3 *(Continued)*

ACTION: in a small "relaxing room," provide comfortable chairs, and headphones and tape players, with relaxation routine tapes for participants to sample.

GIVE-AWAYS: short jokes, funny sayings, or cartoons to be withdrawn from a "crabbiness cure" box.

Rest/Recreation/Renewal

BACKGROUND: travel posters or scenic photos.

ACTION: new games.

GIVE-AWAYS: sing-along song sheets; small flowers (for buttonhole or lapel).

The number of activities in each area depends on space and funds available, size of the crowd, and goals of the fair. Other health-focused activities can also be incorporated, such as blood pressure checks, vision checks, height/weight/skinfold measurement, etc., with appropriate follow-up protocols.

Other ideas to consider

Recruit a volunteer "snapshooter" to take instant photos of participants as they try the activities; display the best on "The Picture of Health" bulletin board at the fair's entrance and use them later (with permission of the subjects) in publicity for coming healthy lifestyle events. Include options to try out some health promotion ideas that are quite new to most people in your community, as well as many that are somewhat familiar. Offer several team approach activities to demonstrate the value of support in a trusting fellowship group.

Survey participants for interest in upcoming events or ideas for developing healthy lifestyles under consideration (for instance health promotion classes, support groups, retreats) by providing a check list or sign-up sheets; this helps the planning group set priorities for the future.

DELIVERY: Publicize, use all available help, and launch the event!

REVIEW: Following the health fair, schedule a meeting to review the participation and response. Note ideas to use in later activities or to pass on to other groups or persons involved.

FOLLOW-THROUGH: Arrange for communication and follow up with physicians and others responsible for healthy lifestyles, and begin planning for the next event.

(Adapted from Burggrabe J, Miller K [1991]. Developing a Healthy Lifestyle. *San Jose, CA: Resource Publications.)*

Serum cholesterol screenings have greatly increased public awareness of the risk of high serum cholesterol and the effect of diet on the development of cardiovascular disease, still the leading cause of death in the United States.

Skin cancers, particularly melanomas, are on the increase. The American Cancer Society and wellness programs sponsored by hospitals periodically sponsor screenings to catch these cancers in the early stages. Dermatologists and nurses usually volunteer their time for this effort.

In many communities, the local Lions Club sponsors annual screening programs for glaucoma, the second leading cause of blindness in the United States. Glaucoma, like hypertension, is one of the "silent" diseases that cause no symptoms in the early stages. Early detection and treatment can prevent or delay blindness. Many ophthalmologists and nurses volunteer to help with these free screenings.

DISPLAY 5-4
Health Fair Planning Guide

Type:
- ☐ Managing Stress
- ☐ Sound Nutrition
- ☐ Physical Fitness
- ☐ Safe Choices
- ☐ Rest, Recreation & Renewal

Project Manager: Phone:

Date and hours: Estimated Cost:

Goals: What will the Health Fair accomplish?

1. _____
2. _____
3. _____

Organizing the Health Fair
The Health Fair's place in the community Healthy Lifestyle program:

What activities should precede the Health Fair?

_____
_____
_____

What activities should the Health Fair offer?

_____
_____
_____

Theme _____

Estimated Attendance: _____ Space needed: _____

"Special" Effects? ☐ no ☐ yes Decorations, Music, Give-aways or Other (specify): _____

_____

Location: _____

Advertising: (list five ways; eg, flyers, public service announcements)

_____
_____
_____

Volunteers needed

Specify skills or task required (Professional: take pulse, blood pressures; Other: copy forms, enter data)

Name	Responsible for:
_____	_____
_____	_____
_____	_____
_____	_____
_____	_____
_____	_____
_____	_____

Programs for confidential HIV testing are available from local health departments, private physicians, and community clinics concerned about AIDS. These blood tests give fairly reliable results and should be repeated at 3-month, 6-month, and 1-year intervals. The test may need to be repeated if suspected exposure has occurred more

DISPLAY 5-4
Health Fair Planning Guide (continued)

Provided by: (Community organization or individuals)   Service

_____   _____
_____   _____
_____   _____

Equipment or supplies needed (eg, computers, tables)
                    Equipment   From whom?

_____   _____
_____   _____
_____   _____

HOW WILL THE RESULTS OF THE HEALTH FAIR BE EVALUATED?
        Evaluation Factors   By Whom?   Date

_____   _____   _____
_____   _____   _____
_____   _____   _____

FOLLOW-UP ACTIVITIES   Date

With participants:_____   _____

With lifestyles planning group:_____   _____

Notes: Which activities were successful? Which need improvement? What have we learned to do better?

_____
_____
_____

(Adapted from Burgrabbe J, Miller K [1991]. Developing a Healthy Lifestyle. *San Jose, CA: Resource Publications.)*

recently. Often a positive test for one disease suggests testing for other diseases. This is true for tuberculosis, hepatitis, and sexually transmitted diseases, which are indicators to test for HIV in high-risk populations.

Other health screening events may include breast examinations and mammography, Pap tests, testicular examinations, prostate-specific antigen and digital examinations of the prostate, and stool examinations for occult blood. When these examinations are done on an individual basis, the term "case finding" is used. Screening of community populations and individual case finding are secondary prevention measures to detect and treat diseases in the early stages (Table 5-4). Table 5-5 contains recommended time intervals for preventive services for persons over age 50.

Primary prevention measures include immunization programs, teaching about safety and nutrition, and health risk appraisal (Display 5-5). The latter is done to identify persons at risk for certain health problems. This appraisal should always be accompanied by health teaching and any needed referrals for follow-up care.

TABLE 5-3. Classification of Blood Pressure for Adults Age 18 Years and Older*

Category	Systolic (mm Hg)	Diastolic (mm Hg)
Normal	<130	<85
High normal	130–139	85–89
Hypertension†		
Stage 1 (Mild)	140–159	90–99
Stage 2 (Moderate)	160–179	100–109
Stage 3 (Severe)	180–209	110–119
Stage 4 (Very severe)	≥210	≥120

* Not taking antihypertensive drugs and not acutely ill. When systolic and diastolic pressures fall into different categories, the higher category should be selected to classify the individual's blood pressure status. For instance, 160/92 mm Hg should be classified as stage 2, 180–120 mm Hg as stage 4. Isolated systolic hypertension (ISH) is defined as SBP ≥140 mm Hg and DBP <90 mm Hg and staged appropriately (eg, 170/85 mm Hg is defined as stage 2 ISH).

† Based on the average of two or more readings taken at each of two or more visits following an initial screening.

Initial Screening Blood Pressure (mm Hg)*

Systolic	Diastolic	Follow-up Recommended†
<130	<85	Recheck in 2 years
130–139	85–89	Recheck in 1 year†
140–159	90–99	Confirm within 2 months
160–179	100–109	Refer to source of care within 1 month
180–209	110–119	Refer to source of care within 1 week
≥210	≥120	Refer to source of care immediately

* If the systolic and diastolic categories are different, follow recommendation for the shorter time follow-up (eg, 160/85 mm Hg should be evaluated or referred to source of care within 1 month).

† The scheduling of follow-up should be modified by reliable information about past blood pressure measurements, other cardiovascular risk factors, or target-organ disease.

† Consider providing advice about lifestyle modifications.

(1993 5th Report Joint National Committee on Detection, Evaluation, and Treatment of High Blood Pressure. NIH Publication #93-1088.)

Teaching the Client, the Family, and the Community

Methods of health teaching by the community health nurse vary with the client, the setting, and the content of instruction needed. Many times health teaching is best done with groups. Nurses are frequently invited by community groups to teach some aspect of wellness promotion. An illustration, graph, or picture is often helpful; the chart in Figure 5-4 dramatically shows the high risk of cigarette smoking.

The nurse must first assess the client's readiness to learn (Display 5-6) and determine

(text continues on p. 132)

TABLE 5-4. Levels of Disease Prevention and Examples of Activities

Level	Description	Activities
Primary	Prevention of the initial occurrence of disease or injury	Immunization; family planning; retirement planning; well-child care; smoking cessation; hygiene teaching; fluoride supplements; fitness classes; alcohol and drug prevention; seat belts and child car restraints; environmental protection
Secondary	Early identification of disease or disability with prompt intervention to prevent or limit disability	Physical assessments; hypertension screening; developmental screening; breast and testicular self-examinations; hearing and vision screening; mammography; pregnancy testing
Tertiary	Assistance (after disease or disability has occurred) to halt further disease progress and to meet one's potential and maximize quality of life despite illness or injury	Teaching and counseling regarding lifestyle changes such as diet and exercise; stress management and home management after diagnosis of chronic illness; support groups; support for caretaker; Meals On Wheels for homebound; physical therapy after stroke or accident; mental health counseling for rape victims

Some prevention activities listed overlap into health promotion or health protection.
(Hunt R, Zurek E [1997]. *Community-Based Nursing.* Philadelphia: Lippincott-Raven.)

TABLE 5-5. Preventive Care Schedule (Recommended time intervals between preventive services)

Preventive Service	Age 50–65+
Blood pressure	1 year (more often if elevated)
Cholesterol	1 year (more often if elevated)
Flexible sigmoidoscopy	3–5 years (more often if at risk)
Fecal occult blood test	1 year
Hearing test	Assess during regular checkups
Vision test, including glaucoma	2–5 years (more often in people who have eye diseases)
Dental exam	6 months
Women Only	
Breast self-exam	Monthly
Mammogram	1–2 years
Pelvic exam	1 year
Pap test	1–3 years
Immunizations	
Tetanus booster	10 years
Influenza immunization	Yearly in autumn (before age 65, only if at high risk)
Pneumococcal immunization	Once (before age 65 if at high risk; booster may be needed after 6 years or longer)

(Adapted from *Guide to Clinical Preventive Services,* U.S. Preventive Services Task Force, 1996.)

DISPLAY 5-5
Healthstyle—a self-test

All of us want good health. But many of us do not know how to be as healthy as possible. Health experts now describe *lifestyle* as one of the most important factors affecting health. In fact, it is estimated that as many as seven of the ten leading causes of death could be reduced through common-sense changes in lifestyle. That's what this brief test, developed by the Public Health Service, is all about. Its purpose is simply to tell you how well you are doing to stay healthy. The behaviors covered in the test are recommended for most Americans. Some of them may not apply to persons with certain chronic diseases or handicaps, or to pregnant women. Such persons may require special instructions from their physicians.

Cigarette Smoking

If you <u>never smoke</u>, enter a score of 10 for this section and go to the next section on *Alcohol and Drugs*.

	Almost Always	Sometimes	Almost Never
1. I avoid smoking cigarettes.	2	1	0
2. I smoke only low tar and nicotine cigarettes *or* I smoke a pipe or cigars.	2	1	0

Smoking Score: _____

Alcohol and Drugs

	Almost Always	Sometimes	Almost Never
1. I avoid drinking alcoholic beverages *or* I drink no more than 1 or 2 drinks a day.	4	1	0
2. I avoid using alcohol or other drugs (especially illegal drugs) as a way of handling stressful situations or the problems in my life.	2	1	0
3. I am careful not to drink alcohol when taking certain medicines (for example, medicine for sleeping, pain, colds, and allergies), or when pregnant.	2	1	0
4. I read and follow the label directions when using prescribed and over-the-counter drugs.	2	1	0

Alcohol and Drugs Score: _____

Eating Habits

	Almost Always	Sometimes	Almost Never
1. I eat a variety of foods each day, such as fruits and vegetables, whole grain breads and cereals, lean meats, dairy products, dry peas and beans, and nuts and seeds.	4	1	0
2. I limit the amount of fat, saturated fat, and cholesterol I eat (including fat on meats, eggs, butter, cream, shortenings, and organ meats such as liver).	2	1	0

DISPLAY 5-5

Healthstyle—a self-test (Continued)

3. I limit the amount of salt I eat by cooking with only small amounts, not adding salt at the table, and avoiding salty snacks. **2 1 0**
4. I avoid eating too much sugar (especially frequent snacks of sticky candy or soft drinks). **2 1 0**

Eating Habits Score: _____

Exercise/Fitness

1. I maintain a desired weight, avoiding overweight and underweight. **3 1 0**
2. I do vigorous exercises for 15–30 minutes at least 3 times a week (examples include running, swimming, brisk walking). **3 1 0**
3. I do exercises that enhance my muscle tone for 15–30 minutes at least 3 times a week (examples include yoga and calisthenics). **2 1 0**
4. I use part of my leisure time participating in individual, family, or team activities that increase my level of fitness (such as gardening, bowling, golf, and baseball). **2 1 0**

Exercise/Fitness Score: _____

Stress Control

1. I have a job or do other work that I enjoy. **2 1 0**
2. I find it easy to relax and express my feelings freely. **2 1 0**
3. I recognize early, and prepare for, events or situations likely to be stressful for me. **2 1 0**
4. I have close friends, relatives, or others whom I can talk to about personal matters and call on for help when needed. **2 1 0**
5. I participate in group activities (such as church and community organizations) or hobbies that I enjoy. **2 1 0**

Stress Control Score: _____

Safety

1. I wear a seat belt while riding in a car. **2 1 0**
2. I avoid driving while under the influence of alcohol and other drugs. **2 1 0**
3. I obey traffic rules and the speed limit when driving. **2 1 0**
4. I am careful when using potentially harmful products or substances (such as household cleaners, poisons, and electrical devices). **2 1 0**
5. I avoid smoking in bed. **2 1 0**

Safety Score: _____

What Your Scores Mean to YOU

Scores of 9 and 10

Excellent! Your answers show that you are aware of the importance of this area to your health. More important, you are putting your knowledge to work for you by practicing good health habits. As long as you continue to do so, this area should not pose a serious

Healthstyle—a self-test (Continued)

health risk. It's likely that you are setting an example for your family and friends to follow. Since you got a very high test score on this part of the test, you may want to consider other areas where your scores indicate room for improvement.

Scores of 6 to 8
Your health practices in this area are good, but there is room for improvement. Look again at the items you answered with a "Sometimes" or "Almost Never." What changes can you make to improve your score? Even a small change can often help you achieve better health.

Scores of 3 to 5
Your health risks are showing! Would you like more information about the risks you are facing and about why it is important for you to change these behaviors? Perhaps you need help in deciding how to make the changes you desire. In either case, help is available.

Scores of 0 to 2
Obviously, you were concerned enough about your health to take the test, but your answers show that you may be taking serious and unnecessary risks with your health. Perhaps you are not aware of the risks and what to do about them. You can easily get the information and help you need to improve, if you wish. The next step is up to you.

YOU Can Start Right Now!

In the test you just completed were numerous suggestions to help you reduce your risk of disease and premature death. Here are some of the most significant:

Avoid cigarettes. Cigarette smoking is the single most important preventable cause of illness and early death. It is especially risky for pregnant women and their unborn babies. Persons who stop smoking reduce their risk of getting heart disease and cancer. So if you're a cigarette smoker, think twice about lighting that next cigarette. If you choose to continue smoking, try decreasing the number of cigarettes you smoke and switching to a low tar and nicotine brand.

Follow sensible drinking habits. Alcohol produces changes in mood and behavior. Most people who drink are able to control their intake of alcohol and to avoid undesired, and often harmful, effects. Heavy, regular use of alcohol can lead to cirrhosis of the liver, a leading cause of death. Also, statistics clearly show that mixing drinking and driving is often the cause of fatal or crippling accidents. So if you drink, do it wisely and in moderation. *Use care in taking drugs.* Today's greater use of drugs—both legal and illegal—is one of our most serious health risks. Even some drugs prescribed by your doctor can be dangerous if taken when drinking alcohol or before driving. Excessive or continued use of tranquilizers (or "pep pills") can cause physical and mental problems. Using or experimenting with illicit drugs such as marijuana, heroin, cocaine, and PCP may lead to a number of damaging effects or even death.

Eat sensibly. Overweight individuals are at greater risk for diabetes, gall-bladder disease, and high blood pressure. So it makes good sense to maintain proper weight. But good eating habits also mean holding down the amount of fat (especially saturated fat), cholesterol, sugar, and salt in your diet. If you must snack, try nibbling on fresh fruits and vegetables. You'll feel better—and look better, too.

DISPLAY 5-5
Healthstyle—a self-test (Continued)

Exercise regularly. Almost everyone can benefit from exercise—and there's some form of exercise almost everyone can do. (If you have any doubt, check first with your doctor.) Usually, as little as 15-30 minutes of vigorous exercise three times a week will help you have a heathier heart, eliminate excess weight, tone up sagging muscles, and sleep better. Think how much difference all these improvements could make in the way you feel!

Learn to handle stress. Stress is a normal part of living; everyone faces it to some degree. The causes of stress can be good or bad, desirable or undesirable (such as a promotion on the job or the loss of a spouse). Properly handled, stress need not be a problem. But unhealthy responses to stress—such as driving too fast or erratically, drinking too much, or prolonged anger or grief—can cause a variety of physical and mental problems. Even on a very busy day, find a few minutes to slow down and relax. Talking over a problem with someone you trust can often help you find a satisfactory solution. Learn to distinguish between things that are "worth fighting about" and things that are less important.

Be safety conscious. Think "safety first" at home, at work, at school, at play, and on the highway. Buckle seat belts and obey traffic rules. Keep poisons and weapons out of the reach of children, and keep emergency numbers by your telephone. When the unexpected happens, you'll be prepared.

Where Do You Go From Here:

Start by asking yourself a few frank questions: *Am I really doing all I can to be as healthy as possible? What steps can I take to feel better? Am I willing to begin now?* If you scored low in one or more *sections* of the test, decide what changes you want to make for improvement. You might pick that aspect of your lifestyle where you feel you have the best chance for success and tackle that one first. Once you have improved your score there, go on to other areas.

If you already have tried to change your health habits (to stop smoking or exercise regularly, for example), don't be discouraged if you haven't yet succeeded. The difficulty you have encountered may be due to influences you've never really thought about—such as advertising—or to a lack of support and encouragement. Understanding these influences is an important step toward changing the way they affect you.

There's help available. In addition to personal actions you can take on your own, there are community programs and groups (such as the YMCA or the local chapter of the American Heart Association) that can assist you and your family to make the changes you want to make. If you want to know more about these groups or about health risks, contact your local health department or the National Health Information Clearinghouse. There's a lot you can do to stay healthy or to improve your health—and there are organizations that can help you. Start a new HEALTHSTYLE today!

For assistance in locating specific information on these and other health topics: write to the National Health Information Clearinghouse.

National Health Information Clearinghouse, P.O. Box 1133, Washington, D.C. 20013

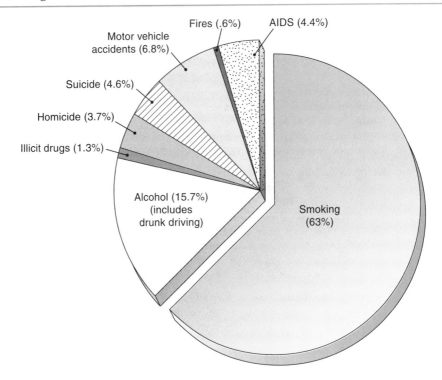

Fires (.6%) AIDS (4.4%)

Motor vehicle
accidents (6.8%)

Suicide (4.6%)

Homicide (3.7%)

Illicit drugs (1.3%)

Alcohol (15.7%)
(includes
drunk driving)

Smoking
(63%)

Number of deaths

Smoking	418,000
Alcohol (including drunk driving)	105,000
Illicit drugs	9,000
Homicide	25,000
Suicide	31,000
Motor vehicle accidents	46,000
Fires	4,000
AIDS	30,000

FIGURE 5-4
Cigarettes kill more Americans than AIDS, alcohol, car accidents, fires, illegal drugs, murders, and suicides combined. Note: All mortality data are for 1990, except alcohol, which is for 1987. (CDC; HIV/AIDS Surveillance Report; National Safety Council Accident Facts; Monthly Vital Statistics Report; SAMMEC; Alcohol-Related Death Index.)

which type of learning is best for that particular client and the subject matter being taught. If health teaching is ineffective, one reason may be that the nurse gave out information he or she thought the client would need without taking the time to assess the client's learning readiness and the learning needs the client considered important. Attention to timing and the learning environment is crucial. Motivation to learn is enhanced by including the client in the planning process.

DISPLAY 5-6
Factors That Affect Readiness to Learn

- Physiologic factors: Age, gender, disease process being treated, intactness of senses (hearing, vision, touch, taste), preexisting conditions
- Psychosocial factors: Sociocultural circumstances, occupation, economic stability, past experiences with learning, attitude toward learning, spirituality, emotional health, self-concept and body image, sense of responsibility for self
- Cognitive factors: Developmental level, level of education, communication skills, primary language, motivation, reading ability, learning style, problem-solving ability
- Environmental factors: Home environment, safety features, family relationships and problems, caregiver (availability, motivation, abilities), other support systems

(Hunt R, Zurek E [1997]. Community-Based Nursing. *Philadelphia: Lippincott-Raven.)*

Types of learning are psychomotor, cognitive, and affective.

Psychomotor learning involves mastering a motor skill (eg, changing a dressing, giving an injection) and is best done with only one person or a small group. The nurse demonstrates the skill, and then the learner practices and gives a return demonstration to ensure that the learning objectives have been mastered.

Cognitive learning involves thinking more than doing. Thinking while reading, discussing, and listening to a lecture are all ways that people learn cognitively. Learning is enhanced by the use of more than one sense, so pictures, charts, and audiovisual materials are beneficial. Some people learn best by writing things down, so clients should be encouraged to take notes if they find that helpful. Because anxiety, fatigue, and distraction block learning to various degrees, it is helpful to offer handout materials to which the client can refer later.

A comfortable atmosphere, free of distractions, promotes learning because it lessens anxiety and makes clients feel free to ask questions. Large groups may be intimidating, so the nurse should be available for one-to-one questions later if the group is large. Sometimes a post-test, presented in a nonthreatening way, is helpful in evaluating if learning has taken place. When working with one or two clients, questions can often be asked in a nonthreatening way. This helps evaluate learning outcomes and determines what needs to be reinforced.

Affective learning, which involves feelings, is the most challenging but the most effective in changing attitudes and behaviors. A classic example is the danger of smoking. Most health professionals who smoke know about the multiple and serious risks of smoking, but they continue to smoke anyway. It is usually an emotional experience, such as the death of a loved one from lung cancer or a plea from their child, that motivates them to take steps to conquer the addiction.

An approach that includes personal experiences, role modeling, and honest discussion is the best way to bring about affective learning and motivate clients to change unhealthy behaviors. Sometimes a crisis presents an opportunity in which the old behavior patterns are no longer adequate and personal changes are needed. To be helpful, the nurse or other health-care provider should be available to give effective guidance at the point of crisis or need. One of the great privileges of the nursing profession is to be involved with clients at points of crisis during their lives when they are most open to change. The nurse must be an active listener to try to understand the client's situation and to communicate empathy and trustworthiness. All nurses must have a good working knowledge of therapeutic communication techniques (Table 5-6).

TABLE 5-6. Therapeutic Communication Guidelines

Methods of Communication	Examples	Explanatory Notes
Approach the client with acceptance and genuine respect.	This is best conveyed by facial expression, tone of voice, posture, and attention to the client's comfort and time constraints. "What concerns you?" "What would you like to talk about?" "Would you like information about . . . ?" "Do you have a plan regarding . . . ?" "What do you think about . . . ?" AVOID: "My advice to you is . . ." "Let me take care of those problems for you." "You shouldn't feel that way." "Being afraid of surgery is silly in this day of high technology." "Don't worry! Everything will be fine!"	Acceptance of the person does not necessarily mean approval of all the behaviors, attitudes, and feelings of the client. It is crucial to distinguish between the person and the behaviors, which may be totally contrary to the nurse's value system. Genuine respect is based on the assumption that each person has value and each person has potential for change. The integrity and the ability of the client to make satisfactory decisions about life, given appropriate help, must be respected. This prevents the pitfalls of giving advice, being glib, attempting to rescue a client, or belittling the client's feelings. Avoidance of clichés and stereotypes is also basic to respect. Statements such as "Don't worry!" do not really reassure. To provide reassurance, be trustworthy and communicate empathy and respect. Also give correct information at the time the client needs it.
Reflect feelings expressed by the client verbally and nonverbally.	"You seem very concerned." "I sense that you are annoyed." "It must be so frightening." "Sounds like you are pretty discouraged." DO NOT SAY: "I understand how you feel." Avoid emotionally charged words until the client uses them—"You must feel so alone" instead of "You feel abandoned." AVOID "You are enraged" (or "depressed") "What a panic you are in!" "You must despise that!" "Are you suicidal?" Instead say: "Do you ever think of hurting yourself?"	Reflections of the client's feelings communicates empathy and builds trust essential to a therapeutic relationship. Reflection seeks to demonstrate understanding of what the client is experiencing. It is rarely appropriate for the nurse to say, "I understand how you feel." Only the client can say, "The nurse understands." The nurse should use gentle terms to assess the degree of feelings initially. Once the client uses a more potent, emotionally charged word, it is appropriate for the nurse to use it. Be aware of cultural and age differences in regard to charged words. For example, elderly American women, often raised to believe that a lady should not get angry, may feel the word "angry" is taboo. People of other cultures, especially Asians, may also be uncomfortable with the word "angry," whereas persons under age 50 raised in the American culture are likely to have no difficulty with it.

(*text continues on p. 137*)

TABLE 5-6. (*Continued*)

Methods of Communication	Examples	Explanatory Notes
Encourage expression of feelings, perceptions, and attitudes by using open-ended questions.	"Tell me about . . ." "What were you feeling (or thinking) when that happened?" "Describe what that was like." "Go on." Wait attentively during periods of silence to give the client time to organize his or her thoughts.	Use of open-ended questions to encourage expression allows the nurse to learn what is important to the client rather than make assumptions based on the nurse's priorities. It also allows the client to verbalize feelings and perceptions and thus begin to identify the cause of vague, inner turmoil and to work on the problem. Even when clients already understand the nature of their problems, the opportunity to ventilate is extremely helpful. 'Talking it out' is a major stress reducer. Persons who talk it out have less need to act it out in socially negative or health-endangering ways.
Focus and structure the discussion.	"Let's get back to what you said about . . ." "Let's see if we can list the reasons . . ." "In exactly what way has . . . been helpful to you?" "Let's try to put things in order of priority." "Go back to the beginning and tell me step by step." "Let's go over the choices you have." "I won't be giving you advice, but if we carefully look at your options together, I think you will have a better sense of what you need to do next." "What happened then?" "Where was that?" "When did you become aware?" "How did that make you feel?" Avoid "Why" questions because they tend to make people feel defensive.	Focusing brings the digressing client back to the main discussion. The nurse should listen for themes, even among the trivia. Similarities and differences in descriptions of events or persons by the client should be pointed out. An over-talkative or aggressively hostile client may present a special challenge. It may be difficult to collect relevant data in a reasonable time unless the nurse firmly focuses on one idea at a time. Remember that all behavior has meaning. Try to determine the reason for the over-talkativeness or hostility to reduce or diffuse it. Courteously interrupt with verbal and nonverbal cues when the discussion persistently wanders. Anxiety may make it difficult for the client to focus on a particular topic for any length of time, and persistence with that topic by the nurse may impede communication, so the nurse must proceed courteously. Recognize that some clients use symbolic language or vague generalities to discuss anxiety-laden information. Try to help the client organize what is being said. Often a client has no idea where to begin to deal with the problems, especially if a number of unmet needs exist. Closed-end questions, worded so that they can be answered with one or two words, are sometimes appropriate in structuring the discussion or filling gaps in the data. Help the client delineate the collaborative role of the nurse and the active participation and basic responsibility of self in his or her own care.

TABLE 5-6. (*Continued*)

Methods of Communication	Examples	Explanatory Notes
Restate to clarify, validate, or confront inconsistencies.	"Am I clear that you said . . . ?" "Could you go over that again?" "Let's see if I have that right. You said . . ." "In other words, you want to . . ." "Did you really mean . . . when you said . . . ?" "What about . . . ?" "You said . . . but now you are saying . . . ?" "Let's see. You did . . . but you say . . . I don't understand." "You were smiling when you said you are so discouraged. How come?" "Do you really believe that?"	Restatement conveys a strong message that what the client says is important, and it conveys empathy. State the implied when the patient makes vague hints. Clarification helps both the nurse and the client understand what has been communicated in greater depth. Voicing doubts and using gentle confrontation to point out inconsistencies promotes realistic thinking in greater depth.
Provide feedback, interpretation, and summary.	"I have the feeling that talking about . . . makes you uncomfortable. Am I right?" "I notice that whenever I mention . . . you change the subject. Is there a reason for this that you would like to talk about?" "Let's explore alternatives." "It sounds like you really want to do . . . Am I correct?" "I would like to review what I think I heard you say. Please correct me if I'm wrong." "Let me summarize what has been said and tell you how I see what is going on in your life." "Here is some information about . . . and a list of resources." "We agreed that you would first do . . . and then contact . . . Am I correct?" "It looks like we've identified the major problems facing you and we talked about how you might begin to tackle them. Do you have any questions?" "It seems to me that some progress has been made today. What do you think?"	Feedback should be descriptive and focus on concrete behaviors. It should not be judgmental. Alternatives should be explored, but giving advice should be avoided. The client should be continually encouraged to give the nurse feedback. Summarizing emphasizes major points, highlights progress, confirms consensual validation, and reinforces important information. It may be in written as well as verbal form. A plan for problem solving is mutually agreed on and a sense of closure is provided.

(Adapted from Stackhouse J [1997]. Facilitative verbal responses. In Leasia S, Monohan F. *A Practical Guide for Health Assessment.* Philadelphia: WB Saunders.)

A warm, accepting approach facilitates learning. The teacher should be well prepared, because a disorganized teacher is distracting. Good preparation enables a more relaxed presentation. In addition to therapeutic communication techniques, other good educational strategies include the use of examples and humor. Role modeling is equally valuable; for instance, the client is unlikely to take seriously a nurse's teaching about the need to stop smoking if the nurse is seen smoking or smells of tobacco. Teaching–learning principles are shown in Table 5-7.

Client–nurse contracts are valuable tools for behavioral change (Fig. 5-5, Displays 5-7 and 5-8). Client motivation and compliance are complex issues affected by many variables. One major factor is the client's sense of self-efficacy, mentioned earlier in this chapter. A trusting nurse–client relationship and partnership in goal setting are key factors.

The client must understand the prescribed care regimen and how it relates to preventing or treating the health problem. Once the plan and the contract, whether an informal or a formally written contract, are established, the nurse is responsible for keeping the contract agreement and helping the client make the desired behavioral changes. This can be challenging if the undesired behaviors have been longstanding (Humphrey & Milone-Nuzzo, 1996). In Chapter 4, the Clinical Application section dis-

TABLE 5-7. Principles for Maximizing the Teaching–Learning Process

Teaching Principles	Learning Principles
1. Adapt teaching to clients' level of readiness.	1. The learning process makes use of clients' experience and is geared to their level of understanding.
2. Determine clients' perceptions about the subject matter before and during teaching.	2. Clients are given the opportunity to provide frequent feedback on their understanding of the material taught.
3. Create an environment conducive to learning.	3. The environment for learning is physically comfortable, offers an atmosphere of mutual helpfulness, trust, respect, and acceptance, and allows free expression of ideas.
4. Involve clients throughout the learning process.	4. Clients actively participate. They assess their needs, establish goals, and evaluate learning progress.
5. Make subject matter relevant to clients' interest and use.	5. Clients feel motivated to learn.
6. Ensure client satisfaction during the teaching–learning process.	6. Clients sense progress toward their goals.
7. Provide opportunities for clients to apply material taught.	7. Clients integrate the learning through application.

(Spradley B, Allender J [1996]. *Community Health Nursing*. Philadelphia: Lippincott-Raven.)

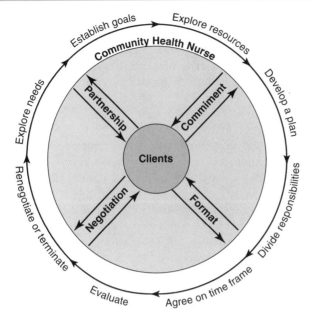

FIGURE 5-5
The concept and process of contracting. Contracting is based on four distinctive features shown here as spokes that support a wheel. These features form the basis for a reciprocal relationship between nurse and clients. This relationship is not static; it is a dynamic process that moves through phases, represented here as the outer rim of the wheel. The relationship moves forward, focused on meeting clients' needs, and enables the nurse to facilitate ultimate achievement of clients' goals. (Spradley BW, Allender JA [1996]. *Community Health Nursing Concepts and Practice.* 4th ed. Philadelphia: Lippincott-Raven.)

cussed an informal contract that a nurse made with Sherry, a woman who was afraid she might physically abuse her children.

Sometimes clients need to become disturbed and concerned about a particular health risk to be willing to change and ready to learn what to do about it. Changing behavior is not easy. The nurse may need to give upsetting information, but it should be delivered with an optimistic attitude that learning and behavior change are possible. One example might be teaching sexually active teenagers to practice safe sex to prevent pregnancy, AIDS, and other sexually transmitted diseases.

DISPLAY 5-7
Learning Contract

Steve Hunt agrees to monitor his blood sugar by using the One Touch montor at 8:00 AM and 6:00 PM for 1 week from June 1 through June 8, 1997. If this contract is not abided by, Best Home Healthcare will discharge Steve Hunt back to Dr. Berger of Neighborhood Clinics. This discharge relieves Best Home Healthcare from any further responsibility for the care of Steve Hunt.

Signed _____

Date _____

Signed by Case Manager _____

Date _____

(Hunt R, E Zurek [1997]. Community-Based Nursing. *Philadelphia: Lippincott-Raven.)*

DISPLAY 5-8
Interventions Used With the Noncompliant Client

* Establish a trusting relationship
* Contract at each visit
* Identify the etiology of the noncompliance
* Use a learning contract for specific problems

(Hunt R, Zurek, E [1997]. Community-Based Nursing. *Philadelphia: Lippincott-Raven.)*

The best teaching in the world is not effective if learning has not taken place. Health teaching is never complete until evaluation of the learning objectives demonstrates positive outcomes. Never assume that learning has taken place just because information has been given. It can be humbling to see how little learning has actually occurred sometimes. Learning is seldom accomplished in one session and requires constant reinforcement presented in many ways using the strategies described above. See Chapter 14 for more about client teaching.

Nursing Assessments

The value of a good nursing assessment cannot be overstated; it is the foundation for appropriate action. Without good assessment skills, a nurse may be "scratching where there is no itch." Physical assessments and nursing histories are what nurses usually mean when they talk about assessment, but the needs are much broader. Assessment skills needed by community health nurses are shown in Display 5-9. A women's health

---

DISPLAY 5-9
Assessment Skills Needed by the Community Based Nurse

Interview skills and the ability to listen and formulate appropriate questions help to establish rapport with the client and family.

Interpretation skills allow the nurse to understand what clients mean regarding their concerns.

Nonverbal communication skills permit a nurse to recognize subtle responses that may reflect the client's moods, attitudes, and psychosocial needs.

Relationship and sensitivity skills cut across social, cultural, and lifestyle barriers to promote a climate of trust.

Observational skills allow a nurse to recognize normal and abnormal responses.

Goal-setting skills help a nurse to see beyond immediate needs and identify continuing and long-term goals for care.

(Hunt R, Zurek E [1997]. Community-Based Nursing. *Philadelphia: Lippincott-Raven.)*

DISPLAY 5-10
Nutrition Assessment Guide

When interviewing or assessing your client, you will want to learn about nutritional behaviors, beliefs, and patterns. The following questions will assist you in obtaining information that can influence your client's health and recovery and your care.

Ask the client or family the following questions:

1. What does food and eating mean to you?
2. With whom do you usually eat your meals? What type of food do you eat? Describe what you eat on a typical day. When do you eat?
3. What do you define as food? What do you believe makes up a healthy diet versus an unhealthy diet? Are you able to obtain the foods necessary for a healthy diet? If not, how do you think that can be remedied?
4. Who shops for food? What kind of stores do you shop at? Who prepares the meals?
5. How are foods prepared at your home (length of time cooked, type of cooking, oils and seasonings)?
6. Have you chosen a particular nutritional practice such as vegetarianism or alcohol free?
7. Do religious beliefs and practices influence your diet? Do you abstain from certain foods at regular intervals or at specific times determined by religious dates?
8. Do you "fast"? What does "fasting" mean to you (define what you do and don't eat)? How long do you fast? How often?

(Hunt R, Zurek E [1997]. Community-Based Nursing, Philadelphia: Lippincott-Raven.)

clinic history form is shown in Chapter 6, Display 6-3. A nutrition assessment guide is shown in Display 5-10, and Display 5-11 presents a spiritual assessment guide.

THE NURSE SPEAKS . . .
About a Wellness Education Course

I am a wellness program supervisor for a hospital, and "What to Do With Your Infant or Child Until Help Arrives" is one of my most successful programs. It lasts about 2 hours and is free to the public. I offer the course four to six times a year to 10 to 15 attendees, such as mothers, fathers, grandparents, pregnant women, and older babysitters. My program calendar is published each month in the newspaper and posted around the community, but it seems that most people come because they hear about it by word of mouth.

I've established five learning objectives in terms of behaviors that the learner can do on completion of the program:

1. State when and how to notify emergency medical services.
2. Discuss basic infection control and prevention measures.
3. Repeat the purpose of the Good Samaritan laws.
4. Discuss initial steps to be taken when an infant or child has the following emergencies: respiratory or cardiac arrest; breathing difficulties; sudden infant death syndrome; fever; seizures;

DISPLAY 5-11
Some Questions to Help Assess the Client's Spirituality

1. Would you like to talk about spiritual things?
2. Is spirituality important in your life?
3. What does the term "spirituality" mean to you?
4. What is your faith tradition?
5. Is worship important to you?
6. Do you participate in any religious activities?
7. Do you believe in the power of prayer?
8. What is your method of prayer or meditation?
9. Does your faith play a role in your health or illness?
10. How has your illness influenced your faith?
11. What brings you inner peace and joy?
12. Do you believe each life has meaning and purpose?
13. What do you think is the purpose of your life?
14. How does your illness or health affect your life purpose?

---

poisoning; bleeding; shock; burns; fractures; impaled objects; teeth knocked out; bites and stings; head or spinal injuries; heat- or cold-related injuries.

5. State general safety rules.

I use a lecture and demonstration format with questions and answers and discussion as we go along. I find it helpful to use transparencies I have made; these enhance learning by visualization. I also use handouts to refer to later at home. These enable the learners to listen intently without having to take notes. I give them a slide card of information and a little folding card to carry in their wallets.

The response to this course has been wonderful, and there seems to be an ongoing need to offer this class to the public. The feedback I get is so positive. People have taken the trouble to call me, even much later, to describe situations in which they used what they learned in my class. This is one of the reasons I love this work so much!

Elaine
WELLNESS PROGRAM SUPERVISOR

CLINICAL APPLICATION

A Critical Thinking Case Study About a Client in a Senior Wellness Program

You are a nurse volunteering every Tuesday in a senior center wellness program. While doing hypertension screening one day, you read a blood pressure of 212/120 mm Hg on Florence, age 72. She tells you that she has never had high blood pressure and takes no medications.

and Think!

- Should you do anything about this?
- If so, what and why?

Florence tells you to call her daughter when you instruct her to see a doctor imme-diately. Her daughter readily agrees to take Florence to see her doctor in a week or so, explaining that her own daughter is getting married on Saturday and the family is extremely busy just now. You take a deep breath and instruct the daughter about the serious risk that Florence may have a stroke with such high blood pressure. You strongly urge her to get medical attention for Florence immediately. With undis-guised irritation, the daughter agrees to do so.

The following Tuesday, you see Florence at the senior center again. You take her blood pressure and get the same dangerously high reading. Florence reports that she did indeed see her doctor, who has been treating her since she was a young woman. "He told me my pressure is fine and I don't need medicine. My daughter is furious with you!"

 and Think!

- Now what should you do?

A while later you check Florence's other arm using different equipment. The clear reading is 210/118 mm Hg. Later that day you check it again with the same results. You remember that there has been a slight change in tone at some of the lower read-ings. You decide to ask a nurse friend who lives nearby to come and check it for you. Your friend assures you that your readings seem correct. Efforts to reach Flor-ence's physician are unsuccessful.

 and Think!

- Can you do anything?
- Should you do anything?

You call the daughter again, and she immediately tells you how much you are com-plicating her life at the time of the wedding. You explain that the blood pressure is still very high. She replies, "Well, he's the doctor and he says it's fine!" and hangs up the phone.

You say to yourself, "If only I knew an M.D. nearby who could check Florence to satisfy her daughter." You speak to the senior center director, who says that this would be very difficult to accomplish, but she will see what she can do. Just then the daughter calls back, saying she has reconsidered and decided you might be right. She explains that Florence's doctor is very elderly. He sees few patients these days and may be a little hard of hearing. She adds that she has doubted his judgment and current knowledge a few times, but Florence is very loyal and wants to stay with him. The daughter takes Florence to another physician, who confirms your hypertensive readings and starts her on treatment.

Poor Florence is terribly confused and upset by all of this and continues to need a great deal of attention and support from you, but you may well have prevented a stroke.

Chapter SUMMARY

Most of the factors that determine health are related to lifestyle choices. Total wellness embraces social, mental, emotional, spiritual, and physical factors, all of which are interrelated. Encouraging clients to take responsibility for their own well-being includes building a sense of self-efficacy and an internal locus of control.

In 1990, the U.S. Public Health Service launched an ambitious program of goals to improve the wellness of the nation, *Healthy People 2000*. All segments of the population were asked to participate in establishing relevant goals; some states also set specific goals for their particular population. In 1996, a midcourse review was published, outlining the degree of achievement at midpoint. Obesity, a major American problem, continues to increase because of our increasingly sedentary lifestyle. Health promotion and disease prevention activities by community health nurses include screening and case finding, health fairs, health risk appraisals, and client teaching.

Community health nurses are heavily involved in health teaching. This may be done on an individual, family, aggregate, or community level. Assessment of learning readiness is crucial. The three types of learning are psychomotor, cognitive, and affective. Nurse-client contracts are a valuable tool to help achieve desired behavioral change. Sometimes clients need to become concerned or disturbed before becoming motivated enough to change. Good teaching is meaningless if learning has not taken place.

The value of good nursing assessments cannot be overstated. Such assessments must be holistic, including a physical, mental, and nutritional assessment. To be thorough, spiritual, cultural, and family assessment is important also. Sometimes a community assessment is also required to understand the client as part of a community, especially if he or she is from another culture.

A list of references and additional readings for this chapter appears at the end of Part 2.

6

Health Department and Hospital Wellness Programs

Key Terms

AIDS dementia

bacillus Calmette-Guérin

chlamydia

colposcopy

cryosurgery

early periodic screening diagnosis and treatment program (EPSDT)

ELISA test

endogenous reactivation

ethambutol (EMB)

exogenous infection

hepatitis A, B, C virus (HAV, HBV, HCV)

HIV/AIDS

human papillomavirus (HPV)

infant health assessment program

isoniazid (INH)

Kaposi's sarcoma

La Leche League

Lamaze program

latent infection

Occupational Safety & Health Administration (OSHA)

opportunistic infections

outreach workers

particulate respirator mask

partner notification program

PPD (Mantoux)

public health nurse

pyrazinamide

rifampin (RIF)

sexually transmitted disease (STD)

shared air

test-of-cure

Western blot test

Learning Objectives

1. Identify the primary focus and role of health departments.

2. Compare health promotion and disease prevention activities and give examples of each.

3. Compare the titles public health nurse and registered nurse.

4. List the steps of a well-child assessment.

5. Describe how tuberculosis is acquired, diagnosed, treated, and controlled.

6. List common sexually transmitted diseases and their specific treatments. Describe control programs of health departments.

7. Identify the diseases that require mandatory reporting by health-care providers.

8. Describe hospital wellness programs.

Health Departments

Public health functions are the activities that lay the groundwork for healthful communities. Safeguarding the wellness of communities is basically the role of the local health department, as delegated by the state health department. Each state must provide health promotion and disease prevention services through some form of state health department. States vary in the number and degree of services provided. In some sparsely populated states, local health departments do not exist. Some cities have their own health departments (Fig. 6-1). The focus of health departments is the community as client.

Health promotion services include maternal-child health programs and health education. Disease prevention programs include infectious disease control and immunizations.

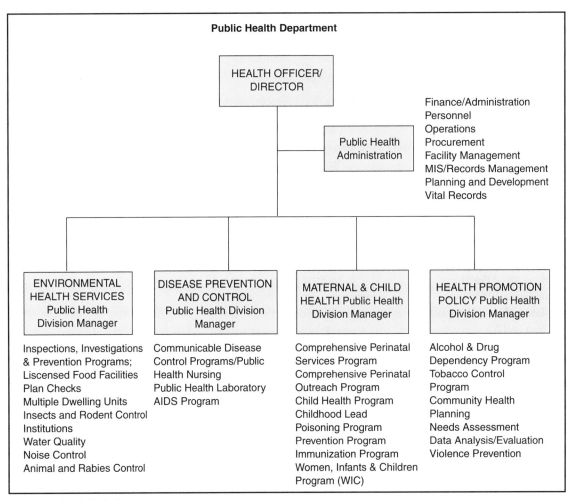

FIGURE 6-1
Some cities have their own health departments, as shown in this diagram of a public health department.

In addition to these wellness services, local health departments fill gaps in personal care services to treat illnesses. This is done when needed services are not provided elsewhere in the community. Personal care might include various ambulatory clinic services (see Chap. 9) or even home care services (see Chaps. 13 through 16). In this case, the person or the family is the client. Local health departments with such comprehensive services are called mixed or combination agencies. Many registered nurses are employed in these programs. Environmental health services are also run by health departments. The health of the community as client is safeguarded by the inspection of restaurants and housing and by the monitoring of swimming pools, lakes, and other potential sources of water pollution. Vector control and air quality also come under their jurisdiction.

The term "public health nurse" is applied to a nurse who works for a health department where the community is the client (Table 6-1). These nurses must complete a state-approved course in public health nursing or have a public health nursing certificate from the state where they practice. Some states require a baccalaureate degree, but some states only require a public health nursing certificate. Some health departments hire experienced registered nurses to work under the supervision of public health nurses until they complete a state-sponsored certification course or a baccalaureate degree with a state-approved course in public health nursing.

Maternal-Child Health Activities

Local health departments provide *prenatal programs* if local obstetricians do not accept Medicaid clients or there are other gaps in prenatal services. Many of the pregnant

TABLE 6-1. Examples of Public Health Nursing Functions

Primary Prevention	Secondary Prevention	Tertiary Prevention
Immunizations	Health screening and referral	Case management for the disabled
Women's health clinics	Case finding for children with disabilities and developmental delays	Home health care
Prenatal clinics		Geriatric evaluations regarding institutional placement
Health education for health promotion	Communicable disease contact investigation	Adult day-care programs
Case finding for communicable diseases	Sexually transmitted disease clinics	Case management for frail elderly persons
Case finding for those at risk for addictions	General medical clinics	
Parental guidance	Tuberculosis clinics	
Home visits for pregnant or new parents or frail elderly persons	Clinics for the homeless	
Safety and environmental education		
School health promotion		
Occupational health promotion		
Wellness classes on diet and exercise		

(Adapted from Smith, CM, 1995)

DISPLAY 6-1
Ten Essential Public Health Services to Promote Maternal and Child Health (MCH)

1. Assess the status of MCH at the local, state, and national levels so problems can be identified and addressed.
2. Diagnose and investigate the occurrence of community health problems and health hazards that affect women, children, youth, and families.
3. Inform and educate the public and families regarding MCH to promote positive health beliefs, attitudes, and behaviors.
4. Mobilize community partnerships between policymakers, health-care providers, and the public to identify and implement solutions to MCH problems.
5. Work with the community to assess the relative importance of MCH needs based on scientific, economic, and political factors and provide leadership for planning and policy development to address priority needs.
6. Promote and enforce laws, regulations, standards, and contracts that protect the health and safety of women, children, and youth and that ensure public accountability for their well-being.
7. Link women, children, youth, and families to needed population-based, personal health and other community and family support services and ensure availability and accessibility by enhancing system capacity, including directly supporting services when necessary.
8. Ensure the capacity and competency of the public health and personal health workforce to address MCH needs effectively.
9. Evaluate the effectiveness, accessibility, and quality of health and population-based MCH services.
10. Conduct research and support demonstrations to gain new insights and solutions to MCH-related problems.

(Excerpted from Public MCH Program Functions: Essential Public Health Services to Promote Maternal and Child Health in America, July 1995.)

---

women participating in these programs are high-risk cases (eg, poverty, teenage pregnancy, HIV infection, drug addiction) (Display 6-1). Many participants are immigrants who come from a different culture and speak a different language. If the clients are not eligible for Medicaid, a fee is charged based on ability to pay. The clinic staff includes prenatal nurses and social workers as well as obstetricians; a nutritionist and an HIV counselor are usually present. Follow-up home visits are made by nurses or social workers as needed.

Some local health departments have received special infant health assessment program grants that provide intensive follow-up care for premature or multiple births and teenage mothers. Usually contracts are made with local hospitals for delivery and postpartum care. Because many hospitals now discharge new mothers 1 or 2 days after delivery, or 3 days after a cesarean section, postpartum home visits are very important.

This is particularly true for a high-risk population whose home environment may be far less than ideal. Follow-up of the babies in well-child clinics is strongly encouraged if the infant has no pediatrician (see Clinical Application case study in Chap. 1).

Programs that use community health nurses to make home maternal-child visits are highly beneficial. Oregon has found nursing visits to new mothers invaluable in improving the status of high-risk children. As Gelfand and colleagues stated in a 1995 article about the effect of maternal depression on children:

> One type of service that holds great promise is home visits by a nurse. Nurses can coach mothers on how to interact with their children, help them with other problems, and help family members recognize their needs. Our research shows that such visits improve both the mother's depressive symptoms and her infant's emotional attachment. (Gelfand D, et al, 1995)

Free *well-child clinics* are provided at various neighborhood locations to make them as accessible as possible to poor people who do no have transportation. Immunizations and routine physical examinations are provided, along with health teaching about child care and developmental milestones. Table 6-2 lists the childhood immunization schedule. Follow-up home visits are often indicated if some risk factor or potential problem is noted. The clinical application case study in Chapter 4 was based on such a situation. Nurses strive to develop a trusting, supportive relationship with mothers so that they will feel free to ask questions and seek help. This may not be easy to achieve if there are indications of illegal drug use, potential neglect, or an unsavory environment. Sometimes nurses must keep their primary goal in mind and be willing to accept certain factors in their clients' lives as long as the child is not being harmed or neglected.

The Medicaid-sponsored early periodic screening diagnosis and treatment program (EPSDT) provides physical examinations, health histories, screening tests, nutritional assessments, immunizations, guidance, and teaching at specific intervals from birth to 18 years of age. Special child rehabilitation programs exist for children who are not necessarily on Medicaid but who have expensive chronic conditions or malformations. For example, the children's cardiac rehabilitation program provides funds for pediatric cardiac specialists, surgeons, and extra nursing and social work services as needed for a child up to age 21. More about children with disabilities is found in Chapters 11 and 15.

Communicable Disease Control

Communicable disease control is a major responsibility of local health departments. The disease surveillance functions of the Centers for Disease Control & Prevention (CDC) were discussed in Chapter 4. Local and state health departments play a critical role in disease surveillance and epidemiologic control. The CDC funds some state and local health departments in their case-finding efforts for contacts of sexually transmitted diseases (STDs), wherever local laws permit these investigations. Funds for childhood immunization programs are also allocated to local and state health departments.

Some state health departments are more powerful than others and have a great deal of regulatory authority within their state. Many people think too much regulatory authority is not only costly but actually inhibits the efficient delivery of good health

TABLE 6-2. Childhood Immunization Update

Because many teenagers and young adults continue to suffer diseases that can be prevented with proper vaccination, the Advisory Committee on Immunization Practices, the American Academy of Pediatrics, the American Academy of Family Physicians, and the American Medical Association have issued immunization guidelines that include adolescents, too. Here's the new schedule.

Vaccine	Birth	1 month	2 months	4 months	6 months	12 months	15 months	18 months	4-6 years	11-12 years	14-16 years
Hepatitis B[1]	Hepatitis B-1	Hepatitis B-2			Hepatitis B-3					Hep B	
Diphtheria and tetanus toxoids and acellular pertussis[2]			DTaP or DTP	DTaP or DTP	DTaP or DTP		DTaP or DTP		DTaP or DTP	Td	
Haemophilus influenzae type b[3]			Hib	Hib	Hib	Hib					
Poliovirus[4]			Polio	Polio		Polio			Polio		
Measles, mumps, and rubella[5]						MMR	MMR		MMR or MMR		
Varicella virus[6]						Var				Var	

Range of acceptable ages for vaccination

"Catch-up" vaccination

1. Infants born to mothers who are hepatitis B surface antigen (HBsAg)-negative should receive the first dose (Hep B-1) of 2.5 mcg of Recombivax HB (Merck & Co.) or 10 mcg of Engerix-B (SmithKline Beecham). The second dose should be administered one month after the first dose. Infants born to HBsAg-positive mothers should receive 0.5 ml hepatitis B immune globulin (HBIG) within 12 hours of birth and either 5 mcg of Recombivax HB or 10 mcg of Engerix-B at a separate site. Infants born to mothers whose HBsAg status is unknown should receiver either 5 mcg of Recombivax HB or 10 mcg of Engerix-B within 12 hours of birth. Blood should be drawn at the time of delivery to determine the mother's HBsAg status. If it's positive, the infant should receive HBIG as soon as possible but no later than one week of age. Adolescents who have not received three doses of this vaccine should initiate or complete the series at age 11-12 years. The second dose should be administered at least one month after the first dose. The third dose should be administered at least four months after the first dose and at least two months after the second dose.

2. DTaP is the preferred vaccine for all doses in the vaccination series, including completion of the series in children who have previously received DTP vaccine. Whole-cell DTP is an acceptable alternative to DTaP. The fourth dose of DTaP may be administered at age 12 months if at least six months have elapsed since the third dose. Tetanus and diphtheria toxoids (Td), absorbed, is recommended at age 11-12 years if at least five years have elapsed since the last dose of DTP, DT, or DTaP. Subsequent routine Td boosters are recommended every 10 years.

3. Dose at six months is not required. After completing the primary series, vaccine can be used as a booster.

4. Inactivated poliovirus vaccine (IPV) is recommended at ages two and four months and oral poliovirus vaccine (OPV) is recommended at ages 12-18 months and 4-6 years. Other possible schedules are: IPV—at ages two, four, 12-18 months, and 4-6 years, or OPV—at ages two, four, 6-18 months, and 4-6 years. IPV is routinely recommended for immunocompromised patients and their household contacts.

5. The second dose of MMR may be administered at least one month after the first one.

6. Varicella virus vaccine can be administered to susceptible children and adolescents at any time after they reach 12 months. Adolescents, who were not vaccinated and don't know whether they had chickenpox, should be vaccinated at age 11-12 years.

(CDC [1997]. Recommended childhood immunization schedule-United States, 1997. MMWR 46(2), 35.)

care because of the amount of time needed to do the paperwork required. Other people insist that more government regulation will improve the quality of service provided.

Core Public Health Functions

Three core public health functions are population-wide, with the community as the client (Display 6-2, Table 6-3, Fig. 6-2):

1. Assessment (health status monitoring and disease surveillance)
2. Policy development (leadership, policy, planning, and administration)
3. Assurance (protection of the community's environment, workplaces, housing, food, and water; health education in the community, targeted outreach, community mobilization for health-related issues, health services quality assurance and accountability, laboratory services, investigation and control of diseases and injuries, training of public health officials).

In addition to the core public health functions are the following personal services that focus on the needs of individuals:

- Primary care for unserved or underserved persons
- Treatment services for targeted conditions (eg, AIDS, drug and alcohol abuse, mental illness)
- Preventive services (eg, immunizations, the Women, Infants, and Children program, women's health services [Display 6-3], family planning, and STD programs).

DISPLAY 6-2
Lead Poisoning Control

- Beware of leaded paint in houses built before 1978.
- Lead pipes may carry water into homes.
- Soil near roads may be contaminated from exhaust fumes before leaded gas was outlawed.

WHAT TO DO?

- Test children under 6 annually for lead poisoning.
- Diets rich in iron and calcium help protect children.
- Wash hands before meals and at bedtime.
- Let water run from the tap for a few moments (use it for watering plants). Boiling water does not remove iron.
- Even if the original paint has been repainted many times, dust from remodeling can be harmful. Keep nonworkers, children, pregnant women, and pets out of the area. Do not use a sander or open flame to remove flaking paint; instead, scrape it.
- Damp-mop weekly to reduce dust in the home.

(National Lead Information Center, 1-800-LEAD-FYI)

(text continues on p. 156)

TABLE 6-3. Environmental Health Programs within Local Health Departments

Categories of Environmental Concern	Programs	Program Purpose
Air	Air quality management	To ensure a community air resource conducive to good health that will not injure plant or animal life or property and that will be esthetically desirable
Water	Water supply sanitation	To ensure the provision of safe public and private water supplies, adequate in quantity and quality for every person
	Water pollution control	To ensure the cooperation with state water pollution control agencies and to ensure that surface and subsurface water supplies meet all state and local standards and regulations for water quality
Waste	Solid waste management	To ensure that all solid wastes are stored, collected, transported, and disposed of in a manner that does not create health, safety, or esthetic problems
	Liquid waste management	To ensure that liquid wastes are treated in such a manner as to prevent problems of sanitation, public health nuisances, or pollution
	Toxic and hazardous waste management	To ensure that toxic and hazardous wastes are stored, collected, transported, and disposed of in a manner that does not create health or safety problems
Food	Food protection	To ensure that all people are adequately protected from unhealthful or unsafe food or food products. This necessitates a comprehensive food protection program covering every facility where food or food products are stored, transported, processed, packaged, served, or sold, and regulating sanitation, wholesomeness, adulteration, advertising, labeling weights and measures, and fill-of-containers
Recreational areas	Swimming pool sanitation and safety	To ensure the safety and sanitation of public, semipublic, and private swimming pools
	Recreational sanitation	To ensure that all public recreational areas are operated so as to prevent health and safety problems
Product safety	Consumer product safety	To ensure that all people are protected from the unhealthful or unsafe substances or products in the home, business, and industry
Radiation	Radiation control	To prevent unnecessary or hazardous radiation exposure from the transportation, use, or disposal of all types of radiation-producing devices and products
Occupational	Occupational health and safety	To ensure, in cooperation with state officials, the health and safety of workers in places of employment, by controlling relevant environmental factors
Vectors	Vector control	To control insects, rodents, and other animals that adversely affect health, safety, or comfort
Noise	Noise pollution control	To prevent hazardous or annoying noise levels in residential, business, industrial, and recreational structures and areas
Accidents	Environmental injury prevention	To influence or regulate planning, design, and construction in such a manner as to reduce the possibility of accidents through proper management of the environment
Buildings	Housing sanitation, safety, and rehabilitation	To ensure programs that will provide decent, safe, and healthy housing for all people
	Institutional sanitation, safety, and rehabilitation	To ensure that institutions such as hospitals, schools, nurseries, jails, and prisons are operated so as to prevent sanitation and safety problems

Modified from American Public Health Association: Position paper on the role of official local health agencies, *Am J Public Health* 65:189–203, 1975; and USDHHS: *Evaluating the environmental health workforce (HRP#0907160)*, Rockville, Md., 1988, USDHHS, p. 3.)

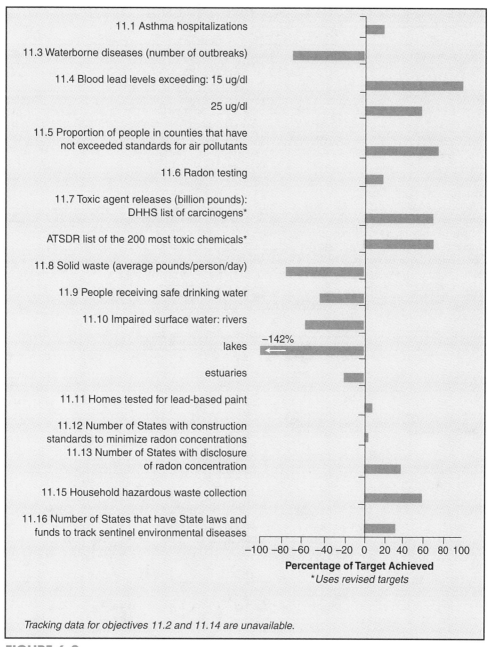

FIGURE 6-2

1995 status of environmental health objectives (*Healthy People 2000*) (see Display 4-4).

Women's Health Service Self Medical History

Name: _____ Date: _____

Please fill out the following form as accurately as you can so that we can help you decide the best method of birth control for you at this time. All information will be kept strictly confidential.

Menstrual History:

First day of last period _____ Was this period normal? _____ Age of first period _____ Are your periods regular? _____ Do you have your period regularly? _____ Do you ever skip a month or have it early? _____ How many days does your period last? _____ Do you have cramps? _____ How many tampons or pads a day are needed? _____ Have you ever noticed vaginal bleeding that is not your period? _____

Intercourse and Birth Control:

Are you having sex now? _____ How frequently? _____

Is your sex experience satisfactory _____ Do you have pain or bleeding during or after intercourse _____

Have you had unprotected intercourse since your last period? _____

What method of birth control are you using now? _____

What method of birth control do you want today? _____

What methods of birth control have you used in the past and have you ever had any problems with them?

_____ Withdrawal _____	_____ Birth control pills	_____
_____ Diaphragm _____	_____ Vaginal foam or film	_____
_____ Condoms _____	_____ Vaginal suppositories	_____
_____ IUD _____	_____ Fertility awareness (rhythm) _____	
_____ Sponge _____	_____ Norplant	_____
	_____ DMPA injections	_____

Do you have any questions regarding birth control methods or the pelvic exam, intercourse, or sexual concerns?

_____

Pregnancy History:

Have you ever been pregnant? _____ How many births? _____ , miscarriages? _____ , abortions? _____ , tubal pregnancies? _____ or cesarean sections? _____ .

Have you had any problems with diabetes _____ , high blood pressure _____ , toxemia _____ , or any other complication? _____

Life Patterns:

Do you smoke? _____ Do you have any problems with weight control? _____

Do you drink milk or eat dairy products on a regular basis? _____

Do you eat red meat, cold cuts, cheese, oils, butter? _____

How often? _____

Do you take vitamins? _____ Do you drink regular coffee? _____ How many cups a day? _____ Do you drink alcohol? _____ How often? _____

Do you have any problems with avoiding cocaine, crack, marijuana, or other substances? _____

Do you need help in this area? _____

Do you ever examine your breasts? _____

Medical History:

Do you have a private physician? _____ Physician's name _____

Are you currently under care for any condition? _____ What is this condition? _____

Date of last doctor visit _____

Have you had any serious illnesses? _____

DISPLAY 6-3 (*Continued*)

Are you abused or treated violently by anyone in your life? _____

Have you had any surgery? _____

List dates for any hospitalization _____

Do you take any medications? _____

List all prescriptions or over-the-counter medications:

_____

Date of your last Pap smear _____ Have you ever had an abnormal Pap? _____ If so, when? _____

Have you had a colposcopy or treatment for an abnormal Pap? _____ If so, when? _____

Check if you have ever had any of the following:

_____ Cancer

_____ Diabetes

_____ Heart disease

_____ Chest pain

_____ Shortness of breath

_____ Coughing spells

_____ Asthma

_____ Rheumatic fever

_____ Dizzy spells or fainting

_____ High blood pressure

_____ Stroke

_____ Frequent headaches

_____ Migraine headaches

_____ Swelling or pain in legs

_____ Blood clot in legs

_____ Varicose veins

_____ Low blood or anemia

_____ Sickle cell anemia or trait

_____ Epilepsy/seizures or fits

_____ Depression

_____ Blurred vision

_____ Frequent indigestion

_____ High Cholesterol

_____ Gallbladder disease

_____ Hepatitis

_____ Mononucleosis

_____ Thyroid

_____ Urinary tract Infection

_____ Kidney problems

_____ Breast pain

_____ Cysts

_____ Nipple discharge

_____ Vaginal infection

_____ Chlamydia

_____ Gonorrhea

_____ Trichomoniasis

_____ Genital warts

_____ Genital herpes

_____ Syphilis

_____ HIV

_____ Tuberculosis

Have you had your German measles vaccine? _____

Family Medical History:

Are your parents, sisters, and brothers alive and well? _____ If not, please explain _____

Do you know the health histories of both sides of your family? _____

Do you know if there are any hereditary diseases? _____

Did your mother take hormones (DES) when she was pregnant with you? _____

Please check if any family members have had or have the following:

Breast cancer	_____	High blood pressure	_____
Ovarian cancer	_____	High cholesterol	_____
Other kind of cancer	_____	Inflammation or blood clot in lower	
Diabetes	_____	extremities	_____
Heart attack or heart disease	_____	Thyroid problems	_____
Stroke	_____	Mental illness	_____
Tuberculosis	_____		

Do you wish to discuss a special problem or concern with the nurse or doctor? _____

Governmental public health services are tax-supported. Information about health department clinics is found in Chapter 9.

Local health departments provide services in varying degrees. They are under the authority of state health departments and their roles and responsibilities are determined by the state legislature. Most local health departments are organized on the county level, but some cities also have their own department of health. Some rural, poorly populated states have only a state health department. Almost 50% of the funding for local health departments comes from federal and state grants. The future of these monies is in serious jeopardy with federal and state efforts to reduce deficit spending.

Tuberculosis Control

Tuberculosis control programs are largely staffed by public health nurses at local health departments or by institutional infection control nurses. The incidence of tuberculosis had been rising from 1985 to 1992, with about 23,000 new cases reported yearly in the United States. A major reason for the increased incidence is the AIDS epidemic, which has produced large numbers of immunodeficient persons vulnerable to infectious diseases. The large influx of immigrants from areas where active tuberculosis is common is another reason for the increased incidence and prevalence of tuberculosis. Because of an aggressive treatment program, with outreach workers tracking clients to ensure treatment compliance and completion, the prevalence of tuberculosis is decreasing again.

Tuberculosis is an air-borne disease—that is, the disease is transmitted by air droplets. Those who share the air with an active case of tuberculosis are at risk of taking the bacillus into their bodies and developing a latent infection. This means they are also at risk for developing active clinical disease if their own resistance is weak. Special disposable masks are worn by health-care workers when in contact with a suspected case of tuberculosis. Attempts are made to cleanse or moderate the shared air by using negative airflow examination rooms or ultraviolet lamps.

Although a vaccination against tuberculosis, called bacillus Calmette-Guérin (BCG), has been used in other countries, it is seldom used in the United States because the immunity that BCG provides is unreliable, and BCG confuses the reading of the Mantoux or purified protein derivative (PPD) screening test for tuberculosis exposure. The latest CDC guideline is to ignore BCG altogether when administering and reading the PPD test.

For the Mantoux or PPD test, 5 TU (tuberculin units) of PPD (0.1 ml) of *Mycobacterium tuberculosis* is injected intradermally in the forearm and the results are read 48 to 72 hours later. Healthy people with no known exposure or other risk factors are read as positive only if the outer area of palpable induration exceeds 15 mm. Persons from high-risk areas or with other risk factors are read as positive with 10 mm of induration. Persons with known exposure to active tuberculosis, or those whose test recently converted, are read as positive with 5 mm of induration. (Some clinics use 10 mm of induration as the cutoff point between negative and positive.) All positive PPD tests should be followed by a chest x-ray. Positive cultures from lung fluids or tissue completes a positive diagnosis for tuberculosis. Bacilli may also be cultured from other fluids and tissues if nonpulmonary tuberculosis is suspected.

If a client has been exposed to tuberculosis, as indicated by a positive PPD in the absence of other findings, prophylactic isoniazid (INH) is usually given for 9 to 12 months to prevent progression to full-blown, active tuberculosis. These persons need monthly clinic visits to monitor compliance and have liver function tests, because INH can be hepatotoxic.

A positive culture and x-ray are indicative of active tuberculosis. This can occur with either a new exogenous infection or the breakdown of an old latent tuberculosis lesion (endogenous reactivation). Aggressive combination drug therapy is given that usually includes four drugs: INH, rifampin (Rifadin), ethambutol (Myambutol), and pyrazina-mide (Tebrazid). Monthly visits to the chest clinic are imperative to monitor for drug side effects, to monitor the disease, and to ensure the drugs are being taken to avoid the development of drug-resistant strains of *M tuberculosis*.

Often clients fail to keep their monthly appointments at the chest clinic and fail to continue taking their drugs. Problems of noncompliance and drug resistance require that outreach workers make home visits for direct observation of therapy compliance. These workers should be conversant in the client's language and should live in the community to do contact investigations. All contacts of clients with active tuberculosis must be tested for their own protection and that of the community as a whole.

The development of a drug-resistant strain of the bacillus is of grave concern because it has only a 50% cure rate and can be fatal. The main reason that drug-resistant strains develop is failure to complete treatment; clients may stop taking the drugs because the active symptoms of tuberculosis subside after 2 to 3 weeks of treatment, and they begin to feel better. Alcoholics and other drug addicts have a high rate of tuberculosis and are particularly unreliable about completing treatment.

U.S. law requires persons with active tuberculosis to comply with treatment or to risk incarceration in hospitals or jails. This law is used only as a last resort by public health officials when efforts to teach and motivate clients fail. The ethical issue of individual freedom vs. protection of the community presents a dilemma between individual rights and societal rights.

HIV/AIDS Control

Several studies have shown that other developed countries have done a better job of educating the public about AIDS prevention. This is particularly true of teenagers, who tend not to use condoms during their first sexual experiences. We need to make condoms readily available to everyone, especially in schools. Although our personal values may be jolted by encouraging condom distribution, as health-care workers we must be objective and professional when facing the reality that most boys and girls are sexually active by age 16. Many teen pregnancies could be prevented with better education and availability of contraception. In the United States, the fastest-growing segment of persons with HIV infection is minority women, many of whom are teenagers.

Local health departments are actively involved in HIV testing and AIDS treatment programs. The number of STD clinics has expanded because of the number of people seeking HIV testing. The enzyme-linked immunosorbent assay (ELISA), a screening test for HIV antibodies, is a highly sensitive test but occasionally gives false-positive results. The Western blot test is then used to confirm and identify the specific HIV antibodies.

Persons with negative ELISA results should be retested at 3 and 6 months because sometimes it takes that long for the HIV antibodies to develop. Nurses staffing these clinics are usually given special HIV counseling training. Confidential or anonymous testing is provided in which the client is known only by a number. In confidential testing, the client is given a copy of the test results. A partner notification program is also offered, with the understanding that the name of the infected contact will never be used. HIV-positive clients are not legally required to notify their partners.

Most local health departments sponsor clinics for AIDS treatment in which medications are provided to clients. The use of a combination drug regimen is very expensive but well worth the cost in increasing the T-cell count and modifying the negative outlook about this disease. Treated persons are showing reduced levels of HIV, and their development of AIDS is being delayed. We do not yet know how long these delays will last, but a few optimists are using the term "cure." However, much work remains to be done to fight AIDS.

Most AIDS clinics are run on a case management basis with medical, nursing, social work, and nutritional services provided. A nurse or a social worker is the case manager. AIDS clients are treated for the various opportunistic infections they develop. Many AIDS clients, most of whom are young, are reluctant to accept a hospice referral when progressive Kaposi's sarcoma or another opportunistic infection not amenable to treatment develops. AIDS dementia is common late in the illness. More and more clients with AIDS are being cared for at home or through hospice programs.

Many ethical issues surround testing and treatment for AIDS. Mandatory testing has been rejected because of the fear and stigma associated with the disease. Without a cure or a vaccine to prevent AIDS, it is likely that testing and partner notification programs will continue on a voluntary basis. States differ in their regulations about AIDS reporting (Table 6-4).

Control of Other Communicable Diseases

Syphilis and gonorrhea have developed drug-resistant strains and are becoming a serious problem. In fact, the epidemic of all STDs is a grave concern. Human papillomavirus and chlamydia are not universally reportable diseases like syphilis and gonorrhea but are thought to be more prevalent. There is no cure for genital herpes, and it can be transmitted to sexual partners and vaginally delivered newborns. It can cause serious infant abnormalities, as evident in the Clinical Application case study in Chapter 1. STD clinics are sponsored by most health departments, are confidential, and are usually free. Community health nurses working in other areas of ambulatory care, such as a physician's office, also deal with these problems professionally. All nurses should teach the public the importance of preventing STDs.

Hepatitis B infection seems to be closely associated with HIV infection, although this is not always the case. Hepatitis B virus is a more infectious organism and is also transmitted in blood and body fluids by infected needles and semen. The hepatitis B virus can live outside the body in dried blood for up to a week (Humphrey & Milone-Nuzzi, 1996). Hepatitis A, B, and C viruses are all lifetime contraindications for blood donation because of the virus's durability. All health-care workers involved in direct patient care should receive the hepatitis B vaccine; the Occupational Safety & Health Administration has mandated that employers offer it free of charge. The hepatitis B

TABLE 6-4. Reporting Requirements for HIV

By Name of Infected Person	Anonymous	Not Required
Alabama	Georgia	Alaska
Arizona	Illinois	California
Arkansas	Iowa	Connecticut§
Colorado	Kansas	Delaware
Idaho	Kentucky	Florida
Indiana	Maine	Hawaii
Louisiana	Maryland*	Massachusetts
Michigan	Montana	New York
Minnesota	New Hampshire	Pennsylvania
Mississippi	Oregon†	Vermont
Missouri	Rhode Island	Washington*
Nebraska	Texas‡	District of Columbia
Nevada	Virgin Islands	
New Jersey		
New Mexico		
North Carolina		
North Dakota		
Ohio		
Oklahoma		
South Carolina		
South Dakota		
Tennessee		
Utah		
Virginia		
West Virginia		
Wisconsin		
Wyoming		

Some of the above states provide opportunities for anonymous testing. Check state health depts. for updated changes.

AIDS is reportable in all states.
* Maryland and Washington require name reporting of people with symptomatic HIV infection.
† Oregon requires name reporting for children 6 and under.
‡ Texas requires name reporting only for children less than 13 years of age.
§ Connecticut requires only reporting by name of children 12 and under.
(National Conference of State Legislatures [1996]. *HIV/AIDS Facts to Consider: 1996.*)

vaccine is now given to newborns and may be required before school entrance. Hepatitis B is a serious disease but can be essentially eradicated with herd immunity.

There is also a vaccine for the hepatitis A virus. It is recommended primarily for persons traveling to countries where hepatitis A exposure is common. Local health departments administer this vaccine in travelers' clinics or special clinics held in areas where there has been an epidemic of hepatitis A. Two injections are required, the second, a booster, given 6 months after the first. Hepatitis A is spread through the oral–fecal route, a major reason why restaurant workers and other food handlers are required to wash their hands carefully after using the restroom. Infection occurs by eating or drinking contaminated food or fluids. A 1997 epidemic among schoolchildren was traced to contaminated frozen strawberries served as part of their school lunch.

There is no vaccine available for hepatitis C virus (formerly known as non-A, non-B hepatitis), a serious virus that often results in cirrhosis or liver cancer.

Measles has been causing renewed concern in recent years. It seems that the measles vaccine, administered to young children as MMR vaccine, does not provide lifelong immunity as previously thought. Many high school and college students need booster injections to avoid measles if their titer is low. One reason for the increase in the incidence of measles may be the casual attitude that has developed about the importance of immunizations. People seem to have forgotten how serious measles can be: in recent years, deaths have occurred, as well as serious, long-term complications. Community health nurses working in immunization clinics or a physician's office must reinforce the importance of keeping immunizations up to date. Local health departments usually hold weekly immunization clinics for children over 5 years old and for adults.

Table 6-5 lists the recommended adult immunization schedule for several communicable diseases.

Hospital-Sponsored Wellness Programs

Hospitals sponsor various wellness programs for inpatients and people in the community. Maternity departments, in particular, hold classes about the perinatal period for clients and their families. Hospital outreach departments sponsor educational programs on health promotion and the three levels of prevention. They also sponsor support groups for clients with diseases such as diabetes, chronic lung disease, or Parkinson's disease. Display 6-4 lists the classes and support groups offered by one 350-bed community hospital; another example is given in "The Nurse Speaks" in Chapter 5. Some hospitals have special programs for senior citizens.

Maternal-child health programs include childbirth preparation, Lamaze training, preparation for cesarean section and anesthesia, newborn care, breastfeeding training and consultation, sibling rivalry, and bereavement support for miscarriage or neonatal death (Display 6-5). Most programs are offered free of charge; some, like the Lamaze classes, have a small fee. Lactation consultation through the hospital or through La Leche League is available for breastfeeding mothers later at home.

Primary prevention activities include subjects such as avoiding heatstroke, preventing lead poisoning, managing stress, reducing the risk of cancer through diet, and offering free flu shots for senior citizens. Secondary prevention programs include screening for blood pressure, cholesterol, blood glucose, and glaucoma and offering school entry physical examinations. Tertiary prevention programs include teaching diabetics how to identify and prevent foot complications, a support group for dialysis patients, a cardiovascular reconditioning program, a lecture on medications that may be risky in elderly patients, a series on helping children with chronic disease lead a normal life, and Alcoholics Anonymous meetings.

TABLE 6-5. Adult Immunization Schedule

Immunization	Who	When
Measles Mumps Rubella (German measles) (MMR)	Persons born in 1957 or later should check with their doctor or health department to see if they are up to date. Persons born before 1957 probably had measles and mumps and do not need to be immunized. Women of childbearing age should check with their doctor to see if they are protected against rubella.	Many adults have only one dose. A second dose may be required in some work settings. Colleges and universities may require that students get a second measles dose.
Polio (IPV)	Health-care and laboratory workers in contact with wild poliovirus or community members where wild poliovirus disease is occurring Travelers to developing countries	Unimmunized adults: IPV 2 doses at 2- to 8-week intervals, third dose 6 to 12 months after second Booster: IPV possible one dose every 5 years OPV: fourth dose with potential exposure
Tetanus—Diphtheria (Td)	Everyone	Booster shots every 10 years. Adults not immunized should get a series of three doses and then a booster every 10 years.
Hepatitis B	Check with your doctor. Some people are more likely to get hepatitis B than others due to their work or lifestyle.	A series of three doses provides lifetime protection.
Influenza	Persons 65 and older People younger than 65 who have health problems such as heart or lung disease, diabetes, asthma, kidney disease, anemia, or a weakened immune system Health-care workers, nursing home residents, or household members who have contact with any of the above people Anyone who wants to lower the chance of catching the flu can get a flu immunization.	Every year in the fall, because flu strains are different each year.
Pneumococcal pneumonia	Person 65 and older People younger than 65 who have chronic illnesses such as those listed above for influenza	One dose for lifetime protection against many forms of pneumonia
Varicella (chickenpox)	Persons who have not had chickenpox and are: • Health-care workers • Family contacts of people with weakened immune systems • Day-care workers or teachers of young children • College students, military staff, prison inmates and staff • Nonpregnant women of childbearing age • Travelers to foreign countries	If you have had chickenpox, you do not need to get the shot. Youth 13 years of age and older and adults receive two doses 1 to 2 months apart. Children 12 months to 12 years of age receive one dose.

(Modified from CDC, Advisory Committee on Immunized Practices, and North Carolina Dept. of Environment, Health and Natural Resources, Immunization Section, July 1997.)

Sample List of Classes and Support Groups Offered at a Hospital

The following groups meet at the hospital:

Alcoholics Anonymous

American Heart Association

*Basic Life Support (BLS)—professional certification by the American Heart Association

Blood pressure screening

*Breastfeeding preparation classes

Crohn's & Colitis Club—provides support and education for those with inflammatory bowel disease (a local chapter of the national foundation)

Diabetes Club

Dialysis group

*Exerflex

Family group

For Families Only—relatives and friends of cancer patients

Heart Club—assists those who have had a heart attack, bypass surgery, or other cardiac problem

Parkinson's support group—for those with Parkinson's disease and their caregivers

Perinatal bereavement (Resolve Through Sharing)—for parents who have lost a baby through stillbirth or newborn death

Postpartum Blues—for parents who have delivered within the past 6 months and feel depressed

*Prepared childbirth class

*Prepared sibling class

Prime Plus/Red Hot Mamas—menopause education and support groups

Recovery group

Sharing—cancer patients, families, and friends

Stop Smoking—American Cancer Society

Transplant recipients

Well Spouse

*Fee involved

Community Hospital Childbirth and Child Care Programs

Lamaze classes—6-week series given by certified Lamaze instructors; includes a tour of the labor and delivery area

Lamaze refresher—for second (or more!) baby

C-Section class—prepares both parents for cesarean experience, should it become necessary

Infant nutrition—breastfeeding and bottle feeding

Infant care—diapering, dressing, bathing, temperature taking, safety in the home

Prenatal and postpartum exercise

Big Brother/Big Sister program—to prepare parents and siblings for the family addition

Disability rehabilitation programs are often sponsored for people who live in the community. Some are in the form of day hospitals and provide coordinated services with physical therapy, occupational therapy, or speech therapy. For more about day hospitals, see Chapters 9 and 11. A wide variety of disorders are treated in these tertiary preventive programs, including spinal cord injuries, head injuries, amputations, strokes, multiple sclerosis, and other neuromuscular disorders. The scope and intensity of these programs may be the same as an inpatient stay, but the clients can remain in close touch with family and home life. When they return home each evening, they can practice their new skills in a familiar environment, making the transition to independent living easier. Many of these clients find outpatient or day hospital programs more satisfying, and these programs are more cost-effective than inpatient care.

THE NURSE SPEAKS . . .
About Tuberculosis Prevention and Control

I work as a communicable disease nurse at a county health department. A major concept to remember about tuberculosis prevention is to avoid or reduce shared air, particularly with tuberculosis suspects. I remember one situation that occurred upstate in a small community hospital. A woman hospitalized for osteomyelitis was receiving irrigations into the wound by use of a Water-Pik. The wound contained, among other organisms, *Mycobacterium tuberculosis* bacilli, and the Water-Pik was aerosoling them into the environment. The nursing staff on that unit, who had previously tested negative for tuberculosis, converted to positive PPD readings! In analyzing how this sudden epidemic of tuberculosis infections had occurred, the presence of *M tuberculosis* in the woman's wound was brought to light. The woman received combination drug treatment, and the hospital staff who were positive converters also were treated prophylactically for 9 months with isoniazid (INH). To my knowledge, none of the hospital staff developed active tuberculosis because they were quickly identified and treated prophylactically.

Donna
COMMUNICABLE DISEASE NURSE

CLINICAL APPLICATION

A Critical Thinking Case Study About Clients With Sexually Transmitted Diseases

You work in a county health department clinic that specializes in women's health needs. Your clinic, which meets daily, serves females of all ages. The goal is to encourage women to learn to value and care for their bodies. You try to raise their consciousness and sense of self-efficacy about the importance of their health and the need to take responsibility for self-care.

You do a great deal of health promotion and disease prevention teaching about women's health issues, consistent with the mission of a public health department.

Your clinic provides contraception as requested and tests for and treats sexually transmitted diseases as well.

 and Think!

- What are all the current methods of contraception?
- Are any of them foolproof?
- Which is the best method?
- On what basis do you define "best?"
- What is the purpose of combined methods?
- If a woman is taking the pill, why does her partner need to wear a condom?
- Do you think that anyone who requests contraception should have access to it?
- Why or why not?

You are appalled at the number of junior high and high school students who are coming to the clinic with sexually transmitted diseases. You believe our society is "missing the boat" in regard to disease prevention in this age group. Several young girls tell you that once girls start menstruating, they should start having sex: this is a common myth among teenagers. The youngsters at the clinic express shock when they become pregnant or catch a sexually transmitted disease so easily. Few of them have used protection because of their attitude that "it can't happen to me."

 and Think!

- What should be done about this problem?
- What can be accomplished realistically?
- When and where should this be done?

The health department where you work recently hired a health educator to visit the schools to talk about the epidemic of sexually transmitted diseases and teen pregnancy. You go with her occasionally to assist. Sometimes you can reach the children, but other times they are very apathetic about these risks. The health educator says that a major nationwide sex education campaign is needed, using mass media and the schools. She blames movies, magazines, television, and celebrities for promoting such a casual attitude about sexual activity. She also blames segments of our society that want to prohibit public sex education and the availability of condoms because of the belief that they encourage sexual activity. In her experience, not enough parents are taking responsibility at an early enough age for their children's sex education, so children are being educated by their peers, with a great deal of dangerous misinformation.

One day, a 15-year-old named Tanya comes to the clinic with her girlfriend Stephanie. Tanya complains of profuse, malodorous, uncomfortable vaginal discharge. She insists that Stephanie stay with her for emotional support. As usual, you conduct an extensive teaching session and take a comprehensive health history. You discuss menses, hormones, breast care, good nutrition, and sexuality. You answer the girls' questions and talk about what they should do to protect their health. You ask about Tanya's family and their health history and habits. You discuss Tanya's symptoms. Both girls say they are having sex with "a few guys." Therefore, a test for pregnancy is done, as well as tests for HIV, chlamydia, gonorrhea, syphilis, trichomoniasis, candidiasis, and bacterial vaginitis. You do a Pap smear for human papillomavirus as well as malignant cells.

 and Think!

- What should a nurse teach young teenagers about sexuality?
- What should a nurse say about abstinence when a teen says he or she is having sex?
- How effective is it to tell teenagers, once they have started having sex, to wait until they are more mature, are married, or at least have stable relationships?
- How can desirable behaviors regarding sex be communicated to teenagers?
- What do you think would happen if you admonished these girls for being too young to be sexually active?

You inform Tanya that she has trichomoniasis, based on the wet-mount smear that is examined under the microscope. She is not pregnant, so she can be treated with metronidazole (Flagyl). She is given oral Flagyl, 500 mg b.i.d. for 7 days, and is instructed not to drink alcohol because of its adverse interaction with Flagyl. You doubt she uses alcohol but should assume nothing. You tell Tanya you will notify her about her Pap smear results. Because she does not want her home called or her parents to know she has been here, you and she agree that she will get her results when she returns for her next clinic appointment.

 and Think!

- Did you forget something?
- Also, what will you do if Tanya fails to come back and the Pap smear is positive?

It is important to instruct Tanya to tell all her sexual contacts to come to the free clinic or a private doctor for confidential testing and treatment. It is common for males to be asymptomatic, so they are not apt to seek treatment on their own. She needs to understand that all infected persons should abstain from sex until treated, or at the very least should use condoms. If Tanya does not return to the clinic and her results are positive, then a reminder letter is sent in an unmarked envelope simply saying, "Did you forget us? Give us a call!"

When Tanya returns, a test-of-cure is done to be sure she is free of trichomonads. All her other tests are negative except the Pap smear, which shows atypical cells that can be symptomatic of human papillomavirus. You stress to Tanya the importance of a second Pap smear and the need to continue to use condoms or abstain in the meantime. You might describe colposcopy with cryosurgery to her as the best treatment for human papillomavirus, although it is very costly. Colposcopy is a procedure in which a physician observes the cervix through a magnifying instrument to identify any dysplasia or compromised area.

 and Think!

- What is human papillomavirus, and what are the risks associated with it?
- Why not retest Tanya immediately with a second Pap smear?

Human papillomavirus, a serious sexually transmitted disease, is at epidemic level in the United States. It is considered a precancerous virus and can also lead to sterility. It is difficult to eradicate and can haunt infected persons for many years. The diagnosis must be accurate. If Tanya's second Pap smear still shows atypical cells, she should be referred for a colposcopy. If dysplasia exists, cryosurgery using liquid nitrogen is performed; this destroys the virus, along with cervical cells. Within 4 months, new, uninfected cells grow back. Young teens are particularly at risk with human papillomavirus, so aggressive treatment is recommended. However, Tanya will be at risk for reinfection unless she uses condoms whenever she has sex.

Stephanie, Tanya's friend, decided that she also needed to be tested, although she has been involved with different boys than Tanya. This turned out to be a wise decision: her examination revealed chlamydia, the most common sexually transmitted disease and the leading cause of sterility in young adults. Stephanie was treated with oral doxycycline, 100 mg b.i.d. for 7 days, and was advised about the importance of not missing any doses. She was instructed to tell her sexual partners to come for treatment, to abstain from sex during treatment, and to use condoms as well as birth-control pills to be protected both from sexually transmitted diseases and pregnancy.

Although both girls were totally surprised and dismayed to learn they were infected, enough of our health education took root for them to say, "We could have caught AIDS or become pregnant! This is a good warning that we have to be a lot more careful about sex."

Chapter SUMMARY

Health departments deal with the community as the client in promoting and safeguarding wellness. They administer a variety of programs, such as health education, environmental quality control, maternal-child health programs, and infectious disease control. Nurses who complete an approved course in public health nursing earn the title "public health nurse."

Maternal-child health programs include prenatal, well-child, and women's health clinics. Control of communicable diseases is achieved by immunization programs and epidemiologic surveillance. Sometimes control of certain diseases can be a challenge because of noncompliant clients whose diseases may become drug-resistant. Tuberculosis control programs include screenings with PPD tests and x-rays and therapy programs using a four-drug regimen; these clients require monthly clinic visits. Community outreach workers maintain contacts and find noncompliant clients who have failed to keep their appointments. HIV and other sexually transmitted diseases are of epidemic proportions, and health departments play a major role in their diagnosis, treatment, and control. Other communicable diseases that continue to cause periodic epidemics, despite available vaccines, include hepatitis and measles.

Hospitals provide many health education, screening, and other wellness programs. Maternity departments, in particular, have a tradition of health teaching with Lamaze and La Leche League programs. Various support and self-help groups are also sponsored by hospitals.

A list of references and additional readings for this chapter appears at the end of Part 2.

7

Volunteer and Staff Opportunities for Nurses in Wellness Programs

Key Terms

adult rehabilitation centers
American Cancer Society (ACS)
American Heart Association (AHA)
American Red Cross (ARC)
basic life support
parish nursing

Reach to Recovery
Salvation Army
triage
Women, Infants, and Children (WIC)
   programs

Learning Objectives

1. Identify at least 10 agencies where nurses often volunteer their services.

2. Describe the work of the American Cancer Society.

3. Describe how nurses are involved with the American Heart Association as volunteers and as paid staff.

4. Rate the contribution of the American Red Cross to the health and well-being of Americans.

5. Describe how the Salvation Army funds its health and welfare causes.

6. Explain why parish nurse programs are called wellness programs.

7. Contrast the four models of parish nurse practice.

8. Identify ways to secure more information about parish nursing.

9. Describe four types of nutrition programs that promote wellness.

Countless opportunities exist for nurses to become involved in wellness programs, either as volunteers or as paid staff members. At some points in a nurse's life, it may not be convenient, appropriate, or desirable to seek paid employment. However, many nurses like to continue some involvement in their profession on an occasional basis without ongoing, heavy responsibility. Volunteer activities in wellness programs fill that need for many nurses. These activities carry much less liability risk because nurses are not administering medications and treatments. At the same time, nurses have abundant opportunity to practice their skills of assessment, therapeutic communication, and health education.

Volunteer work fills a great need in communities. Even employed nurses enjoy donating their time occasionally. A great deal of valuable work is accomplished by volunteers in the United States, and this has been one of our finest traditions as a nation. In addition, volunteer work brings personal satisfaction and gain. The University of Michigan Survey Research Center conducted a 10-year study of 2,700 people in Tecumseh, Michigan, to determine the impact of social relationships on health. The study found that regular volunteer work, more than any other activity, dramatically increased life expectancy (ACS Newsletter, 1995; Luks & Payne, 1991).

Voluntary Agencies

Many voluntary agencies have been established in the United States to help fight specific disorders. Voluntary agencies are supported financially by donations, not taxes. These private, not-for-profit organizations provide information, education, and referral services for clients and their families to help them cope with day-to-day challenges. Some agencies provide a wide variety of services to clients. Some hold fund-raising events to provide financial support for research into the cause or cure of a disease.

The American Cancer Society (ACS) is the nationwide community-based voluntary health organization dedicated to eliminating cancer as a major health problem. Its goals are to prevent cancer, save lives, and diminish suffering from cancer through research, education, and service (Table 7-1). ACS programs and materials are supported by contributions.

The ACS uses volunteer nurses extensively. Many chapters have a nurses' professional advisory committee that organizes educational programs for nurses on various aspects of cancer care (eg, programs on pain management or screening for cancers). Volunteer nurses help run various early detection programs, such as skin, breast, or testicular cancer screenings. Some nurses volunteer to teach classes on reducing cancer risks or breast self-examination. Nurses often volunteer for cancer support programs, which provide counseling and support on a one-to-one basis to help families and clients cope when cancer strikes. The ACS provides training and ongoing supervision from volunteer psychiatrists and psychotherapists. Some nurses also volunteer to help transport clients to treatments, help with office work, or become involved in fund-raising activities. Nurses who are cancer survivors themselves might lend support to newer patients in programs such as CanSurmount, Reach to Recovery, Life After Prostate Cancer, Lost Cord, or ostomy support groups.

The American Heart Association (AHA) is dedicated to fighting heart disease and stroke. In recent years, the incidence of these disorders in the United States has dropped significantly, largely because of public education about ways to control hypertension and reduce coronary artery disease. Much remains to be done, however: heart disease is still the number-one killer of Americans, and cardiovascular accidents rank third (Display 7-1). Public education about cardiopulmonary resuscitation (CPR) saves lives. The AHA is at the forefront of these educational efforts.

TABLE 7-1. American Cancer Society Guidelines for the Early Detection of Cancer in People Without Symptoms Talk With Your Doctor Ask How These Guidelines Relate to You

Age 18–39	Age 40 and Over
Cancer-Related Checkup Every 3 Years	**Cancer-Related Checkup Every Year**
Should include the procedures listed below plus health counseling (such as tips on quitting tobacco use) and examinations for cancers of the thyroid, testicles, mouth, ovaries, skin, and lymph nodes. Some people are at higher risk for certain cancers and may need to have tests more frequently.	Should include the procedures listed below plus health counseling (such as tips on quitting tobacco use) and examinations for cancers of the thyroid, testicles, mouth, ovaries, skin, and lymph nodes. Some people are at higher risk for certain cancers and may need to have tests more frequently.
Breast	**Breast**
• Exam by a health-care professional every 3 years • Self-exam every month	• Exam by a health-care professional every year • Self-exam every month • Screening mammogram (breast x-ray) at age 40, every 1–2 years for ages 40–49, and every year for age 50 and older.
Uterus	**Uterus**
• Pelvic exam every 1–3 years, with a Pap test	• Pelvic exam every year, with a Pap test • Endometrial tissue sample at menopause, if at high risk
Cervix	**Cervix**
• All women should have an annual Pap test and pelvic examination. After three or more consecutive satisfactory normal annual examinations, the Pap test may be performed less frequently at the discretion of the physician. Remember, these guidelines are not rules and apply only to people without symptoms.	• All women should have an annual Pap test and pelvic examination. After three or more consecutive satisfactory normal annual examinations, the Pap test may be performed less frequently at the discretion of the physician.
	Colon and Rectum
	• Digital rectal exam every year • Stool slide test every year after 50 • Sigmoidoscopy, preferably flexible, every 3–5 years after age 50
	Prostate
	• Age 50 and over, annual digital rectal exam and prostate-specific antigen blood test every year

The AHA uses nurses extensively both as volunteers and as paid CPR instructors (basic life support [BLS] is the newest name for CPR). Community BLS classes are taught by volunteer nurses. BLS training centers are staffed by paid instructors who present all levels of BLS training, including BLS for health professionals (level C), BLS for instructors, and BLS for instructor trainers. In many communities, volunteer nurses from the AHA do hypertension screening on a monthly basis at senior citizen centers and clubs. They also perform occasional hypertension screening requested by organizations or businesses. As part of the AHA speakers' bureau, volunteer nurses

---

DISPLAY 7-1
Possible Heart Attack: Seek Help STAT!

Call 911 or other emergency services immediately if chest pain is crushing (feels like some-one is sitting on your chest) or squeezing, increases in intensity, or occurs with any of the following symptoms of a heart attack:

- Pain that radiates to the arm
- Shortness of breath
- Rapid or irregular pulse
- Nausea or vomiting
- Lightheadedness and loss of consciousness

After you call 911, begin rescue breathing and CPR if the person stops breathing or has no pulse.

---

speak to groups about risk factors for heart disease, hypertension prevention, and related topics.

The American Red Cross (ARC) was founded during the Civil War by Clara Barton, who tended wounded soldiers on the battlefield. The ARC has served the public during many disasters and emergencies in the ensuing years (Display 7-2). During the past 5 years, the ARC has had to respond to more major disasters than at any time in its 100-year history. Volunteer nurses are vitally important in staffing its first aid and emergency field centers during emergencies. The ARC is collaborating with the American Nurses Association to prepare disaster training protocols for volunteer nurses. In local communities, ARC volunteers conduct first aid and CPR training. Local chapters offer waterfront safety and other safety programs. The ARC is best known for its blood collection. Blood banks across the nation are organized and managed by the ARC.

The Salvation Army has served poor and homeless people for more than 100 years. On any given night, there are 100,000 people receiving drug and alcohol rehabilitation services free of charge at Salvation Army adult rehabilitation centers. At the heart of each Salvation Army center is the firm belief that rehabilitation is part of God's plan for humans (Display 7-3). The programs are sustained by donations of clothing, furniture, and household items refurbished in workshops as part of the work therapy program. The

---

DISPLAY 7-2
Mission of the American Red Cross

The American Red Cross, a humanitarian organization led by volunteers and guided by its congressional charter and the fundamental principles of the International Red Cross Move-ment, will provide relief to victims of disaster and help people prevent, prepare for, and re-spond to emergencies.

Adopted by The American National Red Cross Board of Governors, 1996

DISPLAY 7-3
Salvation Army Mission Statement

The Salvation Army, an international movement, is an evangelical part of the Universal Christian Church. Its message is based on the Bible. The ministry is motivated by love of God. Its mission is to preach the Gospel of Jesus Christ and to meet human needs in his name without discrimination. Its mission is holistic:
* Meeting physical needs
* Meeting emotional needs
* Meeting spiritual needs

Salvation Army sponsors the Booth Homes (for pregnant girls), senior citizen residences, nutrition and feeding programs, hospitals, and homeless shelters. Salvation Army stores sell used and refurbished items, providing employment and inexpensive household goods. The Salvation Army uses nurses as paid staff or as volunteers in its wide range of services to humanity.

The ACS, the AHA, the ARC, and the Salvation Army are only a few of the excellent voluntary groups in the United States involved in fighting disorders and promoting wellness. For example, some of the groups involved in just one area, neurologic disorders, are the Alzheimer's Association, the American Parkinson Disease Association, the Amyotrophic Lateral Sclerosis Association, the Epilepsy Society, and the Multiple Sclerosis Foundation. These national organizations help educate the public, lend support to clients and families, and raise funds for research into the cause and cure of these disorders. Later in this chapter, a nurse speaks about her experience establishing a group for persons with myasthenia gravis, a neuromuscular disorder.

Nurses helped found many of these voluntary and self-help organizations, and nurses continue to be active in them, either as volunteers or as paid staff. Appendix C lists the toll-free telephone numbers for many of these organizations.

Hospices

Hospices use volunteers extensively. Of the 115,000 persons involved in hospice care in the United States, about 95,000 are volunteers. Nurses, in particular, are drawn to hospice volunteer opportunities and function in various ways according to their preferences. Some nurses assist staff in making home visits and delivering nursing care. Other volunteers function as spiritual caregivers or bereavement counselors. Some volunteer nurses prefer just to spend social time with hospice clients and offer respite to their families. Hospices provide excellent training for all these volunteer roles.

Hospice volunteers are always needed for fund-raising activities as well. Although Medicare reimburses hospices for skilled care on a daily capitation basis, many hospice supportive care services are not reimbursable, so volunteer help is greatly needed. Hospices are not-for-profit agencies.

Health Ministries

Parish nursing (congregational care nursing), a relatively new movement, seeks to recapture the ancient role that faith communities provided in delivering health care holistically. Spiritual, physical, mental, and emotional aspects of health are emphasized, with a focus on health promotion and disease prevention. Parish nursing's roots in the healing traditions of faith communities and in the nursing and health sciences places it at the forefront of current partnerships focusing on disease prevention and wellness promotion for groups. This movement is also called "health ministries" (Display 7-4).

The modern parish nurse movement was founded in the Chicago area by Granger Westberg, a Lutheran pastor who taught courses in health and religion and medical ethics at the University of Chicago Medical School. Parish nursing began among Lutheran congregations but rapidly become ecumenical. The movement developed into four major models:

1. Volunteer nurses who work part-time within their own congregations (church- or synagogue-sponsored volunteer congregational nurses)
2. Paid nurses who work full- or part-time for large congregations or a few smaller congregations within a community (church- or synagogue-sponsored paid congregational nurses)
3. Hospital staff parish nurse coordinators who hire and train congregational nurses. Each nurse is assigned to several churches or synagogues that contract with the institution. Nurses are not usually members of those congregations (institution-sponsored paid congregational nurses).

DISPLAY 7-4
Parish Nursing Resources

- The National Parish Nurse Resource Center
  205 West Touhy Avenue, Suite 104, Park Ridge, IL 60068; (800) 556-5368
Offers documentation and assessment tools, videos, and a curriculum for parish nurse education.
- The Health Ministries Association
  PO Box 7853, Huntington Beach, CA 92646; (800) 852-5613 or (714) 965-0085
Nearly 30 chapters across the country provide information–including how to start a new program–and networking opportunities.
- The International Network for Interfaith Health Practices
  Saint Francis Hospital, 355 Ridge Avenue, Evanston, IL 60202; (847) 316-4040;
  E-mail: interaccess.com/ihpnet
An electronic form lists job openings and provides networking and training opportunities. The network is accessible through an E-mail gateway to the Internet that's available through several online services.

(Adapted from Dunkle R [1996]. Parish nurses help patients–body and soul. RN 59(5):55-57.)

4. Hospital staff congregational nurse coordinators who recruit, train, and support volunteer congregational nurses in their churches or synagogues, who are in partnership with the institution (institution-sponsored volunteer nurses)

The University of Kentucky College of Nursing and one local Presbyterian church have a unique collaborative agreement that involves aspects of both the church- and institution-based models of parish nursing. This parish nurse, Ruth Berry, continues to draw her full salary as a professor of nursing at the college, but the church reimburses the college for the hours she spends each week working as a parish nurse.

Depending on the model used, parish nurses perform in a variety of ways, but their actions always emphasize total wellness (Display 7-5). Parish nurses provide health education through church newsletters, bulletin boards, and classes. They have unique opportunities to provide personal health counseling. The Clinical Application section in this chapter gives an example based on actual experience. Parish nurses visit homes, hospitals, or long-term care facilities to bring support. They help coordinate and train volunteers within the congregation to provide food, custodial care, child care, or transportation as needed. They work closely with institutional discharge planners to ensure that all needed and available community resources, including those within the congregation, are used (Display 7-6).

The National Parish Nurse Resource Center can provide information and help with programs. Several colleges and universities are including parish nursing as part of their community health nursing curriculum. The number of master's degree programs specializing in parish nursing is growing. Annual conferences provide additional training. Several hundred nurses attend the Westberg seminar each September in Chicago. The Health Ministries Association, an inclusive, interfaith group that includes religious leaders and health providers, is held each summer. Each June the Presbyterian Church sponsors a parish nurse conference in Santa Fe. The emphasis is on "Nurturing the Spirit, Mind, and Body: Caring for the Caregiver."

DISPLAY 7-5
Traditional Congregational Nurse Roles

Counselor for personal health

Aware of the faith—health relationship

Referral source and liaison to community

Educator regarding wellness for persons and groups

Support group facilitator and volunteer trainer

DISPLAY 7-6
Get Online With The Global Information Superhighway! Announcing the *International Network for Interfaith Health Practices*

The International Network for Interfaith Health Practices (IHP-NET) is an Internet electronic forum for dialogue and resource sharing among persons of all religious traditions, regarding the dynamic relationship between spirituality and health, especially its practical expression in the advancement of human wellness. IHP-NET is a joint project of The Interfaith Health Program of The Carter Center and the Congregational Nurse Program of Saint Francis Hospital of Evanston, Illinois.

To join, you don't even need a full-service connection to the Internet! IHP-NET is accessible to anyone with only an E-mail gateway to the Internet. This is available through a number of popular commercial on-line services, including CompuServe, America Online and Delphi. There is **no charge** specifically for subscribing to HIP-NET; you pay only those fees, if any, otherwise charged by your on-line vendor.

- Share your experience with subscribers from Georgia to Germany, already self-selected for their interest in faith and health—more than 500 persons are now subscribed.
- Share your thoughts and best practices with the world! Post your newsletters, project descriptions, and professional papers as electronic files, which subscribers can retrieve free from the IHP-NET website at http://www.interaccess.com/ihpnet/
- Announce your symposia, training sessions, and other events.
- Network with peers and announce position openings.
- Collaborate with others acting in faith and working on health.
- Organize actions on key issues among a diverse, international membership.

This forum welcomes community and spiritual leaders, health care providers, health promoters, policy advocates, and educators the world over. These include public officials and community builders; clergy and non-ordained; physicians, nurses, congregationally-based and public health practitioners; and university faculty and students.

*TO SUBSCRIBE **FREE**: Type ONLY the word "subscribe" (no quotes) in the body of a new email message and send this message to: IHP-NET-REQUEST@synasoft.com*

(Reprinted with permission. International Network for Interfaith Health Practices.)

Parish nurses must be mature spiritually and have a good knowledge of community health nursing. The following examples provide a good overview of the scope of parish nursing:

Deanna Koch serves a church of 400 members in Iowa. She has an office at the church and receives a salary. In addition to the traditional aspects of parish nursing (assessing needs, finding resources, visiting, and offering advocacy), she runs a grief-support group, a single-parent support group, and a parenting group for mothers of preschoolers. She works with the coordinator of the Alliance for the Mentally Ill, which meets in her church. In Deanna's "clown ministry," she dresses up in a clown suit and a purple wig to become demure "Violet," who presents wellness lessons in a fun way and brings laughter to children, shut-ins, and nursing home residents.

Sue Mooney, another paid parish nurse, serves a 1,000-member congregation in Ohio. She also works with student nurses in a senior community health nursing class. Her goal is to sensitize her students to the health needs of underserved minority populations. They focus their efforts on four African-American churches in the inner city. They first assess the church members' perceptions of their health needs. For example, one church's health committee determined that their people needed more information on diabetes. The church selected 10 women to attend classes on diabetes education, taught by the nursing students (with Sue present as a resource person). On completion, these women were given "health trainer" badges and a supply of literature and resources. They then became the health education facilitators on diabetes for their congregation, and their assistance has been very well received and used.

Another congregation wanted to put on a neighborhood health fair. Again, Sue and her students had the members identify what they thought was important to include in the health fair. They chose the subjects, and Sue and the students offered them the teaching and resources to do the whole fair themselves (again, with Sue present as a resource person). It was a highly successful health fair, and they can repeat it in the future.

Bobbie Del Sol and Judy Gamarello, who have young families, both work full-time as community health nurses in New Jersey. Bobbie works for a health department, Judy for a visiting nurse association. Together they volunteer as parish nurses for their congregation. They make themselves available by phone or after worship services for health counseling. They provide resource information to the congregation and promote wellness by writing articles for the monthly church newsletter, preparing exhibits for the bulletin board, and distributing literature. Occasionally they visit shut-in or hospitalized members of the congregation. They provide hypertension and other health screenings. Again, their emphasis is always on total wellness, mind, body, and spirit.

Deborah Benada works full-time as a parish nurse coordinator at a medical center in the Los Angeles area. She promotes the growth of parish nursing in 16 congregations. She provides education and spiritual nurture to parish nurses through one-on-one consultations, monthly support groups, and quarterly educational sessions. She keeps in close touch with local health agencies and congregations and edits and distributes "Parishes in Partnership," a newsletter. She also works within the medical center, attending team meetings and serving on the advisory board. Her work is ecumenical, serving Catholic, Lutheran, Methodist, Episcopal, and Presbyterian churches. She and her colleagues developed a certificate program for parish nurses that helps them expand their health ministries.

Nutrition Programs

Nutrition programs are vital in health promotion and disease prevention. Even though Americans are becoming more conscious of the value of good nutrition and the importance of reducing the amount of fat in our diet (Table 7-2, Display 7-7), obesity is on the increase. Poor nutrition is especially prevalent in low-income groups and among the elderly, some of whom are susceptible to food myths (Table 7-3).

Many communities have nutrition centers for the elderly or the homeless. Most of these programs are sponsored by volunteer community groups such as the Salvation Army, churches, or other community-minded agencies. Senior nutrition centers, which are popular, may also be tax-supported. These centers provide socialization and health education as well as nutritious meals to senior citizens, who often live alone and spend little time and energy on meal preparation. At these centers, health professionals may present wellness programs such as health education and screenings. Volunteers, including professional nurses, assist with these programs.

Volunteers for Meals on Wheels deliver food to the homes of shut-ins. This valuable program provides a hot lunch and a cold supper. Fees are on a sliding-scale basis and are low because of the large number of volunteers who help deliver the meals.

Food pantries that give a week's supply of groceries to those in need are sponsored by many community and religious groups and are usually staffed by volunteers. More and more middle-class families who struggle with the financial consequences of unemployment from corporate downsizing are using these services. Some groups include other services in addition to food, such as résumé writing and job search assistance, literacy training, and volunteer counseling.

Women, Infants, and Children (WIC) programs are usually administered by local health departments' maternal-child health clinics and prenatal clinics. WIC programs are funded by the Department of Agriculture and state health departments. Nutritious foods are provided to pregnant and lactating women, infants, and children under 5 years of age who meet certain criteria (income, residency, and nutritional risk requirements). The WIC program has proved to be cost-effective. Medical costs are reduced because adequately nourished pregnant mothers have fewer low-birthweight babies. According to a Harvard University study, for every $1 spent on the prenatal component of WIC, up to $3 was saved in hospital costs for low-birthweight babies (The Nutrition Consortium, 1994a). A study done by the New York State Department of Health showed that for every $1 spent on the prenatal component of WIC, $2.35 in health-care costs was saved in hospitalization costs associated with births (The Nutrition Consortium, 1994b, p. 12).

Although some states dispense food directly, most states provide vouchers so clients can buy the food through participating vendors, usually supermarkets. Available foods include milk, eggs, juice, iron-fortified cereal, and cheese (not reduced-fat cheese) (Table 7-4). Infant formulas are usually required to be iron-fortified or soy-based unless the baby's physician states that a different formula is needed. Some states add canned tuna, peanut butter, beans, and carrots to this list. Staff nurses or other health professionals interview the family to determine nutritional risk; the assessment involves measuring height and weight and testing hemoglobin, hematocrit, and blood lead levels.

(text continues on p. 182)

TABLE 7-2. Fat Content of Some Foods

Foods	Fat Content (Grams)	Total (Kcal*)
Milk and yogurt	Per cup	Per cup
Skim milk (milk solids added)	1	90
Low-fat milk (1%)	3	100
Low-fat milk (2%)	5	120
Whole milk (3.3%)	8	150
Low-fat yogurt, plain	4	145
Low-fat yogurt, fruit-flavored	3	230
Table fats	Per tbsp	Per tbsp
Butter	12	100
Margarine	12	100
Whipped butter or margarine	8	65
Mayonnaise	11	100
Cream	Per tbsp	Per tbsp
Half-and-half	2	20
Sour cream	3	30
Nondairy whipped topping (frozen)	1	15
Liquid nondairy coffee lightener	1	20
Powdered nondairy coffee lightener	1 (per tsp)	10 (per tsp)
Desserts	Per ½ cup	Per ½ cup
Ice cream (11% fat)	7	135
Ice cream, soft serve	12	188
Ice milk (4.3% fat)	3	93
Sherbet	2	135
	Per portion	Per portion
Apple pie, ¼ of 9″ pie	15	345
Danish pastry, 4¼ diam × 1″ deep	15	275
Doughnut, glazed, 3¾″ × 1¼″ deep	11	205
Cheese	Per 1 oz	Per 1 oz
Cheddar	9	115
American processed cheese	9	105
Part-skim mozzarella	5	80
Cottage cheese (4% fat)	5 (½ cup)	118
Cottage cheese (1% fat)	1 (½ cup)	82
Meat, fish, poultry	Per 3-oz serving	Per 3-oz serving
Ham, lean and fat	19	245
Shrimp	1	100
Rib roast, lean and fat	33	375
Ground beef, 21% fat	17	235
Ground beef, 10% fat	10	185
Turkey, light meat	3	150

* Total kilocalories represent the kilocalories not only from fat but also from the protein and carbohydrate the food may contain.

(Source: Nutritive Value of Foods, USDA Home and Garden Bulletin No. 72. Washington DC: U.S. Dept. of Agriculture, 1981.)

DISPLAY 7-7
Check Your Cholesterol and Heart Disease

Are you cholesterol smart? Test your knowledge about high blood cholesterol with the following statements. Circle each true or false. The answers are given on the back of this sheet.

1 High blood cholesterol is one of the risk factors for heart disease that you can do something about.

_____ T F

2 To lower your blood cholesterol level, you must stop eating meat altogether.

_____ T F

3 Any blood cholesterol level below 240 mg/dl is desirable for adults.

_____ T F

4 Fish oil supplements are recommended to lower blood cholesterol.

_____ T F

5 To lower your blood cholesterol level, you should eat less saturated fat, total fat, and cholesterol, and lose weight if you are overweight.

_____ T F

6 Saturated fats raise your blood cholesterol level more than anything else in your diet.

_____ T F

7 All vegetable oils help lower blood cholesterol levels.

_____ T F

8 Lowering blood cholesterol levels can help people who have already had a heart attack.

_____ T F

9 All children need to have their blood cholesterol levels checked.

_____ T F

10 Women don't need to worry about high blood cholesterol and heart disease.

_____ T F

11 Reading food labels can help you eat the heart healthy way.

_____ T F

1 **True.** High blood cholesterol is one of the risk factors for heart disease that a person can do something about. High blood pressure, cigarette smoking, diabetes, overweight, and physical inactivity are the others.

2 **False.** Although some red meat is high in saturated fat and cholesterol, which can raise your blood cholesterol, you do not need to stop eating it or any other single food. Red meat is an important source of protein, iron, and other vitamins and minerals. You should, however, cut back on the amount of saturated fat and cholesterol that you eat. One way to do this is by choosing lean cuts of meat with the fat trimmed. Another way is to watch your portion sizes and eat no more than 6 ounces of meat a day. Six ounces is about the size of two decks of playing cards.

3 **False.** A total blood cholesterol level of under 200 mg/dl is desirable and usually puts you at a lower risk for heart disease. A blood cholesterol level of 240 mg/dl is high and increases your risk of heart disease. If your cholesterol level is high, your doctor will want to check your level of LDL cholesterol ("bad" cholesterol). A high level of LDL cholesterol increases your risk of heart disease, as does a low level of HDL cholesterol ("good" cholesterol). An HDL cholesterol level below 35 mg/dl is considered a risk factor for heart disease. A total cholesterol level of 200–239 mg/dl is considered borderline-high and usually increases your risk for heart disease. All adults 20 years of age or older should

DISPLAY 7-7
Check Your Cholesterol and Heart Disease (continued)

have their blood cholesterol level checked at least once every 5 years.

4 **False.** Fish oils are a source of omega-3 fatty acids, which are a type of polyunsaturated fat. Fish oil supplements generally do not reduce blood cholesterol levels. Also, the effect of the long-term use of fish oil supplements is not known. However, fish is a good food choice because it is low in saturated fat.

5 **True.** Eating less fat, especially saturated fat, and cholesterol can lower your blood cholesterol level. Generally your blood cholesterol level should begin to drop a few weeks after you start on a cholesterol-lowering diet. How much your level drops depends on the amounts of saturated fat and cholesterol you used to eat, how high your blood cholesterol is, how much weight you lose if you are overweight, and how your body responds to the changes you make. Over time, you may reduce your blood cholesterol level by 10–50 mg/dl or even more.

6 **True.** Saturated fats raise your blood cholesterol level more than anything else, so the best way to reduce your cholesterol level is to cut back on the amount of saturated fats you eat. These facts are found in largest amounts in animal products such as butter, cheese, whole milk, ice cream, cream, and fatty meats. They are also found in some vegetable oils–coconut, palm, and palm kernel oils.

7 **False.** Most vegetable oils–canola, corn, olive, safflower, soybean, and sunflower oils–contain mostly monounsaturated and polyunsaturated fats, which help lower blood cholesterol when used in place of saturated fats. However, a few vegetable oils–coconut, palm, and palm kernel oils–contain more saturated fat

than unsaturated fat. A special kind of fat, called "trans fat," is formed when vegetable oil is hardened to become margarine or shortening, through a process called hydrogenation. The harder the margarine or shortening, the more likely it is to contain more trans fat. Choose margarine containing liquid vegetable oil as the first ingredient. Be sure to limit the total amount of any fats or oils, since even those that are unsaturated are rich sources of calories.

8 **True.** People who have had one heart attack are at much higher risk for a second attack. Reducing blood cholesterol levels can greatly slow down (and, in some people, even reverse) the buildup of cholesterol and fat in the wall of the coronary arteries and significantly reduce the chances of a second heart attack. If you have had a heart attack or have coronary heart disease, your LDL level should be around 100 mg/dl, which is even lower than the recommended level of less than 130 mg/dl for the general population.

9 **False.** Children from high-risk families, in which a parent has high blood cholesterol (240 mg/dl or above) or in which a parent or grandparent has had heart disease at an early age (55 years or younger), should have their cholesterol levels tested. If a child from such a family has a high cholesterol level, it should be lowered under medical supervision, primarily with diet, to reduce the risk of developing heart disease as an adult. For most children, who are not from high-risk families, the best way to reduce the risk of adult heart disease is to follow a low-saturated-fat, low-cholesterol eating pattern. All children over age 2 and all adults should adopt a heart healthy eating pattern as a principal way of reducing coronary heart disease.

DISPLAY 7-7
Check Your Cholesterol and Heart Disease (continued)

10 **False.** Blood cholesterol levels in both men and women begin to go up around age 20. Women before menopause have levels that are lower than men of the same age. After menopause, a woman's LDL cholesterol level goes up–and so her risk for heart disease increases. For both men and women, heart disease is the number-one cause of death.

11 **True.** Food labels have been changed. Look on the nutrition label for the amount of saturated fat, total fat, cholesterol, and total calories in a serving of the product. Use this information to compare similar products. Also, look for the list of ingredients. Here, the ingredient in the greatest amount is first and the ingredient in the least amount is last. So to choose foods low in saturated fat or total fat, go easy on products that list fats or oil first, or that list many fat and oil ingredients.

(National Cholesterol Education Program, National Heart, Lung, and Blood Institute; U.S. Department of Health and Human Services Public Health Service, National Institutes of Health, NIH Publication No. 95-3794, May 1995.)

TABLE 7-3. Nutrition Myths and Hoaxes

What You Hear	How to Avoid Being Taken In
Certain foods have "magic" medicinal effects.	Question what "they" say: does the belief hold up when the evidence is in?
"Natural" or "organic" foods are more wholesome than ordinary ones.	No one has found a measurable difference; well-cleaned, fresh, conventional produce is healthful and usually much less expensive.
Skipping meals is a good way to lose weight.	Studies show your body stores more fat if you eat only one or two large meals a day than the same calories in smaller and more frequent meals.
Most everyone needs vitamin supplements as "insurance."	Vitamin deficiency is rare unless a person's diet is extremely unbalanced; excesses of some vitamins can be harmful.
Diet pills safely and effectively cause weight loss.	They are medicines that cause short-term limited changes (increased water output, deaden tastebuds, or act as stimulants); they can be dangerous for some people, and rarely work over extended periods of time.
Red meats, aged cheeses, and fine wines are signs of the "good life."	Expensive foods aren't the hallmark of the good life. Enjoying a lovingly prepared dish in good fellowship usually stays in the memory longer!
Nutritional supplements will delay aging, treat or prevent disease, and restore "pep."	They are usually expensive and highly promoted, but claims are mostly unproven. Some contain toxic ingredients; others are dangerous because they encourage delay in seeking medical treatment.

TABLE 7-4. Women, Infants, and Children (WIC) Nutrition Program

Category	Milk* (Quarts)	Eggs (Dozen)	Juice† (Ounces)	Cereal (Ounces)	Legumes‡ (Ounces)
Pregnant women	28	1-½	276	36	16–18
Breastfeeding women§	28	2-½	276	36	16–18
Postpartum women	24	2-½	184	36	0
Children 1–5	24	2-½	276	36	16–18

* One pound of cheese may be substituted for three quarts of milk.
† Only natural fruit juice is allowed. 72 ozs. of frozen concentrate may be substituted for 276 ozs. of liquid.
‡ Participants are offered either one pound of dried beans or 18 ozs. of peanut butter.
§ Women who are exclusively breastfeeding are eligible to receive an enhanced food package. In addition to the foods listed above for lactating women, this enhanced package include one pound of cheese, up to 322 fluid ounces of fruit juice, 29 ozs. of canned tuna, and two pounds of raw or frozen carrots.
(Source: U.S. Dept. of Agriculture.)

THE NURSE SPEAKS . . .
About Forming a Volunteer Health Organization

After I was diagnosed with myasthenia gravis (MG), I could not continue to work as a community health nurse because of my condition. Two years later, we moved back to my hometown, a midwestern city. In my efforts to find a local, experienced physician, I found that each local neurologist or internist I contacted was seeing just one patient with MG. I know that MG isn't common, but this is a city of over 1 million people, with several excellent medical facilities! Something needed to be done to locate MG patients and develop a specialty clinic so that local physicians could gain experience with the disease. This is particularly important for MG because it is such a variable disease; it can be life-threatening and requires sophisticated, experienced care. Sometimes MG patients go undiagnosed or are misdiagnosed for years despite the severity of their symptoms.

I first contacted the national MG foundation. They could not send me their list of patients in this city because of confidentiality issues, but they agreed to circulate my name and address and encourage local patients to contact me. When patients called, I heard some dreadful stories. The realization that many people were receiving inadequate care made me angry and more determined than ever to establish a local chapter and a local MG clinic. The need for education of family members and the lay public about the disease also became clear when I learned that patients had suffered unnecessarily because of family ignorance.

My family members, fellow church members, and friends offered to help because my strength was limited. They helped me secure the assistance of some prominent, respected community leaders who agreed to serve on our board of directors. Several well-regarded physicians agreed to serve on our medical advisory board. I had letterhead printed up with those names, and this helped lend credibility to our fledgling organization. One of those physicians demonstrated special helpfulness and interest in MG because he had cared for several MG patients during his residency. Although I was always careful to give three names when asked for a physician referral, many patients selected him. When we approached him about helping to establish and staff an MG specialty clinic at the medical center where he was affiliated, he readily agreed. We negotiated with the medical center. I wrote a press release, and we secured excellent newspaper publicity when the clinic opened.

With growing interest in the community from the publicity, we approached the United Way and asked for financial support. We were investigated and appeared at several hearings before being declared an official United Way agency. This enabled me to use my limited energy to focus on programs to help patients rather than on fund-raising efforts. Every week brought us the names of additional patients, often newly diagnosed at the MG clinic. They and their families benefited significantly from the educational efforts and emotional support they received from the organization. Many people sent contributions to support our work. I benefited from the effort because it forced me to look beyond myself and my own struggles with the disease; it was good therapy for me.

Four years later, I developed a remission from the disease that continues to the present time. This renewed health has enabled me to return to my work as a community health nurse, which I dearly love. My work as a nurse has been enhanced and sensitized from those 8 years I spent as a patient. The MG foundation continues to grow and now has a paid part-time director as well as many volunteer workers.

Carol
COMMUNITY HEALTH NURSE

CLINICAL APPLICATION

A Critical Thinking Case Study About a Parish Nurse Situation

You are a volunteer parish nurse in a 350-member congregation. You are available for personal health counseling and referrals between Sunday morning worship services and during the coffee hour that follows. People usually stop by to have their blood pressure checked or to talk or ask questions. One morning Hazel, who is in her late 70s, stopped by, looking quite distressed.

"Please don't tell George I spoke to you. He's made me promise not to talk to anyone about this, but I must talk to someone. I think he's getting Alzheimer's! He says he's seeing things and I know the things he sees just aren't there. He's not himself at all! I don't know what to do. I never thought that it would happen to us so sudden like this—his getting so confused, I mean. He always had such a sharp mind."

 and Think!

- How will you handle this situation?
- Hazel does not want you to tell George she spoke to you.

You find George talking with another man. You assess him while waiting to speak with him and notice that he stands quite rigidly and has a small tremor when he moves his hands. The other man leaves and you see that George propels himself forward quickly as you walk together down the hall. He has a masklike expression. You tell George that he doesn't look quite himself and ask if something is going on with his health. He confides that he is different and comments on your discernment.

"Tell me in what ways you are feeling different, George. We've known each other a long time. Possibly I can help in some way. You seem quite worried," you say.

"I'm worried about what will happen to Hazel, and I guess I'm worried about what's happening to me. I'm seeing things. Right now, for example. I suppose you aren't seeing those squirrels running around the edge of the ceiling? That's the kind of thing I'm experiencing. At times I feel very confused too. It's embarrassing. I don't want anyone to know."

 and Think!

- Do you agree that George may be developing Alzheimer's disease?
- What do you make of his physical symptoms?
- What might be happening?

You suspect that George may have Parkinson's disease, based on his physical symptoms. You ask what medications he is taking; sure enough, he tells you he started taking carbidopa-levidopa (Sinemet) not long ago, which you know is used in the treatment of Parkinson's disease. You are not surprised to learn that George has been taking Sinemet only a few weeks, and you explain that some of the side effects of the medication are confusion and hallucinations. You explain that the medication can be changed or the dose altered. It takes a few minutes for the impact of this information to sink in, and then George's face registers great relief. Later, Hazel calls to thank you profusely and adds that George was so ashamed of his hallucinations that it is unlikely he would have told anyone but you. He never connected his symptoms with his medications.

 and Think!

- How should you follow up on this situation, and why?

You ask George if he feels comfortable telling the doctor about his side effects, and he says yes. You want to maintain client autonomy and responsibility as much as possible. You also suggest that George can have the doctor call you if the doctor thinks you can be helpful.

Chapter SUMMARY

There are abundant opportunities for nurses to serve as volunteers or work as staff in private not-for-profit health agencies. The ACS, the AHA, the ARC, and the Salvation Army make major contributions to the health and welfare of the American people. In addition, nurses serve in a variety of volunteer and self-help groups. Many nurses volunteer for hospices, which use almost 100,000 volunteers nationwide.

The parish nurse or congregational care movement (also called health ministry) promotes wellness from a holistic perspective. Several models of parish nursing practice exist. Parish nurses define their roles creatively in response to the needs of their congregations. A parish nurse must be mature spiritually and knowledgeable and up-to-date about health issues. The role of the parish nurse is one of health promotion and disease prevention and entails a great deal of health education, counseling, and support in a holistic way.

An important aspect of wellness promotion is nutrition. Programs that provide and teach sound nutrition for the elderly, the homeless, and the poor support wellness. Meals on Wheels provides meals to shut-ins. The WIC program provides nutritious foods to poor pregnant women, infants, and children. Senior center nutrition programs provide both meals and socialization to lonely elderly persons. The Salvation Army has provided meals to the homeless for 100 years. Food is donated and dispensed to the needy by religious and community groups across the nation using volunteers.

A list of references and additional readings for this chapter appears at the end of Part 2.

8

School and Occupational Health Nursing

Key Terms

Americans With Disabilities Act of 1990
carcinogenic
dysfunctional families
early and periodic screening, diagnosis, and treatment program
employee assistance programs
environmental surveillance
ergonomic
Family Leave Act of 1993
family resource and service centers
impetigo

latchkey children
mainstreamed
National Institute for Occupational Safety and Health (NIOSH)
Occupational Safety and Health Administration (OSHA)
pediculosis
proactive
school-based health centers
Social Security Act of 1935
worker's compensation

Learning Objectives

1. Identify the three traditional components of school and occupational health nursing.

2. Describe each component in detail.

3. Discuss the challenges of school nursing today.

4. Explain the pros and cons of doing sex education in the schools.

5. Identify the problems of keeping immunization records up-to-date.

6. Explain the impetus for increased certifications and education for school nurses.

7. Trace the history of occupational health programs.

8. List the four categories of causative agents of occupational illnesses and injuries.

9. Identify at least six specific examples under each category.

School Nursing

Nurses care for children in schools in the United States in day-care programs, elementary, junior high, and high schools, and colleges and universities. As in the past, school nurses continue to provide first aid, care for minor ailments, and carry out health screening programs as part of their health services. The three traditional components of school health are nursing service, health education, and maintenance of a safe, healthy school environment. This has been the role of school nurses since Lillian Wald established school nursing in 1902.

In 1990, Nader proposed a modified model that recognizes the influence of family, friends, and the mass media on children's health and education (Fig. 8-1). Children are not influenced only by their school experience, nor do schools have the primary responsibility for raising and educating children, even though that seems to be the attitude of some parents. Some parents are too preoccupied with demanding careers or too weary to do the daily teaching that children require from their parents. Some are working single parents who have little or no outside support to help guide and supervise their children while they are working. Some parents are so controlled by

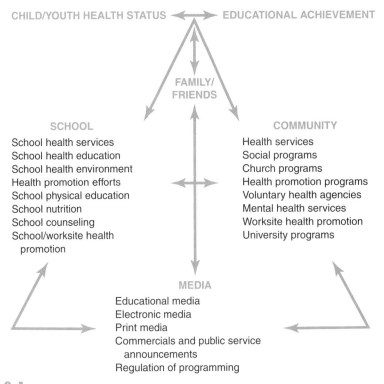

FIGURE 8-1
A school health model. (Adapted from Nader PR [1990]. The concept of "comprehensiveness" in the design and implementation of school health programs. *Journal of School Health,* 60[4], 133–138.)

stress or addictions that they cannot focus on their children's needs. There are many latchkey children who come home from school and watch television until their parents return home in the evening. Some parents welcome television watching because it keeps the children quiet, off the street, and out of trouble; however, these parents seldom monitor what the children are watching. Television is a major influence on children: children in the United States watch an average of 28 hours of television per week. Teaching about values and health, which is ideally supplied by parents, is not always provided. Many of these parents expect, or at least hope, that moral and health teaching will be supplied by schools and churches.

Nader's model also focuses on the close connection between children's health and their educational achievement: when health is deficient, education is hindered. That is why the school nurse is vitally important.

School Health-Care Services

One of the primary goals of school nurses is to keep children well so they can focus on their education instead of being distracted and sidelined by illnesses. "The Nurse Speaks" in this chapter discusses how careful planning by a school nurse enabled a boy with labile diabetes to avoid frequent hypoglycemic or hyperglycemic crises. Often the school nurse assumes the role of case manager, as this situation demonstrates.

School nursing service is challenging because today many children in regular classrooms are medically fragile. The nurse must administer medications to and monitor children with disorders such as attention deficit disorder, seizure disorders, asthma, diabetes, and upper respiratory infections. Federal law mandates that children with disabilities must be offered free and appropriate education in the least restrictive environment. Many children who previously would have been taught at home or in special education classes are now mainstreamed into regular classrooms. "The Nurse Speaks" case study in Chapter 15 is based on the true story of an adolescent quadriplegic who attends school regularly despite being ventilator-dependent with a tracheostomy. Of course, school nurses are involved with special education programs, as well as children in regular classrooms. One of their functions is to maintain the rights of the disabled.

Challenges Presented by Society's Problems

Accidents have surpassed infectious diseases as the leading childhood cause of death in the United States. Because of the escalating violence of our society, homicide and suicide are the second and third leading causes of death among 15- to 19-year-olds. Teen homicides increased by 74% from 1985 to 1990 in the United States. Adolescents have a mortality rate 2.5 times higher than that of younger children (USDHHS, 1993a) (Fig. 8-2).

Drug abuse among children is again on the increase, according to a 1996 federal report (see Figure 10-4), with alcohol and potent marijuana being the most widely abused substances. Other social problems include adolescent pregnancy (although the rate is dropping), sexually transmitted diseases, HIV infection, eating disorders, and suicide attempts. These problems are no longer limited to high school and college

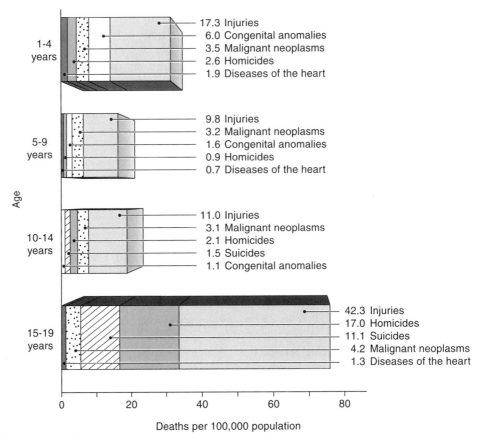

FIGURE 8-2
Leading causes of childhood deaths by age groups: 1990. (Adapted from USDHHS [1993]. *Child Health USA '92.* Washington DC: U.S. Government Printing Office.)

populations: nurses working in middle and even primary schools are seeing these problems and developing programs to deal with them.

Nurses must watch for and report signs of child abuse. This is not an easy problem to identify and deal with because abused children tend to protect the abusing parent or caretaker. Many children feel deep guilt and think the abuse is their own fault, so they are not ready to admit it occurs. School nurses must be alert to subtle signs of abuse (Display 8-1). They must also be proactive and deal with potential abuse and neglect.

Children from dysfunctional families often act out in school. These behaviors require careful assessment, analysis, and intervention or referral without delay. These angry, needy children require professional attention and limit setting, not punishment. Parents need to be referred for family therapy. Programs to promote emotional wellness are included in school nurses' health education programs.

Because of divorce and family breakdowns, many children live in single-parent fami-

DISPLAY 8-1
Indicators of Actual or Potential Abuse

1. An unexplained injury
   a. Skin: burns, old or recent scars, ecchymosis, soft tissue swelling, human bites
   b. Fractures: recent or ones that have healed
   c. Subdural hematomas
   d. Trauma to genitalia
   e. Whiplash (caused by shaking small children)
2. Dehydration or malnourishment without obvious cause
3. Provision of inappropriate food or drugs (alcohol, tobacco, medication prescribed for someone else, foods not appropriate for the child's age)
4. Evidence of general poor care: poor hygiene, dirty clothes, unkempt hair, dirty nails
5. Unusually fearful of nurse and others
6. Considered to be a "bad" child
7. Inappropriately dressed for the season or weather conditions
8. Reports or shows evidence of sexual abuse
9. Injuries not mentioned in history
10. Seems to need to take care of the parent and speak for the parent
11. Maternal depression
12. Maladjustment of older siblings

(Campbell J, Landenburger K [1996]. Violence and human abuse. In Stanhope B, Lancaster J, eds. Community Health Nursing. St. Louis: Mosby.)

lies. Single parents who are working sometimes send sick children to school or are not readily available to pick up sick children at school and take them home. Missing work frequently means putting a much-needed job in jeopardy. A job change by the parent may result in a transfer to a new school for the children. Health problems are more common in children who move a great deal. School nurses find it difficult to monitor and provide adequate care to these children; they cannot adequately assess them and develop a plan of care that fits their needs.

The School Nurse as Educator and Counselor

A great deal of informal health teaching occurs on a one-to-one basis when children come to the nurse's office with a health problem. Students are more apt to talk spontaneously with a nurse than to go see a counselor. Often they come to see the nurse with some minor, innocuous question as an excuse to talk. Then, if they sense an empathetic listener, they share some of their deep anxieties and problems. School nurses must learn when they should simply listen, when they can provide appropriate counseling, and when a referral for further counseling is required.

School nurses also teach health classes on a multitude of subjects and supply classroom teachers with health information to use in the classroom. Another important part of their job is to plan the health curriculum.

Sex Education in the School

Children need to know about themselves, how their bodies function, how to keep themselves healthy, and how to seek help from the health-care system. Healthy principles must be instilled, and children need to be guided toward healthy behaviors that will stay with them throughout their lives. If information about sex is not presented at school, beginning at an early age, children are apt to receive inaccurate information from "the street" or their peers.

Sex education in the schools remains a controversial subject in some communities. Many parents and community leaders are horrified at the idea of children being taught about condoms in junior high and elementary school. They believe that such knowledge encourages sexual activity and promiscuity, or they believe that sex education should be done by families and churches in a moral and spiritual context. In an ideal world, all parents would take on this important responsibility. In an ideal world, such information would not be needed until children approach adulthood. But this is not an ideal world; the high rates of pregnancy and sexually transmitted diseases in teens attest to this. Surveys indicate that by age 16, most adolescents are sexually active. The first experience is usually unprotected, making them vulnerable to pregnancy and HIV or other sexually transmitted diseases.

Immunizations and Health Records

Children are supposed to have up-to-date immunizations and a physician's or nurse practitioner's signed form attesting to their health and completed immunization status before starting school. Many school nurses complain that this is not enforced. Says one school nurse

> A lot of kids just show up on the bus, no parents, no health records! The children can't give their medical history. Phones are disconnected; messages to parents are ignored. Parents are working two jobs or are single parents. They feel hassled when the nurse contacts them. This is a problem that puts nurses—and all the other children and teachers—in jeopardy in the event of an epidemic.

This illustrates the challenge nurses face in keeping good health and immunization records on children in today's mobile society. A good health record is essential to serve as a baseline when illnesses and accidents happen, even years later. Keeping current, accurate health records is a major responsibility of the school nurse, and it is not easy. Accurate and up-to-date health records with immunization compliance must be kept on all teachers and staff also.

Health Screenings

Routine health screening programs are another important function of a school nurse. Speech, hearing, and vision screening and needed follow-up should be initiated as early as possible to prevent the child from feeling self-conscious and being teasing by other children. The earlier that corrective measures are instituted, the less time that the child's self-esteem and education are at risk. Dental screening is very important. The teeth of poor children are often badly neglected. Children need to be taught regular oral hygiene practices and the role of candy and other concentrated carbohydrates in promoting tooth decay. They need to be taught thorough handwashing and its vital importance in preventing the transmission of pathogens.

Screening programs for diseases such as tuberculosis are important, especially if someone at the school has converted from a negative to a positive PPD, indicating the presence of new, possibly contagious disease. Scoliosis screening is important for preadolescents.

Safeguarding the School Environment

School nurses are responsible for the safety and health of the school environment, monitoring for risks such as fires, lead poisoning, contaminated water, vermin, asbestos, toxic chemicals in science courses, unsafe playground equipment, and inadequate lighting. Plans for prevention or prompt correction of these problems are essential. Reliable infection control measures are part of this responsibility. Problems such as pediculosis, impetigo, and conjunctivitis are not rare, and children often come to school with them. Universal precautions regarding blood and body fluids are essential. Children with AIDS have the right to come to school and do not pose a threat to others if universal precautions are maintained.

Expanding Responsibilities

Teachers and other school personnel are not trained in health care and find it difficult to know how to care for the increasing number of disabled and chronically ill children in the classroom. School nurses have taken on the added role of educator to other school personnel. They also have responsibility for the health of teachers and staff and act as liaisons to community agencies in health matters.

School-Based Health Centers

Some communities have learned that school-based health centers are useful ways to provide primary health services. There are several hundred across the United States, and this number is expected to grow because these centers provide easy access to primary health care for children and are cost-effective. The centers are staffed by school nurse practitioners in addition to registered nurses. In several states, these centers are expanding into family resource and service centers for comprehensive care of the whole family.

Credentials, Certifications, and Advanced Education for School Nurses

Many states, such as Massachusetts, require all newly hired school nurses to have at least a baccalaureate degree in nursing. Massachusetts also requires completion of a state certification program for all school nurses. Many states require certification. Given the many demanding responsibilities of school nurses, many nurses are striving to upgrade state qualifications for certification in states where it does not exist.

The increasingly complex role of the school nurse involves case management, curriculum development, and policy-making functions. These high-level responsibilities, as well as the complex social requirements of school nursing, lead some school nurses to feel that they need more education. One of their dilemmas is that they are financially unable to stop working to pursue advanced courses. Bachman (1995) has proposed the establishment of accessible programs that allow school nurses to receive advanced education while continuing to work. Certified practitioner roles for school nurses include school nurse practitioner, pediatric nurse practitioner, family nurse practitioner, and community health nurse specialist for schoolchildren. Some nurses pursue a second degree in school guidance and counseling, but this subject matter is now included in graduate nursing programs also.

School nurses who work in preschool settings or special education programs or at colleges and universities also seek additional education pertinent to their subspecialty. This includes courses such as early childhood development or extra training to implement the early and periodic screening, diagnosis, and treatment program sponsored by Medicaid programs around the country. Advanced education is helpful for screenings on the college level in areas such as contraception, pregnancy, sexually transmitted diseases, and emotional disorders.

Goals for the 21st Century

Healthy People 2000 established many goals involving school health in the United States (Display 8-2). A midcourse review in 1995 showed that in some areas, there was movement in the right direction; some had even achieved 50% improvement by 1995. However, in other areas, there was movement in the wrong direction; note goals 13.2 and 13.12 in Figure 8-3.

In 1990, the National State Governors' Association (U.S. Department of Education, 1990) established goals for education for the year 2000 that are relevant to school nurses:

1. All children will start school ready to learn.
2. The high school graduation rate will increase to at least 90% for all groups.
3. All children will leave grades 4, 8, and 12 having demonstrated competency in challenging subject matter in English, mathematics, science, history, and geography.
4. U.S. students will be the first in the world in mathematics and science achievement.
5. Every student will be literate and possess the knowledge and skills necessary to compete in a global economy and to exercise the rights and responsibilities of citizenship.
6. Every school in America will be free of drugs and violence and will offer a disciplined environment conducive to learning.

In his State of the Union address in 1997, President Clinton declared that improvement in educational achievement and school environments was the priority goal of his administration into the 21st century. Thus, the role of the school nurse will take on even greater importance in the future.

DISPLAY 8-2

National Health Objectives Related to School Health

By the year 2000:

1. Increase to at least 50% the proportion of children in grades 1 to 12 who participate in daily physical education activities at school.

2. Increase to at least 90% the proportion of school lunch and breakfast programs with menus consistent with nutritional principles contained in Dietary Guidelines for Americans.

3. Increase to at least 75% the proportion of the nation's schools that provide nutrition education from preschool through twelfth grade.

4. Include tobacco-use prevention in the curricula of all elementary, middle, and secondary schools.

5. Provide children in all primary and secondary schools with educational programs on alcohol and other drugs.

6. Increase to at least 85% the proportion of people 10 to 18 years of age who have discussed human sexuality with their parents or received information from parentally endorsed sources, such as schools.

7. Increase to at least 50% the proportion of elementary and secondary schools that teach nonviolent conflict-resolution skills.

8. Provide academic instruction on injury prevention and control in at least 50% of public school systems.

9. Increase to at least 95% the proportion of schools that have age-appropriate HIV education curricula for children in grades 4 to 12.

10. Include in all middle and secondary schools instruction on preventing sexually transmitted diseases.

(Healthy People 2000: National Health Promotion and Disease Prevention Objectives. *Washington DC, 1991, USDHHS Public Health Service.*)

Occupational Health Nursing

Occupational health nursing has the same three basic components as school nursing: nursing service, health education, and maintenance of a safe, healthy environment. The goal is to maintain the optimal wellness of the employees, similar to school nursing.

Nursing service includes direct care such as first aid and care of minor illnesses and emergencies. Periodic health assessments are performed, including preemployment examinations. Other scheduled screening examinations may include mammograms and blood pressure and cholesterol tests. Nurses evaluate when employees can return to work after injuries or illness and process worker's compensation claims. Employee assistance programs offer confidential counseling for a variety of problems. The nurse's health education role includes offering individual teaching and formal classes about the health risks that exist both on and off the job. Lunch-hour walks or other exercise

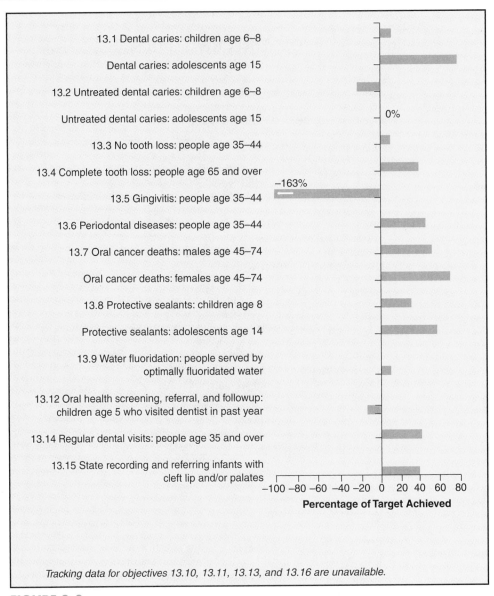

FIGURE 8-3
Status of oral health objectives. (Source: National Institutes of Health, Centers for Disease Control and Prevention.)

activities are often scheduled. Environmental surveillance programs usually include collaborative efforts with safety officers and other members of the occupational work team. Occupational nurses need to keep abreast of all complex health issues (Display 8-3).

DISPLAY 8-3
Scope of Services Provided Through an Occupational Health and Safety Program

Health assessments
  Replacement
  Periodic: mandatory, voluntary
  Transfer
  Retirement/termination
  Executive
  Health risk appraisal
Preventive health screening with education
Employee assistance programs
Lifestyle classes: smoking cessation, weight control, stress management, physical fitness, and conditioning
Rehabilitation
Treatment of illness and injury
Primary health care for workers and dependents
Fitting of protective equipment
Worker safety and health education related to occupational hazards
Job analysis and design
Prenatal and postnatal care and support groups
Medical self-help and consumerism classes
Safety audits and accident investigation
Plant surveys and environmental monitoring
Workers' compensation and processing of OSHA claims and reports
Health-related cost-containment strategies, such as medical care, utilization review, case management, and advice on benefit use
Risk management, loss control
Emergency preparedness
Preretirement counseling

(Stanhope M, Lancaster J [1996]. Community Health Nursing. *St. Louis: Mosby.)*

Future expectations for the profession (Lusk et al, 1990) include analyzing trends in health promotion, risk management, and expenditures and conducting research to determine more efficient, cost-effective alternative operations. "Produce, produce, produce, as inexpensively as possible. That's the name of the game today," says one occupational health nurse.

History of Occupational Health Nursing

Occupational nursing has come a long way, as has the quality of life for workers. In the middle of the 19th century, almost 50% of all New England's full-time factory workers were children ages 7 to 16. Massachusetts enacted a child labor law in 1836, the first state to do so (Felton, 1976). Unsafe and unhealthy conditions characterized workplaces throughout the nation. The working conditions of slaves in the South varied, depending on the cruelty or benevolence of their owners. Years ahead of its time, the Vermont Marble Company provided many worker benefits, and in 1895 it hired Ada Mayo Stewart, the first industrial health nurse in the United States. The John Wanamaker Company in New York hired Anna B. Duncan in 1897, and the specialty of industrial (occupational) nursing was born (Pinkham, 1988).

The first major report on occupational safety was issued in 1903 by the federal government (U.S. Department of Labor, 1977). This report and the work of Alice Hamilton, M.D., spearheaded the public's awareness of the hazards and diseases that workers were subject to at that time. Dr. Hamilton, known as the founder of occupational medicine in this country, devoted her long, remarkable life to improving the health of America's workers.

In 1911, New Jersey passed a Workmen's Compensation Act to cover the medical expenses of workers injured on the job; it was the first state to do so. Not until 1948 did all states enact workmen's compensation legislation. The Social Security Act of 1935 helped give workers security through programs such as unemployment insurance and old age benefits (McGrawth, 1945). In 1970, the Occupational Health and Safety Act became law and the Occupational Safety and Health Administration (OSHA) and the National Institute for Occupational Safety and Health (NIOSH) were born. OSHA sets policies; NIOSH identifies and researches safety and health hazards (Display 8-4). Other significant legislation includes the Americans With Disabilities Act of 1990 and the Family Leave Act of 1993. The former law protects the rights of disabled workers; the

DISPLAY 8-4
Functions of Federal Agencies Involved in Occupational Health and Safety

OSHA

Determine and set standards for hazardous exposures in the workplace.
Enforce the occupational health standards (including the right of entry for inspection).
Educate employers about occupational health and safety.
Develop and maintain a database of work-related injuries, illnesses, and deaths.
Monitor compliance with occupational health and safety standards.

NIOSH

Conduct research and review of research findings to recommend permissible exposure levels for occupational hazards to OSHA.
Identify and research occupational health and safety hazards.
Educate occupational health and safety professionals.
Distribute research findings relevant to occupational health and safety.

(Stanhope M, Lancaster J [1996]. Community Health Nursing. *St. Louis: Mosby.)*

latter protects the jobs of workers who must care for a sick family member (unpaid leave for up to 12 weeks is allowed).

Objectives of Occupational Health Nursing

Healthy People 2000 cited occupational health as a priority area, and the 1995 midcourse review of those goals shows variable progress. Excellent progress was achieved in two areas: hepatitis B infections among occupationally exposed workers have been reduced, and the number of states with occupational lung disease exposure standards has increased. See Figure 8-4 and Display 8-5 for the status of other goals, including the poor showing for trauma and skin disorders.

Today, employers and workers alike recognize that healthy, satisfied workers are the most productive and therefore the most cost-effective. This is why occupational health nurses work so hard to prevent disease and injury and keep workers on the job. Most work-related illnesses and injuries are preventable. Categories of causa-

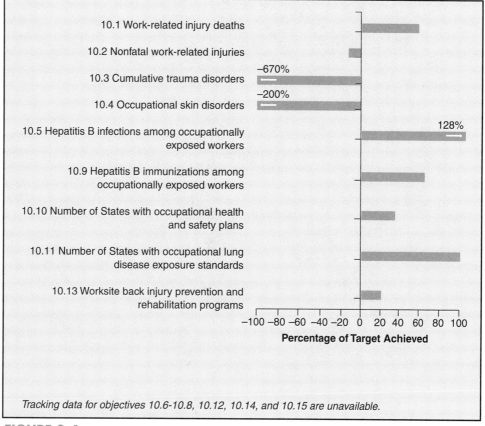

Tracking data for objectives 10.6-10.8, 10.12, 10.14, and 10.15 are unavailable.

FIGURE 8-4
Status of occupational safety and health objectives. (Source: Centers for Disease Control and Prevention.)

DISPLAY 8-5

Occupational Safety and Health: *Healthy People 2000* Objectives

HEALTH STATUS OBJECTIVES

1. Reduce deaths from work-related injuries to no more than 4 per 100,000 full-time workers.
2. Reduce work-related injuries resulting in medical treatment, lost time from work, or restricted work activity to no more than 6 cases per 100 full-time workers.
3. Reduce cumulative trauma disorders to an incidence of no more than 60 cases per 100,000 full-time workers.
4. Reduce occupational skin disorders or diseases to an incidence of no more than 55 per 100,000 full-time workers.
5. Reduce hepatitis B infections among occupational exposed workers to an incidence of no more than 1,250 cases.

RISK REDUCTION OBJECTIVES

6. Increase to at least 75% the proportion of worksites with 50 or more employees that mandate employee use of occupant protection systems, such as seat belts, during all work-related motor vehicle travel.
7. Reduce to no more than 15% the proportion of workers exposed to average daily noise levels that exceed 85 dBA.
8. Eliminate exposures that result in workers having blood lead concentrations greater than 25 ug/dl of whole blood.
9. Increase hepatitis B immunization levels of 90% among occupationally exposed workers.

SERVICES AND PROTECTION OBJECTIVES

10. Implement occupational safety and health plans in 50 states for the identification, management, and prevention of leading work-related diseases and injuries within the state.
11. Establish in 50 states exposure standards adequate to prevent the major occupational lung diseases to which their worker populations are exposed (Byssinosis, asbestosis, coal workers' pneumoconiosis, and silicosis).
12. Increase to at least 70% the proportion of worksites with 50 or more employees that have implemented programs on worker health and safety.
13. Increase to at least 50% the proportion of worksites with 50 or more employees that offer back injury prevention and rehabilitation programs.
14. Establish in 50 states either public health or labor department programs that provide consultation and assistance to small businesses to implement safety and health programs for their employees.
15. Increase to at least 75% the proportion of primary care providers who routinely elicit occupational health exposures as a part of patient history and provide relevant counseling.

(USDHHS [1991]. Healthy People 2000: Health Promotion and Disease Prevention Objectives for the Nation, *full report, with commentary. Washington DC: U.S. Government Printing Office.)*

tive agents include:

1. Biologic: Bacteria, fungi, insects, molds, parasites, animals, plants, raw sewage, contaminated water and foods
2. Chemical: Fumes, dusts, gases, liquids, vapors, particles, mists, solvents, lead
3. Ergonomic: Fatigue, monotony, boredom, poor work flow, unrealistic standards, confusing or unjust leadership, low pay, crowded space, ethical dilemmas
4. Physical: Noise, heat, cold, pressure, vibration, radiation (electromagnetic and ionizing)

Table 8-1 lists the 10 leading work-related diseases and illnesses in the United States, according to the Centers for Disease Control and Prevention (CDC). Carcinogenic industrial substances and their related cancers, as identified by the CDC, are listed in Table 8-2.

Occupational nursing staffs vary with the employer and the number of employees being served (Display 8-6). One pharmaceutical and chemical research facility with 3,000 employees has five full-time-equivalent nurses, but most facilities have only one nurse. Many small businesses contract with outside health agencies for occupational health services; this seems to be a trend. One such agency lists the following services: asbestos physicals, audiology, back assessments, back-to-work evaluations, electrocardiography, fitness-for-duty physicals, NIOSH physicals, immunizations, laboratory analysis, mammography, medical review officer services, muscle and nerve conduction studies, drug and alcohol screening, orthopedic consultations, physical therapy, preemployment physicals, preplacement physicals, specialist referrals, spine evaluations, spirometry, stress tests, surgery, VIP corporate physicals, and X-rays.

TABLE 8-1. The 10 Leading Work-Related Diseases and Injuries—United States

Diseases/Conditions	Examples
1. Occupational lung diseases	Asbestosis, byssinosis, silicosis, coal workers' pneumoconiosis, lung cancer, occupational asthma
2. Musculoskeletal injuries	Disorders of the back, trunk, upper extremity, neck, lower extremity; traumatically induced Raynaud's phenomenon
3. Occupational cancers (other than lung)	Leukemia, mesothelioma; cancers of the bladder, nose, and liver
4. Traumatic injury and death	Amputations, fractures, eye loss, lacerations
5. Cardiovascular diseases	Hypertension, coronary artery disease, acute myocardial infarction
6. Disorders of reproduction	Infertility, spontaneous abortion, teratogenesis
7. Neurotoxic disorders	Peripheral neuropathy, toxic encephalitis, psychoses, extreme personality changes (exposure-related)
8. Loss of hearing	Noise-induced hearing loss
9. Dermatologic conditions	Dermatoses, burns (scaldings), chemical burns, contusions (abrasions)
10. Psychological disorders	Neuroses, personality disorders, alcoholism, drug dependency, stress reactions

(CDC [1983]. Leading work-related diseases and injuries. *MMWR*, Jan. 21; and USDHHS. *Healthy People 2000* [1991]. Washington DC: U.S. Govt. Printing Office.)

TABLE 8-2. Occupational Carcinogens

Carcinogen	Cancer Site	Examples of Exposed Occupations
4-Aminodiphenyl Auramine B-naphthylamine Magenta Benzidine	Bladder	Dye manufacturing, rubber manufacturing
Arsenic	Skin, lung, liver	Metal smelting, arsenic pesticide production, metal alloy workers
Asbestos	Lung, mesothelium, gastrointestinal tract	Asbestos miners, insulators, shipyard workers
Benzene	Leukemia (blood-forming organs)	Petrochemical workers, chemists
Bischloromethyl ether (BCME)	Lung	Organic chemical synthesizers
Cadmium	Prostate	Cadmium alloy workers, welders
Chromium/Chromates	Lung, nasal sinuses	Chromate producers, metal workers
Coke oven emissions	Lung, kidney	Coke oven workers
Foundry emissions	Lung	Foundry workers
Leather dust	Nasal cavity, nasal sinuses, bladder	Shoe manufacturing
Nickel	Lung, nasal passages	Nickel smelting, metal workers
Radiation (x-rays)	Leukemia (blood-forming organs), skin, breast, thyroid, bone	Radiologists, industrial radiographers, atomic energy workers
Radon gas	Lung	Uranium and feldspar miners
Soots, tars, and oil (aromatic hydrocarbons)	Skin, lung, bladder, scrotum	Roofers, chimney sweeps, petroleum workers, shale oil workers
Ultraviolet light	Skin	Outdoor workers
Vinyl chloride	Liver, brain, lung	Polyvinyl chloride synthesizers, rubber workers
Welding fumes	Lung	Welders
Wood dust	Nasal passages	Hardwood workers, furniture makers

(Blumenthal, D., Rutenber, J. [1994]. *Introduction to Environmental Health,* 2nd ed. New York: Springer.)

Occupational Health Services of New Mexico, an example of such an agency, is a specialist company that provides occupational health services to more than 3,000 businesses around the state using many satellite centers. The company employs many occupational health nurses and claims high efficiency and cost-effectiveness.

THE NURSE SPEAKS . . .
About School Nursing

In the third grade, Ryan transferred to the elementary school where I work. I received a rather sketchy report about him—that he had diabetes mellitus and seizures and had required several

---

DISPLAY 8-6

Staffing Recommendations for an Effective Occupational Health Nursing Program

- One occupational health nurse for up to 300 employees in an industrial setting and up to 750 in a nonindustrial setting
- Two or more occupational health nurses for up to 600 industrial employees
- Three or more occupational health nurses for up to 1,000 employees in an industrial setting

- One occupational health nurse for each additional 1,000 employees in either setting
NOTE: Larger and more hazardous occupational settings require more nursing personnel. Smaller organizations can implement an effective program with part-time nursing services.

(American Association for Occupational Health Nurses [1991]. Occupational Health Nursing: The Answer to Health Care Cost Containment. Atlanta: The Association.)

---

trips to the emergency room by ambulance. I met with Ryan's mother, who is a single parent and works full-time. She explained that Ryan is a brittle diabetic and is prone to frequent "insulin reactions." Sometimes he has seizures with these reactions; the doctor is not sure whether he has a separate seizure disorder or if the seizures are caused by the hypoglycemia. She added that they moved because she had to take so many days off work to care for him that she lost her previous job.

I immediately knew that my first goal would be to prevent those emergency episodes. They are emotionally damaging to children and terribly disruptive to their educational process. A school nurse's primary goal is to keep children at optimal wellness so they can attend school and attend *to* school.

I conferred with Ryan's endocrinologist and set up a plan for better control of his diabetes. I ordered glucagon and a glucometer for the school and trained other personnel how to use them if I am away or unavailable. I taught his teacher the signs and symptoms of high and low blood sugar. With Ryan, we developed a schedule for him to measure his blood sugar before lunch and before gym class, when extra activity might cause hypoglycemia. Ryan learned to do his own blood sugar testing and write the results on a chart, with my supervision. I gave him extra regular insulin as needed and began teaching him how to administer it. I kept orange juice and sugar tablets all around the school for quick access—in the classroom, the playground, the gym. I prepared a teaching plan about diabetes for his peers, which Ryan and I presented together in the classroom. I also ordered books for the school library so children could read about diabetes, seizure disorders, and other chronic conditions.

School field trips presented a very big challenge. The key to juvenile diabetes management is a good balance of insulin, food, and exercise, and this is easier to plan with a regular, predictable schedule. I discussed the uncertainty of field trip activities and timetables with his mother and tried to get her to go along whenever she could. I made up a "field trip bag" of emergency supplies and trained the bus drivers to be sure to keep the supplies in the bus at all times.

On days when extra activity was planned, I had Ryan's mother give him less insulin before school, and we always took his blood sugar just before leaving school. At a meeting with Ryan's teachers, we decided to do a blood sugar measurement just before all major examinations and give treatment as needed so that Ryan could do his best on examinations. This was also done for school plays and sports contests in which Ryan participated.

Another challenge was that this 8-year-old was a latchkey child who went home to an empty house. His mother always had a snack waiting for him. She arranged for a neighbor to check on him and to be available if he needed her. He also carried his mother's work phone number with him at all times.

I'm proud to say that in the 2 years since we started the program, he has had no seizures or hypoglycemic crises. At times his blood sugar dipped very low, but it was discovered and treated immediately. Ryan has performed well in school and is very popular with his peers, who seem to understand and accept his disease. By age 10, Ryan and his mother have become very knowledgeable about how to manage his disease.

Louise
SCHOOL HEALTH NURSE

CLINICAL APPLICATION

A Critical Thinking Case Study About Occupational Nursing

As an occupational health nurse, your goal is to maintain your workers at their optimal level of wellness. However, sometimes accidents happen on the job, regardless of strong preventive measures. When that happens, you must have policies in place to deal with emergencies and to protect coworkers should bleeding occur. Sometimes the accidents are extremely traumatic, such as the amputation of a body part. What is your responsibility to the client and coworkers in that instance?

 and Think!

- What policies should be in place ahead of time?
- What legal guidelines should be followed?
- What procedures are necessary to protect coworkers from blood-borne pathogens?
- What specific follow-up is important for coworkers?

You develop an emergency policy based on OSHA and NIOSH regulations. All workers are trained in the emergency policy, and it is posted throughout the building. It indicates priority life-saving measures such as maintenance of an open airway and basic life support. It indicates when to call the occupational health nurse and when to call 911 for an ambulance. It requires universal precautions when handling, or potentially handling, blood and body fluids. Latex gloves are readily available to workers.

Once the emergency is handled, or the injured worker has been sent to the hospital, the coworkers who witnessed or were involved in helping during the accident must be considered. Counseling is needed to prevent posttraumatic stress disorder. Listen and talk with the coworkers, tell them about the need for counseling after a traumatic event, and describe the employee assistance program at your company.

Frank, a 61-year-old employee, sustained a crushing injury to his right thumb. He is brought to your office by coworkers. You know that Frank has a history of moderately severe diabetes mellitus and hypertension. He also has borderline cardiac disease.

 and Think!

- What will you do first?
- How will you fix his thumb?
- Can you handle his care in your office?
- What do you need to do about his other health problems?

Using aseptic technique, you dress Frank's hand and pack it in ice and call an ambulance to take him to the emergency room of the general hospital nearby that is associated with your company's health maintenance organization. Frank should travel by ambulance because this is company policy and because his other medical problems could be exacerbated by the trauma. Ambulances are equipped to deal with emergencies en route. While awaiting the ambulance, you take Frank's vital signs and do a fingerstick to test his blood sugar with your glucometer. You speak calmly with Frank. You realize that he will probably need surgery to amputate the rest of his thumb. You call the hospital emergency room to communicate your observations about his traumatized hand, his vital signs and blood sugar, and his medical history. You also call his wife.

 and Think!

- What complications might you expect after the amputation of Frank's right thumb?
- What kind of therapy will he need?
- Do you think he will be able to work again? If not, where will he find income on which to live?

Frank's hand heals very slowly because of his diabetes. Fortunately, his wound does not become infected, which sometimes happens with a crushing injury such as his, especially when dirty, greasy machinery is involved. For several weeks he experiences phantom pain in his amputated thumb. When adequate healing takes place, the surgeon orders occupational therapy for his right hand. Frank has no grasp in his right hand. He has spasms along with the phantom pain. It is generally assumed that Frank will be unable to work anymore. He will be eligible for disability payments each month until his pension begins at age 65.

You continue to call Frank and his wife regularly. On several occasions, Frank mumbles, "I'm useless." His wife reports that he is depressed and not sleeping or eating well. She explains that he never had hobbies or interests outside of work and adds that he enjoyed working and took pride in being the family breadwinner.

"His job was his life," she says. "Now he just sits and stares out the back window or complains because he can't work."

 and Think!

- Would referring Frank to a psychiatrist for antidepressant medication solve his problem?
- Do you think there is some way Frank could return to work?

Frank is so motivated to work that you decide to confer with his doctor, the manager of his department, and the claims adjuster of his disability insurance to be sure that his insurance will not be jeopardized if Frank attempts a trial period back at work. All agree to try your plan if you will coordinate it and if Frank can pass a functional capacity assessment to be done by a consulting physical therapy group. That group advises that Frank needs a work-hardening program before he can return to a productive work assignment. Again, you work out a plan with Frank's full involvement. You arrange for a temporary workplace with physical therapy where he goes through various motions, learning to reuse his hand and learning to deal with the pain. You ask his manager to have him do some undemanding office work for 2.5 days a week while he attends the work-hardening program the rest of the week at the physical therapy facility. You set 6 weeks as a goal and then plan to reevaluate his status.

Frank is very motivated, and his depression lifts. Suddenly, however, the situation changes when he stops by your office to be checked and you discover that his blood pressure is elevated and his pulse is erratic.

 and Think!

- What should you do, if anything?
- Because Frank is doing so well otherwise, do you really need to report this to anyone?
- This could jeopardize the plan you so carefully devised. So many people have worked hard to make this plan work for Frank. Should you wait a few days and check again?

Frank's total health is the issue, not just his hand. At risk to your current plan, you must report and record this latest development; to do otherwise would be unethical. You call his cardiologist, who sees him the same afternoon, changes his medications, and says that Frank should stay home. Within 6 weeks, the cardiologist determines that Frank can return to work on a light schedule of duty.

Wearing gloves constantly, Frank gradually reaches full work capacity and is extremely pleased with himself. You're proud of him and yourself, too! You advocated for him and engaged the cooperation of his manager, who worked with you at each step of Frank's progression. You secured the cooperation and help of Frank's doctors. Most of all, you helped Frank regain his self-confidence and sense of usefulness.

 and Think!

- What problems do you anticipate for Frank?
- What can you do to help him be proactive about them?

In just 4 years, Frank will reach retirement age. You encourage him to participate in some of the preretirement seminars you schedule as part of your employee education program. He needs to prepare now for the day when his job no longer fills his time and his life. Frank needs to develop hobbies and interests to avoid another episode of psychological trauma and depression. Now he has the time and self-confidence to do that.

(Note: "Frank" is a real person, and his story was reported by a real occupational health nurse. She added that Frank never missed a day's work from the time he resumed full employment).

Chapter SUMMARY

The three traditional components of school health nursing are nursing service, health education, and maintenance of a safe, healthy school environment. Contemporary challenges to school nurses include children of single working parents or children from dysfunctional families. Many children are on medications for chronic disorders, and children with disabilities are mainstreamed whenever possible. These children need the school nurse's close monitoring. Other societal and family problems that affect schoolchildren include escalating violence, drug use, sexually transmitted diseases, and HIV infections. Up-to-date immunization records are difficult to keep because of the problems of contacting some parents. School nurses also function as health educators and counselors, both for children and staff. They hold screening programs and constantly monitor the school environment for safety. Educational requirements for school nurses are expanding in some states, and many school nurses are seeking certifications and advanced degrees.

Occupational health nursing has the same three basic components as school nursing. These nurses provide first aid and treat minor illnesses and emergencies. They do frequent screening programs, including physical examinations, and make referrals to appropriate sources of care. Health education and environmental surveillance programs occupy much of their time. Occupational health nurses work closely with the NIOSH to maintain OSHA standards in the workplace.

A list of references and additional readings for this chapter appears at the end of Part 2.

PART 2

References and Additional Readings

AARP (1996). Physical activity—it's never too late! *Perspectives in Health Promotion and Aging*, vol. 2. November, pp. 1–5.

Achterberg J et al (1994). *Rituals of Healing: Using Imagery for Health and Wellness*. New York: Bantam Books.

Ackley B, Ladwig G (1995). *Nursing Diagnosis Handbook: A Guide to Planning Care*. St. Louis: Mosby.

Adair J, Adair M (1994). *Living in the Bubble: The Model for Wellness and Wellbeing*. Gaitlinburg, TN: The Mountainbrook Foundation.

Adams J et al (1995). Primary care at the worksite: The use of health risk appraisal in a nursing center. *AAOHN J* 43(1):17–22.

Agee B (1996). How to write clear instructions. *RN* 59(11):26–31.

American Association of Occupational Health Nurses (1994). *Standards of Occupational Health Nursing Practice*. Atlanta: The Association.

American Heart Association (1996). *Heart and Stroke Facts: 1996 Statistical Supplement*. Dallas: AHA National Center.

American Nurses Association (1992). *Expanding School Health Services to Serve Families in the 21st Century*. Washington DC: The Association.

Anderson E, McFarlane J (1996). *Community as Partner*, 2d ed. Philadelphia: Lippincott-Raven.

Arnold J (1996). Nursing implications for health promotion. *Home Healthcare Nurse* 14(10):777–783.

Arnold J (1996). Rethinking grief: Nursing implications for health promotion. *Home Healthcare Nurse* 14(10):777–783.

Bachman J (1995). A need for school nurse education. *Journal of School Nursing* 11(3):20–23.

Bailey L (1994). Confined space: Occupational health hazards. *AAOHN J* 42(4):182–188.

Balakas K, Schappe A. (1995). Well baby assessment. *Home Healthcare Nurse* 13(5):82–84.

Bandura A (1997). Self-efficacy. *The Harvard Mental Health Letter,* 13(9):4–6.

Barnes L (1996). Patient teaching: Multidisciplinary time-based protocols. *MCN* 21(4):177.

Barratt A et al (1994). Worksite cholesterol screening and dietary intervention: The staff healthy heart project, steering committee. *Am J Public Health* 84(5):779–782.

Bauer T, Barron C. (1995). Nursing interventions for spiritual care: Preferences of community-based elderly. *J Holistic Nursing* 13(3):268–279.

Bellows J, Rudolph L (1993). The initial impact of a workplace lead poisoning project. *Am J Public Health* 83(3):406–410.

Bender J et al. *Congregational Wellness Manual*. Goshen, Indiana: Mennonite Mutual Aid.

Beneson A. (1995). *Control of Communicable Diseases Manual*, 16th ed. Washington DC: American Public Health Association.

Berggren-Thomas P, Griggs M (1995). Spirituality in aging: Spiritual need or spiritual journey? *J Gerontological Nursing* 21:5–10.

Bernstein L, Bernstein R (1980). *Interviewing: A Guide for Health Professionals*. New York: Appleton-Century-Crofts.

Bielenson PL et al (1995). Politics and practice: Introducing Norplant into a school-based health center in Baltimore. *Am J Public Health* 85(3):309–311.

Bradley J, Edinberg M (1982). *Communication in the Nursing Context*. Norwalk, CT: Appleton-Century-Crofts.

Bragg M (1997). An empowerment approach to community health education. In Spradley B, Allender J. *Readings in Community Health Nursing*, 5th ed. Philadelphia: JB Lippincott.

Braun I (1996). Varicella zoster virus: Trends and treatment. *MCN* 21(4):187–190.

Bromberger J, Matthews K (1994). Employment status and depressive symptoms in middle-aged women. *Am J Public Health* 84:202–206.

Burrell LO (1997). *Adult Nursing: Acute and Community Care.* Stamford, CT: Appleton & Lange.

Callahan E (1994). Quality in occupational health care: Management's view. *J Occup Med* 36(4):410–413.

Campbell J, Landenburger K (1995). Violence and human abuse. In Stanhope M, Lancaster J, eds. *Community Health Nursing.* St. Louis: Mosby.

Canobbio M (1996). *Mosby's Handbook of Patient Teaching.* St. Louis: Mosby.

Carlson L (1995). The next step: Creating healthier communities. *Healthcare Forum Journal* May–June, pp. 14–18.

CDC (1993). *HIV/AIDS Surveillance Report,* 1st quarter ed. Atlanta: CDC.

CDC (March 9, 1984). Leading work-related diseases and injuries. *MMWR.*

CDC (1993). *The Prevention of Youth Violence.* National Center for Injury Prevention and Control. Atlanta: CDC.

Clark C (1996). *Wellness Practitioner,* 2d ed. New York: Springer.

Clemen-Stone S et al (1995). *Comprehensive Community Health Nursing.* St. Louis: Mosby.

Clinebell H (1995). *Counseling for Spiritually Empowered Wellness. A Hope-Centered Approach.* New York: The Haworth Pastoral Press.

Consumers Union (1996). Facing our fears: Risks, health & environment. *Consumer Reports* 61(12):50–53.

Consumers Union (1996). Weight control: Do diet pills work? *Consumer Reports* 61(8):15–17.

Djupe A et al (1994). *Reaching Out: Parish Nursing Service, An Institutional/Congregational Partnership.* Park Ridge, IL: Parish Nurse Resource Center.

Doheny M et al (1997). *The Discipline of Nursing.* Stamford, CT: Appleton & Lange.

Donnelly E (1993). Health promotion, families, and the diagnostic process. In Wegner, Alexander, eds. *Readings in Family Nursing.* Philadelphia: JB Lippincott.

Dossey B (1996). Help your patient break free of anxiety. *Nursing '96* 26(10):52–54.

Dossey L (1993). *Healing Words: The Power of Prayer and the Practice of Medicine.* San Francisco: Harper.

Drury-Zemke L (1997). Mutual support groups. In Sprad-ley B, Allender J, eds. *Readings in Community Health Nursing.* Philadelphia: JB Lippincott.

Dunkle R (1996). Parish nurses help patients—Body and soul. *RN* 59(5):55–57.

Eckler J (1996). About Immunizations. *Nursing '96* 26(10):60.

Editors (July, 1994a). The Nutrition Consortium.

Editors (July, 1994b). Hunger in New York State. *The Nutrition Consortium.* p. 12.

Editors (1995). How to achieve total wellness. *HEALTH EDCO,* Waco, TX: WRS, Inc.

Editors (1996). Dieting in America. *Nursing '96* 26(9):55–56.

Editors (1996). What you should know about chlamydia. *Nursing '96* 26(9):24f–24h.

Editors (1997). Diet Drugs: Redux weighs in. Health After 50. *Johns Hopkins Medical Letter* 9(1):1–2.

Felton LJ (1976). 200 years of occupational medicine in the U.S. *J Occup Med* 28:809–814.

Fitchett G (1993). *Assessing Spiritual Needs: A Guide for Caregivers.* Minneapolis: Augsburg Press.

Fitzpatrick J, Shinners M (1996). How to make assessing as easy as ABC. *Nursing '96* 26(8):51.

Forbes E (1994). Spirituality, aging, and community dwelling caregiver and care recipient. *Geriatric Nursing* 15(6):297–302.

Girgis A et al (1994). A workplace intervention for increasing outdoor workers' use of solar protection. *Am J Pub Health* 84(1):77–81.

Grajny AE, Christie D, Tichy AM et al (1993). Chemotherapy: How safe for the caregiver? *Home Health Nurse* 11(5):51–58.

Gray J (1996). Meeting psychosocial needs. *RN* 59(8):23–28.

Green T (1994). *Bright Futures: Guidelines for Health Supervision on Infants, Children And Adolescents.* Arlington, VA.: National Center for Education in Maternal and Child Health.

Haag AB, Glazner LK (1992). A remembrance of the past, an investment for the future. *AAOHN J* 409(2):56–60.

Health Care Resources (1996). *Handbook of High-Risk Perinatal Home Care.* St. Louis: Mosby.

Health: United States, 1995, USDHHS Pub N (PHS) 73-1232. Washington DC: USDHHS.

Hoffman C, Turner T (1994). Strategies for using university health services for cholesterol screening. *J Am Coll Health* 43(2):86–89.

Hopkins E et al (1995). *Working with groups on spiritual themes.* Duluth: Whole Person Associates.

Huber H, Spatz A (1994). *Homemaker/Home Health Aide,* 4th ed. Albany, NY: Delmar Publishers.

Humphrey C (1996). Public health and home care—Coming closer together? *Home Healthcare Nurse* 14(10):753.

Humphrey C, Milone-Nuzzo P (1996). Client teaching in the home. In *Manual of Home Care Nursing Orientation.* Gaithersburg, MD: Aspen.

Hunt R, Zurek E. (1997). *Community-Based Nursing.* Philadelphia: JB Lippincott.

Igoe JB, Giordano BP (1992). *Expanding School Health Services to Serve Families in the 21st Century.* Washington DC: American Nurses Publishing.

Igoe JB, Speer S (1996). Community health nurse in the school. In Stanhope B, Lancaster J, eds. *Community Health Nursing.* St. Louis: Mosby.

Irvine J. (1995). *Sexuality Education Across Cultures: Working With Differences.* San Francisco: Jossey-Bass.

Iverson D (1990). Comprehensive school health education programs. In Matarazzo et al. *Behavioral Health.* New York: John Wiley & Sons.

Jaffe M, Skidmore-Roth L (1997). Assessments. In *Home Health Nursing Care Plans,* pp. 1–49. St. Louis: Mosby.

Jeffrey RW et al (1993). The healthy worker project: A worksite intervention for weight control and smoking cessation. *Am J Public Health* 83(3): 395–401.

Kang R (1995). Building community capacity for health promotion: A challenge for public health nurses. *Public Health Nursing* 12(5):312–318.

Katz E et al (1994). Exposure assessment in epidemiologic studies of birth defects by industrial hygiene: Review of maternal interviews. *Am J Industrial Med* 26(1):1–11.

Kelly L, Joel L (1995). *Dimensions of Professional Nursing,* 7th ed. New York: McGraw-Hill.

Kelsey M (1995). *Healing and Christianity,* 3d ed. Minneapolis: Augsburg Press.

Kimball M (1995) *Religion, Spirituality and Aging: A Handbook.* Minneapolis: Fortress Press.

Kimbrough R et al (1995). Survey of lead exposure around a closed lead smelter. *Pediatrics* 95(4): 550–555.

King E, Cheatham D (1995). Health teaching for people with disabilities. *Home Healthcare Nurse* 13(6): 52–58.

King J, Striepe J (1990). *Wholistic Nursing Curriculum: Models for Parish Nursing Education and Nursing Practice.* Sioux City, Iowa: Northwest Aging Association.

Klinger C, Jones M (1994). The OSHA standard-setting process: Role of the occupational health nurse. *AAOHN J* 42(8):374–378.

Knollmueller R (1993). *Prevention Across the Life Span: Healthy People for the 21st Century.* American Nurses' Publishing.

Koenig H (1997). Use of religion by patients with severe medical illness. *Journal of Clinical Behavioral Medicine* 2(1):31–36.

Kristjanson L, Chalmers K (1993). Preventive work with families: Issues facing public health nurses. In Wegner, Alexander, eds. *Readings in Family Nursing.* Philadelphia: JB Lippincott.

Kub J, Steel S (1995). School health. In Smith C, Maurer F, eds. *Community Health Nursing.* Philadelphia: WB Saunders.

Lapp C et al (1993). Family-based practice: Discussion of a tool merging assessment with intervention. In Wegner, Alexander, eds. *Readings in Family Nursing.* Philadelphia: JB Lippincott.

Larson D (1997). Making the case for spiritual interventions in clinical practice. *Journal of Clinical Behavioral Medicine* 2(1):20–30.

Levin J (1996). How prayer heals: A theoretical model. *Alternative Therapies* 2(1):66–73.

Lewis P (1996). A review of prayer within the role of the holistic nurse. *Journal of Holistic Nursing* 14(4):308–315.

Lloyd R, Solari-Twadell A (1994). Organizational framework, functions and educational preparation of parish nurses: A comparison of national survey results. In *Proceedings of Eighth Annual Westberg Symposium,* pp. 107–115. Park Ridge, IL: The National Parish.

LoBiondo-Wood GD, Haber J (1994). *Nursing Research: Methods, Critical Appraisal, and Utilization,* 3rd ed. St. Louis: Mosby.

Luks A, Payne P (1991). *The Healing Power of Doing Good.* New York: Fawcett Columbine.

Lusk SL et al (1990). Corporate expectations for occupational health nurses' activities. *AAOHN J* 38(8): 368–374.

Lusk SL et al (1995). Health-promoting lifestyles of blue-collar, skilled trade and white-collar workers. *Nursing Research* 44(1):20–24.

Maier S et al (1994). Psychoneuroimmunology: The interface between behavior and immunity. *American Psychologist* 49(12).

Marwick CD (1995). Should physicians prescribe prayer for health? Spiritual aspects of well-being considered. *JAMA* 273(20):1561–1562.

Matthews D, Larson D (1997). Faith and medicine: Reconciling the twin traditions of healing. *Journal of Clinical Behavioral Medicine* 2(1):3–9.

Maurer F (1995). Teenage pregnancy. In Smith B, Maurer F, eds. *Community Health Nursing.* Philadelphia: WB Saunders.

Mayo Clinic (1996). Health and spirituality. *Mayo Clinic Health Letter* 14:(11).

McGrawth BJ (1945). Fifty years of industrial nursing in the United States. *Public Health Nursing* 37:119–124.

McKenna B (1994). The Americans With Disability Act and the health care worker. *Healthwire.* Washington DC: Federation of Nurses and Health Professionals.

Metler M, Kemper D (1996). *Healthwise for Life.* Boise, ID: Healthwise.

Modesti PA et al (1994). Comparison of ambulatory blood pressure monitoring and conventional office measurement in the workers of a chemical company. *Int J Cardiol* 46(2):151–157.

Moore D (1995). Most Americans say religion is important to them. *Gallup Monthly Poll* 353, 16.

Morris S (1994). Academic occupational safety and health training programs. *Occup Med* 9(2): 189–200.

Moskowitz E, Jennings B (1996). *Coerced Contraception? Moral and Policy Changes of Long-Acting Birth Control.* Baltimore, MD: Georgetown University Press.

Narrigan D (1994). Postcoital contraception: Has its day come? *J Nurs Midwifery* 39(6):363

National Association of School Nurses (1993). *School Nursing Practice: Roles and Standards.* Scarborough, ME: The Association.

Noden PR (1990). The concept of comprehensiveness in the design and implementation of school health programs. *J School Health* 60(4):133–138.

Norman E et al (1994). Rural–urban blood lead differences in North Carolina children. *Pediatrics* 94(1):59–64.

Osler C et al (1996). Community health nurse in occupational health. In Stanhope M, Lancaster J, eds. *Community Health Nursing.* St. Louis: Mosby.

Paskett ED et al (1994). Breast cancer screening education in the workplace. *J Cancer Educ* 9(2): 101–104.

Payling K (1994). A hazard we can no longer ignore: Effects of excessive noise on well-being. *Prof Nurse* 9(6):418–421.

Pender N (1996). *Health Promotion in Nursing Practice,* 3d ed. Stamford, CT: Appleton & Lange.

Pickett G, Hanlon J (1994). *Public Health Administration and Practice,* 10th ed. St. Louis: Times Mirror/Mosby.

Pimomo J, Salazar M (1995). Environmental issues: At home, at work, and in the community. In Smith C, Maurer F, eds. *Community Health Nursing.* Philadelphia: WB Saunders.

Pincus H (1997). Commentary: Spirituality, religion, and health. *Journal of Clinical Behavioral Medicine* 2(1):49.

Pinkham J (1988). 100 years of industrial nursing has vastly improved workplace safety. *Occupational Safety & Health* 57(4):20–23.

Platt J (1993). Radon: Its impact on the community and the role of the nurse. *AAOHN J* 41(11):547–550.

Pope D (1995). Music, noise, and the human voice in the nurse–patient environment. *Image: J Nursing Scholarship* 27(4):291–296.

Porru S et al (1993). The utility of health education among lead workers: The experience of one program. *Am J Industrial Med* 23(3):473–481

Poster E, Ryan J (1994). A multiregional study of nurses' beliefs and attitudes about work safety and patient assault. *Hospital and Community Perspectives* 45(11):1104–1108.

Postol R (1993). Public health and working children in 20th-century America. *J Public Health Policy* 14(3):348–354.

Project India (1996). Call for Volunteers. *MCN* 21(4):176.

Rabinowitz S et al (1994). Teaching interpersonal skills to occupational and environmental health professionals. *Psychological Reports* 74(3):1299–1306.

Ragland G (1997). *Instant Teaching Treasures for Patient Education.* St. Louis: Mosby.

Ram E, ed. (1995). *Transforming Health: Christian Approaches to Healing and Wholeness.* Monrovia, CA: Marc Publications.

Rigotti N et al (1994). Do businesses comply with a no-smoking law? *Preventive Medicine* 23(2):223–229.

Rogers B, Cox A. (1994). Advancing the profession of occupational health nursing. *AAOHN J* 42(4): 158–163.

Rogers B et al (1993). Employee satisfaction with occupational health services. *AAOHN J* 41(2):58–65.

Roper M (1996). Assessing orthostatic vital signs. *AJN* 96(8):46.

Ross P (1994). Ergonomic hazards in the workplace: Assessment and prevention. *AAOHN J* 42(4): 171–176.

Savage N et al (1996). Nursing on your own time. *RN* 59.

Savitz DA (1994). Magnetic field exposure in relation to leukemia and brain cancer mortality among electric utility workers. *Am J Epidemiology* 14(2): 123–134.

Sax NI (1994). *Dangerous Properties of Industrial Materials*, 5th Ed. New York: WB Saunders.

Schank M et al (1996). Parish nursing: Ministry of healing. *Geriatric Nursing* 17(1):11–13.

Schauffler H (1994). *Educated Guesses: Making Policy About Medical Screening Tests.* Berkeley: University of California Press.

Schneider M et al (1995). Stated and unstated reasons for visiting a high school nurse's office. *J Adolescent Health* 16:35–41.

Schwab N, Hass M (1995). Delegation and supervision in school settings. *J School Nursing* 11(1):26–34.

Sepkowitz K (1994). Tuberculosis and the health care worker: A historical perspective. *Ann Intern Med* 120(1):71–79.

Shames K (1996). Harnessing the power of guided imagery. *RN* 59(8):49–50.

Sherwen L, Scoloveno M, Weingarten C (1995). *Nursing Care of the Childbearing Family.* Norwalk, CT: Appleton & Lange.

Silverstein M. Analysis of medical screening and surveillance in 21 Occupational Safety and Health Administration standards. *Am J Indust Med* 26(3): 283–295.

Smeltzer S, Bare B. (1996). *Brunner and Suddarth's Textbook of Medical-Surgical Nursing*, 8th ed. Philadelphia: JB Lippincott.

Smith C (1995). Public health nursing services by levels of prevention. In Smith and Maurer, eds. *Community Health Nursing.* Philadelphia: WB Saunders

Smith J, Hanks C (1994). Reaching out to mothers at risk. *RN* 57 (Oct):42–46.

Snyder M et al (1994). Environmental and occupational health education: A survey of community health nurses' need for educational programs. *AAOHN J* 42(7):325–328.

Solari-Twadell P et al (1990). *Parish Nursing: The Developing Practice.* Park Ridge, IL: National Parish Nurse Resource Center.

Solari-Twadell P et al (1994). *Assuring Viability for the Future: Guideline Development for Parish Nurse Education Programs.* Park Ridge, IL: National Parish Nurse Resource Center.

Sorensen G et al (1993). Promoting smoking cessation at the workplace: Results of a randomized controlled intervention study. *J Occup Med* 35(2):121–126.

Spear H (1996). Anxiety: When to worry, what To do. *RN* 59(7):40–46.

Spector R (1996). *Guide to Heritage Assessment and Health Traditions.* Stamford, CT: Appleton & Lange.

Spradley B, Allender J (1996). *Community Health Nursing.* Philadelphia: JB Lippincott.

Stackhouse J (1994). Death, dying, bereavement and spiritual distress. In Monahan F, Neighbors M, eds. *Nursing Care of Adults*, 2d ed. Philadelphia: WB Saunders.

Stackhouse J (1997). Facilitative verbal responses. In Leasia S, Monahan F, eds. *A Practical Guide for Health Assessment.* Philadelphia: WB Saunders.

Stanhope M, Knollmueller R (1996). *Handbook of Community and Home Health Nursing.* St. Louis: Mosby.

Stellman J (1994). Where women work and the hazards they face on the job. *J Occup Med* 36(8):814–825.

Stolte KM (1996). *Wellness Nursing Diagnoses for Health Promotion.* Philadelphia: JB Lippincott.

Stone DJ (1997). *Occupational Injuries and Illness.* St. Louis: Mosby.

Talbot L, Curtis L (1996). The challenge of assessing skin indicators in people of color. *Home Healthcare Nurse* 14(3):168–173.

Turnock B et al (1994). Local health department effectiveness in addressing the core functions of public health. *Publ Health Rep* 109(5):653–658.

U.S. Statistical Abstracts of the United States (1995). Washington DC: U.S. Govt. Printing Office.

U.S. Department of Labor (1977). *Labor Firsts in America.* Washington DC: U.S. Govt. Printing Office.

USDHHS (1991). *Healthy People 2000: Health Promotion and Disease Prevention: Objectives for the Nation*, full report with commentary. Washington DC: U.S. Govt. Printing Office.

USDHHS (1993a). *Child Health USA.* Washington DC: U.S. Govt. Printing Office.

USDHHS (1996). *Healthy People 2000: Midcourse Review and 1995 Revisions.* Washington DC: U.S. Govt. Printing Office.

USDHHS, Office of Disease Prevention and Health Promotion (1993). *Preventive Services in the Clinical Setting: What Works and What It Costs.* Washington DC: ODPHP, May.

Vahldieck R et al (1993). A framework for planning public health nursing services for families. In Wegner, Alexander, eds. *Readings in Family Nursing.* Philadelphia: JB Lippincott.

Wallis C (1996). Faith and healing. *Time* 147(26):58–70.

Wassel M (1995). Occupational health nursing and the advent of managed care. *AAOHN J* 43(1):23–28.

Wells-Federman C (1996). Awakening the nurse healer within. *Holistic Nursing Practice* 10(2):13–29.

Westberg G, McNamara JD (1990). *The Parish Nurse.* Minneapolis: Augsburg-Fortress Press.

Wills E (1996). Nurse–client alliance. *Home Healthcare Nurse* 14(6):455–459.

Winslow E (1996). Should children with mild illness be vaccinated? *AJN* 96(8):48.

Yates S (1994). The practice of school nursing: Integration with new models of health delivery. *J School Nursing* 10(1):10–19.

Zhou C, Roseman J (1994). Agricultural injuries among a population-based sample of farm operators in Alabama. *Am J Indust Med* 25(3):385–402.

Part 3

Nursing Practice in Ambulatory Care

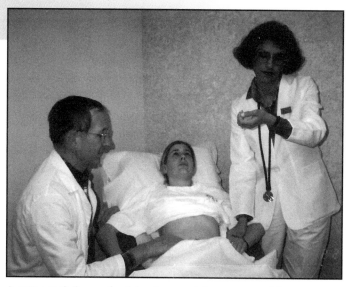

A nurse assisting a physician in examining a young girl.

9

Ambulatory Treatment Settings

Key Terms

biofeedback
Blue Cross and Blue Shield
cognitively impaired
community health centers
conscious sedation
continuing care communities
contraception
contractual agreements
cranial electric stimulation
deinstitutionalized
dialysis
emergicenters
epidemiologic functions

health maintenance organization
indemnity plans
independent practice association
Meals on Wheels
migrant workers
Office of Aging
Office of Economic Oppor-
   tunity
point-of-service plans
preferred provider organization

prospective payment
pulse oximetry
rehabilitative
retrospective fee-for-service
   basis
RU-486
surgicenters
transcutaneous electrical
   nerve stimulation
triage
underserved designation

Learning Objectives

1. Identify the various ambulatory treatment settings where nursing practice takes place.

2. Describe the role of the nurse in these settings.

3. Explain how some of these settings relate to managed-care systems.

4. Identify the settings primarily designed to serve the uninsured and underinsured.

5. Describe the benefits of day hospitals, school-based health centers, and continuing care retirement communities.

Ambulatory care refers to health services rendered to clients who *come to* health-care providers, usually for treatment of health problems. Some are referred to as clinic services. Ambulatory care occurs in a wide variety of settings, and nurses work in all the ambulatory care settings described in this chapter. The American Academy of Ambulatory Care Nursing was established in 1978 with the goal of promoting high standards of ambulatory care nursing. An annual convention and a bimonthly newsletter are benefits of membership. To contact the organization, see the resource directory in Appendix B.

Physicians' Offices

Traditionally, most people go to physicians' private offices when they need medical care. The vast majority of medical care provided by physicians is on an ambulatory basis; only a few clients are admitted to hospitals and long-term care facilities, and this is happening less and less often. This trend in ambulatory care will accelerate into the 21st century and will include a wide variety of health-care settings.

The number of physicians in solo practice in the United States has dropped significantly. Partnerships, small group practices, and multiple physician conglomerates are replacing the "Marcus Welby, M.D." image of medical practice as the American model. However, most physicians are still in private practices and are still paid mainly on a fee-for-service basis, either by their clients directly or by third-party payments from insurance companies, Medicare, or Medicaid. Traditional health insurance plans are called indemnity plans. Some insurance plans, such as Blue Cross and Blue Shield, often are not-for-profit; others, such as Aetna and Metropolitan, are for-profit. About 1,500 insurance companies are involved in health-care coverage in the United States. Because of increasing competition, more physicians are joining managed-care organizations and charging on a prospective payment basis while still continuing to use the retrospective fee-for-service system for clients who are not enrolled in managed-care programs.

Physicians and Managed Care: HMOs and PPOs

The classic model of a health maintenance organization (HMO) is a storefront ambulatory care center or clinic with hired physicians and other health-care workers who agree to a set salary as employees of the HMO. A hospital and long-term care facility, part of the system, may be owned by the HMO or may be affiliated by contractual agreement.

In independent practice associations, another type of HMO, physicians continue to practice in their private offices and charge fees in a prepaid plan that delivers care to enrolled members. Alternatively, a group of physicians might provide care to enrolled clients at more than one location. Sometimes an HMO contracts with several group practices to form a network to provide care. The various styles of HMOs demonstrate that HMOs are not just a place, but an organizational system of care (Table 9-1). An HMO combines delivery of health care into one system. Clients enrolled in the system must seek health care within that system (if the care is to be paid). "The Nurse Speaks" section of Chapter 2 discusses a nurse's work in the office of a physician who is a managed-care provider.

HMO clients or their employers prepay a fixed monthly premium to receive comprehensive health care. HMOs have historically emphasized preventive services to keep enrollees healthy and to avoid expensive hospitalizations and other costly care. Clients must use the physicians and agencies within the HMO, and many complain about

TABLE 9-1. Various Models of Health Maintenance Organizations (HMOs)

Independent Practice Association	Group	Network	Hired Staff
Contract physician service in solo or partnership practice	Contract physician service in a multispecialty group practice	Contract physicians from many group practices	Salaried physicians, nurses, and others at HMO facility.
Pays on discounted fee-for-service basis	Pays at negotiated rate/cap to the group	Pays at negotiated rate to all groups	HMO assumes all financial risks.

limitations in HMO services. Case managers seek the most cost-effective ways to deliver quality care, and there are strong incentives for physicians to keep costs down. In the past, this led to criticism of some HMOs whose physicians were not allowed to recommend or even tell clients about expensive treatments or specialty referrals. The Health Care Financing Administration has prohibited HMOs from muzzling physicians in this way. When physicians join HMOs, they must agree to work for reduced rates. This is one of the reasons why HMOs are unpopular with physicians.

A federally qualified HMO is one that has gained approval from the federal office of prepaid health care for compliance with quality assurance and financial standards. HMOs are expanding at a rapid rate and advertise many benefits, not all of which are forthcoming. HMOs vary in the quality and amount of service they render. HMO care is more economical than traditional fee-for-service systems, however. Display 9-1 lists questions to ask to evaluate an HMO.

More recently, point-of-service plans or riders have been added to some HMO plans, at an additional charge. These plans allow clients some freedom to select physicians outside the HMO, thus addressing a major criticism of HMOs.

Preferred provider organizations (PPOs) are not HMOs but are similar to point-of-service plans in that clients can choose to go to physicians outside the system by paying higher charges. Physicians in PPO plans must agree to discount their usual fees for enrolled clients. Clients then pay only a small copayment for an office visit, and the PPO promptly reimburses the physician for the rest of the reduced fee. Physicians are willing to reduce their fees to join PPOs because they are assured of prompt reimbursement. Clients like PPOs because they are given more freedom of choice of physicians, hospitals, and other services. When clients choose to see physicians outside the PPO system, they must pay the physician personally, and they then receive about 80% reimbursement from the PPO. Until the recent rapid growth of HMOs, PPOs were more numerous than HMOs.

Recent changes in HMO regulations have made them more profitable, and they are now widely advertised and promoted because they have become big business enterprises. Many clients are switching to HMO plans because they aggressively advertise generous benefits. Employers like HMOs because they provide more economic premiums by avoiding waste and duplication in the system. But however nice eyeglass coverage and other fringe benefits sound, some HMOs provide very limited coverage for home care visits and other vital services.

DISPLAY 9-1
What to Ask in Choosing an HMO

1. What are the exact benefits? What is the amount of copayment?
2. What are the benefit limits? Annual and lifetime dollar maximums? Maximum number of hospital days covered per illness? Maximum number of ambulatory, outpatient sessions per illness? Maximum number of home care visits per illness?
3. What services or treatments are not covered?
4. What are the restrictions on mental health benefits?
5. If the benefits cover only "medically necessary treatment," who makes that decision?
6. Are there limits on what drugs can be taken?
7. Are there limits or restrictions about the use of experimental treatment?
8. Is the primary physician assigned or selected by clients, and how large is the provider panel?
9. Is it possible to see a doctor outside the plan? If so, how much extra does that cost?
10. What are the rights of appeal if coverage is denied or cut short?
11. Will the plan add new providers if a client's family doctor or specialist cares to join?
12. How are the HMO's doctors paid? What incentives do they have to spend less on care?
13. Which hospitals and other facilities are approved by the plan?
14. How are family doctors and specialists selected to join the HMO?
15. How many of the doctors are board-certified?
16. Is the HMO accredited by the National Committee for Quality Assurance?

Physicians and Medicare and Medicaid

Most health-care clients are elderly, and those over age 65 are automatically covered for hospitalization by Medicare Part A. Medicare Part B covers 80% of physicians' office fees and other ambulatory care services. Part A is tax-supported; Part B is funded by premiums paid by senior citizens or their previous employers as part of pension benefits. Persons declared disabled and those with end-stage kidney disease are also eligible for Medicare, regardless of age. It is estimated that Part A will be bankrupt after the turn of the century, but Part B is more solvent. Transfer of some of the benefits now provided by Part A to Part B is one recommendation for salvaging the program. However, this will lead to higher premiums for clients. Another recommendation is to increase Part B premiums for wealthy clients on Medicare.

Medicaid is primarily federally funded but is administered by states, with some added state monies. It provides more liberal benefits than Medicare. It was designed primarily for the medically indigent, which includes persons on public assistance (welfare) and senior citizens who have only Social Security on which to live. Today, most Medicaid money supports disabled and elderly middle-class people whose funds have been depleted by the cost of long-term care facilities.

Some physicians dislike having to deal with Medicaid. Community health nurses seeking quality medical care for poor people find it difficult to understand why some physicians refuse to accept Medicaid clients, but physicians cite many hassles, such as cumbersome paperwork, low reimbursement fees, and long delays in being paid, as reasons for doing so. Some physicians provide care to poor people free of charge or at greatly reduced rates rather than deal with Medicaid. Some prefer to give their time free or for a small honorarium to staff public health clinics for poor people rather than accept Medicaid clients as their private patients.

The Role of Nurses in Physicians' Offices

The type of medical practice determines the role of the nurse to some extent. However, most registered nurses are employed in family practice and pediatric offices. Nurses who work for medical specialists are often nurse practitioners or nurse clinicians. Telephone triage, to determine the nature and urgency of the client's problem, is an important nursing function. Taking health histories, monitoring vital signs, performing electrocardiograms, taking throat cultures, doing venipunctures for laboratory tests, administering injections, and doing pulmonary function tests are some of the duties required. Nurses sometimes assist with office surgical procedures and scrub in hospital surgery. They assist with physical examinations, especially gynecologic examinations. Client and family teaching is a vital part of the role, including aspects of health promotion and disease prevention.

In large, multispecialty group practices, where clients are apt to be seen by various specialists, office nurses usually function as case managers. In most medical offices, nurses play an important management role. This includes hiring and supervising other office personnel and scheduling clients and staff. Many nurses who work well with their physician employers have considerable autonomy in developing office protocols and ways to improve the delivery of quality care.

The mission of the American Association of Office Nurses (AAON) is to provide continuing education specific to the needs of nurses to enhance the delivery of quality care in physicians' offices. *The Office Nurse*, a bimonthly journal, and *Nurses Exchange Office News*, a bimonthly newsletter, are periodicals published by the AAON for its members. Regional, national, and home study continuing education programs are available. See the resource directory in Appendix B for information about this organization.

Hospital Outpatient Clinics

Over the years, hospitals have developed outpatient clinics to serve the needs of ambulatory clients. The type and scope of clinics depend on the population being served. The large Vanderbilt Clinic of Columbia-Presbyterian Medical Center in New York City serves about 500,000 clients a year and operates a wide range of specialty clinics, as well as basic adult and pediatric care. The Vanderbilt Clinic was established in 1888 and primarily serves the poor of New York who have no private physician.

Small-town community hospitals offer a limited variety of outpatient clinics depending on the needs of the community. Many hospitals offer rehabilitation services such as physical, occupational, and speech therapy as outpatient services. Tests such as endoscopy and diagnostic imaging and treatments such as electroconvulsive therapy and radiation therapy are done on an outpatient basis. At some small-town hospitals, the emergency department is used as an outpatient clinic because the community lacks such a service.

Intravenous conscious sedation for procedures such as endoscopy used to be administered only by anesthesiologists. Today, in accordance with standards set by 15 speciality nursing organizations as well as the Joint Commission on Accreditation of Healthcare Organizations, nurses are administering conscious sedation during various outpatient procedures. Pulse oximetry, in which arterial blood oxygen saturation is monitored, is an example of high-tech equipment that is being used increasingly in community settings such as outpatient clinics, emergency departments, ambulatory surgicenters, and even home care settings. The oximeter allows medical intervention to be provided before the client becomes hypoxemic.

Famous Clinics

The ambulatory diagnostic and treatment clinics at various centers around the country have become world-famous for quality care and draw clients from around the globe. Most are centered in large medical centers or they developed into large medical centers from small private clinics founded by physicians. They include the Mayo Clinic in Minnesota, the Lahey Clinic in Massachusetts, and the Cleveland Clinic in Ohio. Other famous ambulatory care centers are well known for specialty care, such as the Joslyn Clinic in Boston for diabetes mellitus. These are just a few of the well-known centers offering quality ambulatory care in the United States.

Emergency Departments

Hospitals developed emergency departments to care for accident victims and clients with a sudden, acute need for medical care. They are open 24 hours a day, 7 days a week. Nurses play a vital role in triage, because only 10% of the clients who come to the emergency department need to be admitted to the hospital.

Some people abuse emergency departments; they go to there instead of making an appointment with a private physician or public clinic. Often they do not need immediate care, or they delay seeking care until an emergency exists. This results in extremely busy emergency rooms so full of clients that waiting periods are long (except for those with actual emergencies). Generally, emergency department care costs two to three times that of care in other settings.

Proprietary Walk-In Centers

Walk-in centers or ''emergicenters'' developed in response to the overuse and the long waiting times of hospital emergency departments. First established in 1976, these facilities are among the most rapidly growing systems of health-care delivery. They are usually located conveniently in shopping centers. They can exist on a for-profit or not-for-profit basis. Some are part of managed-care systems. Nurses work in these walk-in centers. Some emergicenters employ various medical specialists as well as providing primary-care personnel for routine medical problems. Costs are usually 30% to 40%

lower than in hospital emergency departments, and the waiting time is about 15 to 30 minutes. Occasionally, emergicenters are hospital-owned and operate as hospital satellites.

Public Health Personal Care Clinics

Health departments provide personal care clinic services in accordance with their mandate to fill gaps in local services for the unserved and underserved in the community. Health departments primarily exist to serve the community with health promotion, disease prevention, and epidemiologic functions. However, health departments also provide services to meet the health-care needs of people. These personal services usually take the form of clinics and sometimes even include home care if no home care agency exists in the community.

Treatment services sponsored by health departments include general medical clinics, orthopedic clinics, pediatric clinics, women's health clinics, and clinics for persons with special needs such as AIDS (Display 9-2) and sexually transmitted diseases. Nurses usually manage these clinics with part-time or volunteer physicians. A social worker is

DISPLAY 9-2
Who Should Be Tested for HIV/AIDS?

1. Persons having one of the signs and symptoms (see below)
2. Past or present users of intravenous drugs
3. Men who have had sex with another man, even one time, since 1977
4. Persons with hemophilia or related clotting disorders who have received clotting factor concentrates
5. Men and women who have engaged in sex for money or drugs and persons who have been their heterosexual partners
6. Persons who engaged in unprotected sex with multiple partners since 1977
7. Persons testing positive in a test for HIV in the past
8. Persons who have spent more than 72 hours in prison in the last 12 months
9. Sexual partners of any of the above categories

The main signs and symptoms of AIDS:

- Fever of unknown cause that persists longer than 10 days
- Persistent white spots or unusual blemishes in the mouth
- Unexplained sweating, particularly at night
- Persistent diarrhea
- Unexplained weight loss of more than 10 lb
- Persistent sore or swollen lymph nodes or glands lasting more than 1 month
- Unexplained red, purplish, or blue spots in the skin or mucous membranes that fail to heal
- Persistent cough and shortness of breath

(Adapted from City of Hope Blood Bank, DAC96.FRM.)

present when a sliding-scale fee is charged based on the client's income and ability to pay. Social workers also do counseling. Nurses and nutritionists perform health teaching. Many of the clients are poor and have multiple health and social problems.

Disease prevention clinics include flu clinics held in the autumn for the elderly and chronically ill. Strains of influenza constantly mutate, so carry-over immunity is unreliable from year to year. These clinics are sometimes free. Monthly child health clinics provide regular, free check-ups and immunizations for children under 5 years of age. These clinics are usually held in donated space at neighborhood churches or schools to make them more accessible to poor clients. Travelers' clinics provide immunizations and health guidance for those traveling overseas, especially to Third World countries. A fee is charged for these clinics. Prenatal clinics are widely sponsored by health departments in an effort to prevent complications in both mothers and infants. A nutritionist is also usually present to teach mothers how to eat properly for their health and the health of their infants.

Health promotion clinics include women's health or family planning clinics. Counseling, laboratory work, a physical examination, and a careful health history are done, along with health teaching. Various options for contraception are explained, and the one the client chooses is provided. Gynecologic conditions are treated, including sexually transmitted diseases. Nurse practitioners or nurses certified in that specialty are often hired to work in women's health clinics. Ethical issues arise about serving young teenagers in these clinics without their parents' consent. In 11 states, parental consent is required for treatment. Young girls who come for contraception are already sexually active. This, in itself, constitutes adult status in most states. Girls say that if parents were called, they would not come to the clinics, and they need protection and guidance if they are sexually active. These clinics help prevent teen pregnancies and sexually transmitted diseases, including AIDS. A true case study about work in a women's health clinic is presented in Chapter 6's "Clinical Application."

The Development of Community Health Centers

A wide variety of community health centers (CHCs) have developed in the past 30 years. Some are owned by hospitals and operate as satellites. Some are owned by HMOs. Some are privately owned by other health-care businesses. Some not-for-profit centers were started and initially funded by charitable or religious groups, health foundations, or philanthropists. Some were started with federal or state grants. Some target specific aggregates. All came into being in response to unmet health needs in a particular community. Community health nurses staff these centers and usually manage them.

Government-sponsored neighborhood health centers emerged from the social concerns of the 1960s. The government's Office of Economic Opportunity initially funded them during President Lyndon Johnson's administration. They provided full-salaried health-care providers, usually nurses, in community ambulatory care settings. Gradually these neighborhood centers came to be known as CHCs. Funds to maintain government-sponsored centers were secured under the Public Health Service Act to provide both primary health care and case management services to underserved populations. Designation of a population as "underserved" is based on the percentage of the population below the poverty line in that geographic area. Additional data include the area's infant mortality rate and the number of physicians practicing there per 1,000 persons. Currently, some 2,000 CHCs operate in the United States, serving about 6 million people in urban and rural areas (Kelly & Joel, 1995).

The philosophy of the CHC movement is a good one. There is strong emphasis on community involvement, with representatives from the area on the governing board and among the staff. The health needs identified by the community are addressed. This promotes better communication, especially when the aggregate being served is an ethnic group with distinct cultural practices and language patterns. For back-up special services, these centers are affiliated with hospitals or health departments. CHC services are less expensive than hospital emergency departments or outpatient clinics because of lower overhead expenses. Services are more holistic. Care focuses on health promotion and disease prevention as well as treatment. Use of community workers as part of the health team promotes a friendly atmosphere of understanding and caring.

Despite their strengths, many CHCs have been closed because of financial problems. Few can be self-supporting because of the low incomes of the clients they serve. When government or other subsidies end, client fees and Medicaid and Medicare reimbursements are not enough to maintain these centers. Reductions in personnel and services diminish the quality of service provided. Some health planners are critical, saying that CHCs lead to and perpetuate a separate, second-class system of health care for the poor. For these reasons, the future of CHCs in the United States is in question.

Nursing Centers and Clinics

Nursing centers are described in detail in Chapter 12. Many provide health care to underserved aggregates. Nursing centers are considered a contemporary development in nursing practice, but pioneers such as Lillian Wald, Mary Breckenridge, and Margaret Sanger established nursing centers early in the 20th century.

Migrant Worker Clinics and Centers

In 1962, the Migrant Health Centers Grant was established by Public Law 87-692, which authorized government money for clinics and health centers for agricultural migrant workers and their families. Farming is a very high-risk occupation. Migrants are seasonal workers who travel wherever temporary farm help is needed. The temporary nature of their work, poor housing conditions in migrant worker camps, low wages, and the lack of continuity of schooling for the children all lead to potential health and social problems. These centers are a variation of CHCs. They are usually staffed by registered nurses and part-time physicians, nurse practitioners, and social workers.

Services provided at the more than 100 migrant worker centers in the United States include prenatal, pediatric, dental, and medical treatment. Mental health, substance abuse, and other social services are included. Emergency care is available also.

Clinics and Shelters for the Homeless

Old "bag ladies" and chronic alcoholic men living on Skid Row are outdated stereotypes of the homeless population. In the United States, the fastest-growing group of homeless people (33%) is families with small children (Mihaly, 1991).

There are many causes of homelessness in the United States. Some people are temporarily or episodically homeless. The growing number of long-term homeless people is a grave concern. Growing poverty among certain groups, such as unskilled workers, and a shortage of affordable housing are obvious causes. The drug epidemic is a major cause. Deinstitutionalized mentally ill persons make up more than a third of the homeless population. Homeless persons often carry a dual diagnosis of addiction and serious mental illness.

There is concern that changes in welfare benefits may result in increased homelessness. New laws that require persons on welfare to find employment after 2 years on public assistance may be beneficial if there are enough employment opportunities and if back-up services, such as child care and low-cost housing, are provided by society. If not, the problems of homelessness will increase greatly.

Homelessness creates complex, multidimensional problems. Homeless people have physical needs related to chronic diseases, malnutrition, poor hygiene, and exposure to bad weather and violence. Community health nurses work as volunteers or paid staff in clinics and shelters for the homeless.

Community Mental Health Centers, Group Homes, and Halfway Houses

Mental health facilities are described in Chapter 10. Although grouped separately, this is an artificial categorization: mental, physical, emotional, and spiritual divisions do not exist separately in human experience, only in textbooks.

School-Based Clinics and Family Centers

As described in Chapter 8, school-based clinics and family health centers are proving to be popular and effective health-care locations. Schools provide convenient treatment centers. These locations are familiar, friendly, and easily accessible. These factors lead to improved compliance and motivation for clients to address their health-care needs.

The Indian Health Service

The Indian Health Service has existed for many years and falls under the jurisdiction of the U.S. Public Health Service. Its aim is to provide, in cooperation with the various tribes, a comprehensive health-care system to Native Americans and Alaskan Natives. One problem is that few Native Americans who become nurses and physicians return to work on the reservations, and outsiders are seldom familiar enough with the language and culture. Most physicians and nurses in the Indian Health Service work on a reservation, providing ambulatory care for a relatively short time before moving on. Lack of continuity and cultural understanding leads to less-than-optimal health care.

Planned Parenthood

Planned Parenthood, a private, not-for-profit organization, was founded in the early 1900s by Margaret Sanger, a nurse (Display 9-3). As a community health nurse working among the urban poor, Ms. Sanger came to know many women who died because of septic, ''back room'' illegal abortions. The only other course open to these women was bearing multiple children. Frequent pregnancies and many births resulted in worn-out, prematurely aged women and high infant mortality. Inadequate provisions for all the children led to high childhood morbidity and mortality rates. Ms. Sanger became committed to providing birth control for women in such circumstances. Contraceptive devices were then illegal and considered obscene in the United States, so she had to travel to Europe for supplies and education on how to use them. She suffered a great deal of harassment by some groups when her work began, and she was imprisoned several times as a result of her efforts. But she improved the lives of hundreds of thousands of women through her legacy, Planned Parenthood Services of America.

Abortion Clinics

Abortion clinics are usually privately owned. They are highly controversial. Tax-supported clinics do not do abortions because some taxpayers oppose abortion; federal funding for abortion services was eliminated for the same reason. Some states that fund abortions for the medically indigent must assume all the costs without federal funds.

DISPLAY 9-3
Facts About Planned Parenthood

- Each year more than 4 million Americans are served by 922 Planned Parenthood centers.
- Each year Planned Parenthood helps avert over 500,000 unintended pregnancies.
- A recent survey found that one in four women, age 16 to 49, says she is a current or former Planned Parenthood client.
- Each year 1,300,000 tests for sexually transmitted diseases are performed at Planned Parenthood centers.
- All Planned Parenthood clinics provide HIV/AIDS testing and safer sex counseling and education.
- Over 9,000 women receive prenatal care, of whom 87% are Medicaid recipients.
- Of the 130,000 women who had abortions performed at 63 Planned Parenthood affiliates, 54% had incomes at or below *the poverty level.*

(Modified from Planned Parenthood Fact Sheet.)

Abortion centers are sometimes picketed by antiabortion groups. Staff and clients coming for care are sometimes harassed to the point of violence and even homicide. Consequently, some health-care professionals are no longer willing to work in these facilities, and centers are closing. This is just one reason that the number of abortions is decreasing each year among teenagers. More likely, the steady decrease in abortions is due to more accessible contraception. Possibly, fear of contracting AIDS is a factor leading to less sexual activity.

Release of "the abortion pill" (RU-486) by the Food & Drug Administration (FDA) will reduce the number of abortion clinics needed. With RU-486, women will not need to go to an abortion clinic or a hospital; the procedure can be done in the privacy of a physician's office. The abortion pill was developed and used safely and effectively for many years in France. Antiabortion groups in the United States fought for many years to keep it out of the United States until the FDA decided to study it for recommendation that it be licensed. This pill will enable women to have abortions much earlier than they do now and will avoid late-term abortions.

Teen-age pregnancy is a serious problem in the United States, even though the number of teenage births has decreased since 1991. Pregnant teenagers often choose to have abortions. Even before the advent of RU-486, about 40% of all teen pregnancies were terminated by abortion (Smith & Mauer, 1995). Until 1993, nurses could not, without parental consent, legally give pregnant teenagers any information about the advantages and disadvantages of having abortions or where abortion services might be found. This is still true in a few states. This "gag rule" causes an ethical dilemma for nurses involved in family planning services, the majority of whom have come to believe that abortion is a positive alternative to teen-age pregnancy, especially in 13- and 14-year-olds with poor support systems. The dilemma about whether to obey the restrictive law or to follow one's personal professional beliefs is a difficult one for many women's health clinic nurses. The rate of teen pregnancy has been slowly decreasing over the past few years.

Day Hospital Programs

Day hospitals are very popular and serve a variety of needs. Programs include ambulatory surgery, rehabilitation services, and services for clients with Alzheimer's and other dementias and serious mental illnesses. Social day-care programs for the elderly also exist.

Ambulatory Surgery

Day hospitals for surgical clients have developed in an effort to reduce the number of costly inpatient days. Newer arthroscopic, laparoscopic, and other techniques have helped make some surgeries less invasive. Anesthesia times have been shortened and postoperative problems have lessened. Therefore, in many cases clients can leave the hospital the same day.

Same-day surgical units are staffed with nurses for about 12 hours a day. The history, physical examination, x-rays, and laboratory testing are done on an ambulatory basis several days before the scheduled surgery. A nurse from the unit meets with clients beforehand to take a careful nursing history and explains in detail what will happen on the day of surgery; this way, clients know what to expect and can ask questions. When appropriate, the nurse sets up interviews with the anesthesiologist and additional information time with the surgeon. When the client returns from the recovery room and all bodily functions have returned to normal, including the ability to void, the client can go home. Before leaving, the client and the friend or family member escorting him or her home are given verbal and written instructions by the nurse. Any needed prescriptions are supplied by the surgeon, along with careful instructions about when to call and when to go to the physician's office to have stitches removed, if necessary. If the client develops a problem requiring a longer hospital stay, he or she is transferred to another unit in the hospital when the ambulatory surgical unit closes at the end of the day.

Some surgeons or groups of surgeons have established their own freestanding ambulatory surgery centers, called surgicenters, in separate locations from hospitals; they have admitting privileges to a hospital if clients should need a longer stay to recuperate. Some centers specialize in plastic or ophthalmologic surgery. These independent surgicenters perform as many as 6,000 procedures a year and claim to be able to do up to 40% of all surgical procedures (Kelly & Joel, 1995). Some ambulatory day hospitals are part of managed-care systems.

Rehabilitation Day Hospitals

Intensive rehabilitative services are offered at day hospitals. In scope and intensity, these services may be the same as inpatient hospital stays, but without the overnight stay, clients can benefit from a structured therapeutic program and still stay in touch with family and home life. By returning home each evening, clients can test their new skills in a familiar environment, making the transition from hospital life to independent living easier and ensuring a continuum of care. These programs usually operate Mondays to Fridays from 8 PM to 5 PM. Lunch is often provided, offering an opportunity for occupational therapy instruction in eating skills as needed. Some clients attend the program daily; others attend part-time.

To be eligible for a rehabilitation day hospital program, the client must be able to manage at home but must require at least two of the following services: physical therapy, occupational therapy, or speech therapy. The client must be medically stable, must be able to tolerate the daily commute to and from the program, and must have a caregiver to help on evenings and weekends. Day hospital programs treat clients with a wide spectrum of disabilities, including cerebrovascular accident, amputation, head and spinal cord injury, multiple sclerosis, Parkinson's disease, and other neuromuscular disorders.

Experienced nurses, often certified in rehabilitative nursing, coordinate the interdisciplinary treatment team, led by a physiatrist. Diagnostic services include cardiovascular and cardiopulmonary stress testing, electroencephalography and electromyelography, gait analysis, and functional capacity evaluations. Neurologic and psychiatric and sensory integration evaluations are performed, along with many other tests. Therapeutic services range from speech and language therapy, audiology, dysphagia treatment, cognitive therapy, nutritional counseling, and pulmonary and cardiac rehabilitation to aquatic therapy and hydrotherapy, seating and wheelchair mobility, use of orthotics and prosthetics, driver evaluation and training, and vocational and industrial rehabilitation.

Nurses play a valuable role in these ambulatory care facilities. They do intake assessments to determine if clients meet eligibility requirements and how they can best be helped. They develop an individualized plan of care for each client. They function as case managers and have heavy responsibilities in client and family teaching. The "Clinical Application" case study in this chapter discusses this type of nursing.

Therapeutic Senior Day-Care Programs for the Cognitively Impaired

Day-care programs exist for older adults suffering from Alzheimer's disease and related disorders such as Parkinson's disease and cerebrovascular disorders that cause dementia. These programs provide enjoyable activities for cognitively impaired persons and give their caregivers a chance to perform everyday tasks without worry. These programs can prevent early institutionalization.

After the initial assessment, including brief psychological and physical testing and family interviews, the client's remaining strengths are identified. A comprehensive treatment program is then designed and implemented. Goals include promoting social interaction, maintaining self-dignity, and promoting physical well-being. The focus is on accentuating the client's strengths to maintain integrity and promote hope in the face of ongoing loss. Safety is always a priority.

Caregivers for clients with dementia suffer overwhelming daily demands, 24 hours a day. Spouses, usually elderly, have chronic health problems of their own. In addition to physical demands, constant caregiving produces isolation, depression, anger, and greater susceptibility to physical illness. Many day-care centers sponsor weekly support groups for caregivers to learn more about dementia and techniques to solve many day-to-day problems. In addition, a support group provides a forum to express feelings related to caregiving.

Sponsors and funding vary for these important services. Some centers are privately sponsored, and some are publicly sponsored. For example, the graduate school of psychology of Fuller Theological Seminary sponsors and staffs such a program in the Los Angeles area. Meals on Wheels programs in New York sponsor similar programs, with partial funding by the state and the local Office of Aging. In some places, these programs are sponsored by mental health grants and are part of regional mental health programs. Fees are usually based on the client's ability to pay. United Way organizations and other community and religious groups often provide supplemental funding.

There are also social day-care programs for senior citizens who do not suffer from dementia. They provide socialization activities and lunch. They are often sponsored by the local Office of Aging and staffed by volunteers as well as paid staff. These are primary prevention programs to provide mental stimulation, socialization, and good nutrition to the elderly.

Specialty Programs Functioning on an Ambulatory Basis

Nurses work in various special ambulatory programs such as dialysis centers and biofeedback, stress, and pain management centers.

Dialysis Centers

Outpatient or freestanding dialysis centers serve clients with end-stage renal disease. These are often open-staffed facilities, meaning that nephrologists may apply for privileges to refer clients to the centers. If a pediatric nephrologist is on staff, both pediatric and adult clients are accepted for treatment. Services are provided for clients who are visiting from another area but need to continue their regular dialysis regimen. These facilities offer comfortable reclining chairs, televisions and video cassette recorders, and laptop computer outlets.

In hemodialysis, a machine removes waste from the bloodstream and returns the cleansed blood to the client. Dialysis becomes necessary when the kidneys can no longer perform this function. Dialysis centers contain hemodialysis stations, which provide constant blood pressure monitoring and computerized recording of dialysis sessions. Stations also provide conventional, high-efficiency, and high-flux dialysis. The centers also can train eligible clients to self-administer treatments at home. Training is available for both home-based hemodialysis and peritoneal dialysis. In peritoneal dialysis, the peritoneal membrane performs the cleansing process through a catheter into the abdomen.

Nurses are responsible for administering treatments prescribed by physicians and for coordinating other members of the team. Nurses also handle home-care training and counsel patients on participating in their dialysis regimens. These clients are highly stressed physically, socially, emotionally, spiritually, and economically, and need a great deal of support and counseling from nurses.

Strict state and federal licensing requirements and practice standards are required in these centers, and they are frequently inspected for recertification. Nurses play a vital role in ensuring that all protocols and staff adhere to these requirements.

Stress, Pain Management, and Biofeedback Centers

Ambulatory programs that provide relief of chronic pain or stress and anxiety may exist as separate clinics or as one program. In these centers, teams of professional specialists combine their talents with state-of-the-art pain and stress management techniques to produce relief. These treatment methods decrease or eliminate the need for pain medication, lessen dependence on the health-care system, and enable clients to return to a more productive, active lifestyle. Conditions that respond well to these treatments include migraine and tension headaches, chronic neck and back pain, temporomandibular joint problems, bruxism and facial pain syndromes, post-traumatic stress disorders, Raynaud's disease, hypertension, arthritic pain, fibromyalgias, radiculopathies, premenstrual syndrome and menstrual pain, torticollis, neuralgia, hyperesthesia, muscles spasms and tics, depression, anxiety, stress, and phobic disorders.

Clients are evaluated when they enter these programs to determine their condition and needs. A comprehensive, individualized treatment plan is developed; more than one modality may be used to provide relief. A popular treatment method is biofeedback, a noninvasive, clinically proven method for the relief of chronic pain and stress-related disorders. Through relaxation techniques and biofeedback training, clients learn how to respond more positively to stress and minimize its impact on their health. Clients learn to identify and control autonomic physical responses to stress such as muscle tension, sweating, and temperature changes. They can then learn to modify the responses that provoke or exacerbate pain, tension, and anxiety.

Clients with chronic pain are offered several types of mild electrical stimulation techniques to break the pain cycle. Cranial electric stimulation provides high-frequency, low-intensity, delicate stimulation to abort or decrease the pain cycle and cause an increase in endorphin levels, especially serotonin, the body's own painkiller. Transcutaneous electrical nerve stimulation (TENS) provides electrical cutaneous stimulation that blocks pain messages to the brain, according to the gateway theory of pain transmission. The stimulation provided to muscles in spasm encourages them to relax. Progressive relaxation training is used to ease the mind and the body's reaction to stress.

Other stress management techniques include exercise and behavioral and attitudinal changes. Cognitive therapy helps clients identify and restructure underlying beliefs and behaviors that contribute to stress, anxiety, and pain. Finally, medications are used as appropriate to help relieve depression and anxiety. Nurses help to administer and teach clients about all these modalities. Display 15-1 in Chapter 15 suggests nonpharmacologic methods to deal with pain.

Correctional Facilities

To provide health care to inmates, local jails and state and federal prisons hire registered nurses as well as nurse practitioners and clinical nurse specialists. The latter two groups are particularly well qualified to provide the primary care and counseling needed by inmates.

Laws mandate that physical examinations be done on all inmates after they are sentenced and begin serving their time. Illnesses are treated. Basic care is provided according to the regulations, but any extra services that inmates may request, such as new dentures, new eyeglasses, and elective surgery, are usually denied.

Most incarcerated persons are poorly educated and come from backgrounds of poverty. Many have some type of mental illness, especially personality disorders. The prevalence of sexually transmitted diseases, including AIDS, is fairly high in prison populations. Homosexual activity, both voluntary and involuntary, among the incarcerated puts inmates at high risk for contracting HIV infection. When prison officials insist that homosexual activity is not allowed, and therefore condoms cannot be distributed, nurses may experience ethical problems about client confidentiality and the transmission of HIV.

Retirement Community Clinics and Health Services

More and more middle-class senior citizens choose to enter retirement communities that offer progressive levels of health services and living arrangements. Retirees commonly enter in their mid-70s and live independently in small houses or apartments. For health care, they visit ambulatory clinics on the grounds, which may be open 1 to 5 days a week, depending on the size of the community. A registered nurse is usually on duty 24 hours a day to help triage and refer clients to appropriate care. Primary care clinics are staffed by physicians or nurse practitioners.

As residents become more frail, they may need to transfer to assisted living units in the retirement community. These residents live in large private rooms; all meals are provided in the dining room, and a nurse is on duty at all times to offer assistance with medications and other needs. Assisted living residents must be well enough to go to the dining room independently and dress themselves with minimal assistance. A slight to moderate degree of memory loss may have occurred; the nurse offers reminders and monitoring.

Some retirement communities have special units for clients with Alzheimer's disease and other dementias. These units provide close supervision, assistance with activities of daily living, and constant monitoring because of severe memory loss. These units provide safe places where residents may wander, even outdoors in fenced areas.

If and when residents become so ill that they require skilled nursing care, they transfer to a facility on the grounds, either temporarily or permanently. Many of these units provide hospice services. The advantage of these facilities is that senior citizens who need care are still surrounded by their friends. Residents can avoid having to make a major move to a distant location when their level of need changes. Also, many elderly couples age at a different rate: one spouse may need more advanced care while the other can still live independently in their apartment or cottage. In these multilevel care communities, couples remain close enough geographically to spend most of each day together; the sicker partner may even visit their home for several hours each day.

Retirement communities can be quite costly, depending on the sponsors. Many are privately owned, profitable businesses. Some are sponsored by churches and other not-for-profit groups. Financial arrangements vary. Many operate on a "pay-as-you-go" basis, in which residents pay for whatever service or level of care they need. Other retirement communities, known as continuing care communities, have a different financial arrangement. Residents pay a large entrance fee that guarantees them free health-care services as long as they live. Fearing years of expensive nursing home care, some elderly people elect to enter a continuing care community for the financial security it provides. More about the needs of elderly clients, the predominant users of health care, is found in Chapter 11.

THE NURSE SPEAKS . . .
About Her Work at Planned Parenthood

I work at a Planned Parenthood center that provides family planning and prenatal services. A woman in her 30s came in looking distraught and seeking an appointment to talk about her 14-year-old daughter, whom she had just learned was pregnant. The mother did not know what to do or where to turn for help. She had to work two full-time jobs as a nurse's aide just to make ends meet financially for the two of them. She could not take on the responsibility of caring for a baby, nor did she think her 14-year-old daughter could manage that responsibility. As a single parent, she knew how difficult that can be. She came from Trinidad and had no relatives in the United States to help. She seemed to want someone to tell her daughter to have an abortion. Of course, I couldn't do that, but I did suggest that the mother and daughter come in together to talk.

The three of us sat down to talk together a couple of days later. The daughter started to cry when I asked her to share her thoughts about the pregnancy. She said she had not realized that a girl could get pregnant so easily, and she didn't use protection. She said that she had wanted to go to school, even college, and now she didn't know what to do. She added that she was afraid of an abortion. She didn't know if her mother would think it was right, and some people called it murder. Then she started to cry again.

The mother looked at me and said, "What do you think she should do?" I said that I couldn't tell her what to do, but I could give her some information about what would happen if she had an abortion and what would happen if she carried the baby to term. I added that it sounded like the two of them had not really had a frank talk to discuss this, and suggested that I give them time alone to talk and share their feelings.

The two of them spent about an hour together in the room, and when they exited it was obvious that both had been crying. They had decided that the girl would have an abortion, and asked for information about where to find an abortion clinic. They both seemed more relaxed and resigned to the situation.

A few weeks later, the girl came back to see me to ask for contraceptive help. She was put on the pill and given condoms for protection against sexually transmitted diseases. We discussed at length the epidemic of sexually transmitted diseases and the real danger of AIDS to people who do not use condoms faithfully.

"I learned my lesson about how easy it is to get pregnant, so I'll keep reminding myself the same thing about infections. If my boyfriend won't use a condom, I'll just refuse him, that's all, even if he says he is clean. You never know," she said.

We also discussed her feelings about the abortion. She said it made her sad but she felt sure it was the right thing to do. She added that she and her mother were closer these days because of all they went through together. She said that they talk more openly about lots of things.

Shandra
PLANNED PARENTHOOD NURSE

CLINICAL APPLICATION

A Critical Thinking Case Study About a Client Needing Rehabilitation Services

Russ, a 66-year-old man, is referred to the rehabilitation day-care center where you work. He is in a skilled nursing facility, but his wife Emma wants to bring him home if affordable community day-care services are available to assist with the transition. Russ requires assistance in walking and transfers, as well as constant supervision. He has severe short-term memory loss and can retain new information only about 15 seconds. His medical diagnosis is status postcerebral hemorrhage with left hemiplegia. Russ required a craniotomy to evacuate blood after his hemorrhage. During the procedure, he had a sudden, marked drop in blood pressure that progressed to system shutdown, including renal and heart failure. He was in a coma for 2 weeks.

Before his cerebrovascular accident, Russ lived in a private home with his wife and two unmarried adult children. There are three steps at the front door of his house. There is a bedroom and bathroom on the first floor. Russ is covered by Medicare and Medigap insurance.

 and Think!

- What additional information do you need to determine if this discharge to the community is an appropriate and workable plan?
- Does Russ need skilled physical therapy, as you suspect? If so, the couple will be helped with day-care costs by his Medicare and Medigap insurance, so they can afford that service.
- Has Emma been trained to perform car transfers, and can she drive Russ to and from day care?
- Insurance will not pay for transportation. Has Emma demonstrated ability to ascend and descend the front steps safely with him?
- With severe short-term memory deficits, what safety factors are a consideration, both at home and at day care?
- Does Emma have the stamina to care for her husband on weekends and during the 16 hours each day that he will not be in day care?
- Is there a secondary caregiver available to provide relief for her?

Russ was discharged to home after the couple received training at the skilled nursing facility to manage stairs and car transfers. After admission to the day hospital, Russ required a moderate amount of physical assistance, plus physical and occupational therapy. All the team, but especially the nurses, worked to improve his short-term memory deficit. He needed many environmental reminders, as well as constant cuing.

Russ adjusted very well and seemed to enjoy the program, which he attended 5 full days a week. Emma reported that they were managing well at home. Although she appeared exhausted, she denied it. She did acknowledge that she was awakened two or three times each night to help Russ go to the bathroom or to change his sheets if he did not remember that he needed to void. About 5 weeks later, during a caregivers' support group you were leading one morning, Emma fainted, apparently from exhaustion.

 and Think!

- What should you do first?

You make sure that she is lying safely, cover her, take her vital signs, and examine her for injuries. If a physician or nurse practitioner is available at the facility, you ask that she be further checked. If not, insist that she see her own physician that day. Call her daughter at work to come and drive her. When the daughter arrives, tell her that it is imperative that a family conference be held very soon that includes both the adult children and the couple, because Emma needs assistance and changes in the plan of care are imperative.

The next day, when they arrive for the family conference, it is obvious that the family has already discussed the situation and made some decisions. You try to make everyone feel comfortable and ask each person for input. Emma begins by explaining that the children had offered several times earlier to help her but she had refused because "I was raised to think it is a woman's duty to take care of her husband when he is sick."

She added that she tried to keep her house in the same immaculate condition and cook the same delicious meals because if she didn't maintain her standards, she would lose control of the whole situation and everything would fall apart. "The kids have convinced me that's silly, and I guess they are right. I just can't do it all alone."

You validate her comments, her efforts, and her realization that one person cannot realistically care for a sick loved one who needs constant care and do all the cooking and housework as well. You ask each member what should be done, they reach a consensus, and a new plan of care is established for Russ at home. The son will alternate nights with Emma for helping Russ go to the bathroom. (You recommend use of a urinal, commode, and disposable, waterproof pads under Russ' hips in the bed.) The daughter will cook all meals on weekends and occasionally during the week. Both children will finance a weekly cleaning woman. Russ said he will try to stop asking his wife to fetch him things every few minutes. Emma said she would stop being such a perfectionist about everything and be more willing to accept help. She admitted that she had learned that she has to pace herself to keep Russ at home. Before adjourning, you schedule another family conference in 2 weeks to evaluate how things are progressing.

Chapter SUMMARY

More and more health care is taking place in ambulatory settings. Nurses play an increasingly important role in these settings, particularly in triage and teaching. Advanced practice nurses deliver primary care in several of these settings, but most nursing care is delivered by registered nurses. Traditionally, most clients continue to seek medical care in physicians' offices, with nurses assisting in various ways. The number of doctors in solo practice is decreasing as competition requires them to join managed-care systems. Emergency department abuse is declining with the advent of walk-in centers, which are much less costly. Several ambulatory settings are designed primarily to serve the poor and uninsured. These include public health clinics, CHCs, some nursing centers, migrant worker centers, homeless shelters and clinics, some school-based clinics and family centers, and the Indian Health Service. Day hospitals of various types also employ nurses extensively. This chapter also discussed the benefits of various other ambulatory care settings.

A list of references and additional readings for this chapter appears at the end of Part 3.

10

Mental Health Nursing in the Community

Key Terms

affective disorders
agoraphobia
anticonvulsant medication
autism
benzodiazepines
bipolar disorder
borderline personality disorder
chemical dependencies
cognitive-behavioral therapy
comorbidity
compulsion
custodial care
deinstitutionalized
delirium
delusions
desensitization
detoxification
Diagnostic & Statistical Manual IV
dichotomy
dopamine

dually diagnosed
electroconvulsive therapy
flooding
grandiose thinking
guided imagery
guided mastery
hallucinations
HIV-related dementia
impulsivity
intervention
lithium carbonate
marijuana
meditation
mental retardation
methadone maintenance
monoamine oxidase inhibitors
neuroleptic medications
neuropsychiatric
nicotine
obsession
opportunistic infections

panic attacks
paranoia
phobias
positron emission tomography
posttraumatic stress disorder
progressive muscle relaxation
psychoanalysis
psychosis
recidivism
schizophrenia
selective serotonin reuptake inhibitors
stigmatized
taboo
tardive dyskinesia
tricyclic antidepressants
triply diagnosed
12-step programs
unconscious drives

Learning Objectives

1. Explain why mental illness is no longer considered merely psychogenic.

2. Describe what led to the development of mental health programs in the commu-

nity and the founding of community mental health centers.

3. Identify nursing roles and functions in community mental health.

4. Outline five major mental disorders and their treatments.

5. Identify five high-risk categories of mental health treatment that require case management.

6. List the most common substances abused by the general public.

7. Explain in detail the effects of nicotine and alcohol on health.

8. List the four questions to ask while using the CAGE screening tool.

9. Differentiate between the terms "polyaddiction" and "dual diagnosis."

10. Become familiar with each of the 12 steps of Alcoholics Anonymous.

An artificial dichotomy exists between mental health and physical health services. The agencies involved with mental health services are administered and funded separately and differently. Third-party reimbursements for mental health services are traditionally lower than those for physical illnesses. Health providers separate quite distinctly into mental and physical health personnel in both education and experience. These artificial separations are confusing to clients with mental and physical illnesses.

The 1990s were heralded as "the decade of the brain" by Congress and the National Institute of Mental Health (Simmons-Alling, 1996). Positron emission tomography and other advanced technology provided a better understanding of mental illness resulting from biochemical imbalances in the brain. Brain mapping pinpoints specific areas of the brain's gray matter that become active during particular thoughts or mental states (Fig. 10-1). As our knowledge of brain function and pathology increases, we are coming to understand illnesses such as schizophrenia as neurologic as much as psychiatric, so the term "neuropsychiatric" is more correct. Imbalances of the neurotransmitter dopamine are found in schizophrenia. Too much dopamine in the brain's emotion centers and too little in the seat of reason seems to cause suspiciousness and even the paranoia of schizophrenia. Impulsivity, obsessions, and compulsions are linked to imbalances of serotonin in the frontal lobe and the limbic system. A shortage of norepinephrine seems to rob people of the ability to pay attention, focus their thoughts, and concentrate. Deficiencies in these neurotransmitters have been associated with clinical depression. Psychotropic medications to correct these imbalances are being used successfully. Thus, the artificial separation between mental illness and physical illness is breaking down as medication is used to treat mental illnesses.

Beginning with Freud's remarkable discovery of unconscious drives, treatment of mental illness was dominated by psychological models of treatment through the mid-20th century. Expensive psychoanalysis or other forms of psychotherapy were available in private offices to those who could afford them. Most people did not seek treatment for milder mental illnesses, feeling shame and guilt about their supposed emotional weakness and inability to cope. Lack of resources to pay for private therapy prevented many people from seeking help. When behaviors became socially unacceptable, the mentally ill were committed to mental hospitals, often for the rest of their lives. There was considerable shame connected with commitment. It became taboo for family members to talk about mental illness in the family.

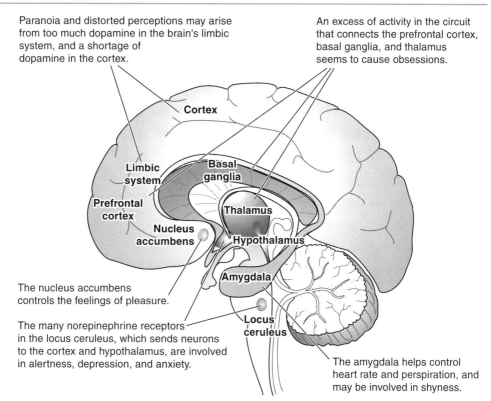

Paranoia and distorted perceptions may arise from too much dopamine in the brain's limbic system, and a shortage of dopamine in the cortex.

An excess of activity in the circuit that connects the prefrontal cortex, basal ganglia, and thalamus seems to cause obsessions.

The nucleus accumbens controls the feelings of pleasure.

The many norepinephrine receptors in the locus ceruleus, which sends neurons to the cortex and hypothalamus, are involved in alertness, depression, and anxiety.

The amygdala helps control heart rate and perspiration, and may be involved in shyness.

Cortex

Limbic system

Basal ganglia

Prefrontal cortex

Thalamus

Nucleus accumbens

Hypothalamus

Amygdala

Locus ceruleus

FIGURE 10-1
Mapping the Mind. Personality traits from shyness to impulsiveness, scientists believe, are produced by particular brain molecules acting on specific brain structures. Through brain mapping and biochemistry, researchers have identified some of them. (Blumrich. © 1994, Newsweek, Inc. All rights reserved. Reprinted by permission.)

A few private mental hospitals existed, but most seriously mentally ill persons were committed to one of the large state institutions. An elaborate system with enormous state institutions for the mentally ill and the mentally retarded developed in each state to house persons with mental retardation, schizophrenia, bipolar mood disorders, or other illnesses causing psychosis. Care was custodial and treatment was minimal, making these institutions large human warehouses. These state institutions housed thousands of people all over the United States; many patients stayed for most of their lifetimes. They lost their civil rights as persons.

The Development of Mental Health Programs in the Community

Several factors led to the need for community mental health programs to replace state psychiatric institutions (Display 10-1). The advent of new psychotropic drugs, beginning with chlorpromazine (Thorazine) in the 1950s, allowed severe psychiatric symptoms

---

DISPLAY 10-1
A Brief History of Community Mental Health

THE 1950s

- Psychotropic drugs were introduced to control psychotic symptoms, facilitating a transition to community care.

THE 1960s

- The Joint Commission on Mental Illness reported to Congress, recommending a shift to community-based care.
- The Community Mental Health Centers Act authorized $150 million in federal matching funds to states to develop services.

THE 1970s

- The National Institute of Mental Health (NIMH) began the community support program and established an Office of Programs for the Homeless Mentally Ill.

THE 1980s

- Congress passed the Omnibus Budget Reconciliation Act, placing services formerly directed by the NIMH in federal block grants to states.

THE 1990s

- The NIMH Epidemiologic Catchment Area Study funded research demonstration programs authorized by the Stewart B. McKinney Homeless Assistance Act.
- The federal task force on homelessness and severe mental illness made recommendations for the expansion of housing and service options to the homeless mentally ill.
- The Americans with Disabilities Act affirmed the rights of those with psychiatric disabilities.

(Adapted from Chafetz L [1996]. The severely and persistently mentally ill in the community. In Wilson H, Kneisl C, eds. Psychiatric Nursing. *Menlo Park, CA: Addison-Wesley.)*

---

such as psychosis to be controlled. Many patients on neuroleptic medications were no longer a threat to themselves or to others and therefore no longer needed to be locked up in mental hospitals. Groups concerned with their unjust loss of civil liberty sued on their behalf, and patients were gradually released to the community. By 1975, almost 500,000 people had been released from state mental hospitals (Worley, 1995).

Although the intention was to create comprehensive community services for the deinstitutionalized mentally ill population, it did not fully happen. Also, the number of services required in addition to mental health services was underestimated. Community services to house and supervise such large numbers of vulnerable people were inadequate and fragmented. That problem still exists. There is still great resistance to the establishment of group homes and halfway houses for the mentally ill or mentally retarded. Neighbors are often hostile and demonstrate against the residences. Most mentally ill persons end up living in substandard housing in the poorest, most crime-ridden urban areas in the United States. An estimated one third of all homeless people are mentally ill. Most chronic mentally ill persons fall below the poverty guidelines listed in the Federal Register. Poverty, homelessness, severe mental illness, substance abuse, and high risk for HIV infection and other communicable diseases make this population extremely vulnerable.

Community Mental Health Centers

President John F. Kennedy signed the Community Mental Health Centers Act into law in 1963. It provided $150 million in matching funds to states to establish community mental health centers throughout the United States. This act followed the 1961 National Mental Health Study by the Joint Commission on Mental Illness and Health. In addition to a shift from institutional to community care, this study called for a new emphasis on easy availability and rapid administration of treatment (eg, secondary prevention). It also stressed primary preventive services.

Community mental health centers received matching federal funds if they provided at least five essential services: emergency services, hospitalization, outpatient services, partial hospitalization, and consultation and education to prevent mental illness. Thus, primary, secondary, and tertiary prevention services are provided to avoid long-term hospitalizations. Both secondary and tertiary prevention are provided by inpatient and outpatient services. Display 10-2 describes nursing roles and functions at the three levels of prevention.

Community mental health centers were successful and stimulated other community agencies to develop similar mental health services. For example, many community general hospitals sponsor both outpatient services and inpatient mental health units within the hospital as well as medical-surgical care. A psychiatric-mental health nurse clinical specialist working at a private hospital's mental health outpatient clinic as a therapist recounts the following case story:

> Andy was brought to me by another of my young clients because of our sliding-scale fees. He had no money and he didn't want to tell his parents what he was experiencing. He was very depressed, even suicidal, because of rejection by his girlfriend. He needed to be hospitalized for suicide monitoring but refused. He denied that he was suicidal. However, he did agree to allow me to call his parents and tell them about his situation. Andy's mother expressed outrage that anyone would suggest that their son might try suicide or that he was depressed. I told her about emergency resources at our hospital and at the community mental health center and advised that they take Andy for care. She told me to stop interfering with other people's business and hung up the phone.
>
> Three days later, Andy slit his wrists but was found in time and brought to the emergency room by his parents. At that time, we had no opening in our in-hospital unit, so he was transferred to the community mental health center crisis unit, where they hospitalized him. I kept in touch with him and learned that he was given antidepressant medication and assigned to group therapy with other suicidal adolescents. He received individual psychotherapy every day.

DISPLAY 10-2
What do Community Mental Health Nurses do?

- Promote mental education and consultation
- Advocate politically regarding mental health issues
- Teach effective-parenting classes
- Identify high-risk populations in the community
- Recognize potentially stressful conditions in the community
- Organize divorce therapy groups for couples, families, and individuals
- Assist with psychotherapy for groups, families, and persons
- Organize suicide hotlines and counseling programs
- Staff crisis intervention programs
- Provide disaster counseling
- Screen, case find, and assess clients
- Provide emergency mental health service
- Counsel victims of violence and other crimes
- Plan discharge for clients from one setting to another
- Coordinate and monitor follow-up care in homes or halfway houses
- Teach self-care activities
- Use psychosocial rehabilitation strategies with clients
- Staff partial hospitalization and outpatient clinics
- Visit clients in their homes as needed

Within 3 weeks, his mood started to lift. After a month, it was determined that he was no longer suicidal and could go back to school during the day, returning to the therapeutic milieu of the hospital the rest of the time. He was not ready to go home and needed partial hospitalization. Family therapy was recommended due to dysfunctional family communication patterns.

After 6 weeks, Andy was discharged to home but continued to return three times a week for psychotherapy. Family therapy continued, and his parents also enrolled in a primary prevention class about dealing with teenagers. The crisis was over. From all that I've heard, Andy was fine after that.

Mental Health Disorders and Their Treatments

Disorders such as depression, anxiety, panic attacks, and phobias are most common (Table 10-1) and can be treated successfully on an outpatient basis unless the client is suicidal. With most disorders, more than one type of therapy is used concurrently. The more serious disorders (schizophrenia, bipolar disorder, and some personality disorders) may require episodic long-term treatment, with hospitalization from time to time. The *Diagnostic & Statistical Manual IV* of the American Psychiatric Society describes all the mental health disorders with criteria for diagnosis. Some *Healthy People 2000* national objectives related to mental health problems are listed in Display 10-3.

TABLE 10-1. Proportion of US Population Affected by Selected Mental Disorders According to the NIMH–ECA Study

Type of Condition	Percent of Population Affected
Anxiety disorders, phobias	8.9
Substance abuse disorders	6.0
Affective disorders	5.8
Dysthymia (mental distress)	3.3
Major depressive disorder	3.0
Schizophrenia	0.8
Bipolar disorder	0.5

(Source: National Institute of Mental Health–Epidemiologic Catchment Area Study, 1990.)

Depression

Depression can rob one of vitality, pleasure, and hope. Sleep disorders (especially early-morning awakening), constipation, and changes in appetite are additional symptoms of depression. Psychomotor retardation results in slow thinking and movement and loss of energy. A sense of hopelessness and despair sometimes leads to suicide.

DISPLAY 10-3
Healthy People 2000: Selected National Health Objectives Related to Chronic Mental Health Problems

6.3   Reduce to less than 10% the prevalence of mental disorders among children and adolescents.

6.4   Reduce the prevalence of mental disorders (excluding substance abuse) to less than 10.7% of adults living in the community.

6.5   Reduce to less than 35% the proportion of people 18 years of age and older who experienced adverse affects of stress in the past year.

6.6   Increase to at least 30% the proportion of people 18 years of age and older with severe mental disorders who use community support programs.

6.7   Increase the proportion of people with major depressive disorders who obtain treatment to at least 45%.

6.8   Increase the proportion of people aged 18 and older who seek help in coping with personal and emotional problems to at least 20%.

6.13   Increase the proportion of primary care providers who routinely assess client's emotional, cognitive, and behavioral functioning to at least 50%.

(Source: U.S. Department of Health and Human Services.)

Medications to treat depression bring relief to 60% to 80% of people within 3 to 6 weeks (National Advisory Mental Health Council, 1993b). The various subgroups of medications are thought to correct neurotransmitter deficits and imbalances. Tricyclic antidepressants such as amitriptyline (Elavil) are the oldest groups and can cause weight gain, drowsiness, constipation, and dry mouth. Monoamine oxidase inhibitors such as phenelzine (Nardil) can cause serious, sudden, high elevation of blood pressure if taken with foods containing tyramine or if taken with certain other medications. Selective serotonin reuptake inhibitors (SSRIs) such as fluoxetine (Prozac) are the newest major subgroup. SSRIs are the most effective and have the fewest side effects of the antidepressant drugs, but some persons respond better to drugs from the other two classifications.

Persons with bipolar mood disorder are usually treated with lithium carbonate, which seems to regulate the manic episodes and prevent the depressive episodes. Carbamazepine (Tegretol), an anticonvulsant, is sometimes used to treat mania. Electroconvulsive therapy can be an effective modality and is used for severely depressed persons who cannot take medications or are not responsive to them.

Psychotherapy, by itself or with medications, can also be effective in the treatment of depression. Cognitive therapy, which teaches clients to correct negative beliefs and assumptions that affect their emotions, has the same success rate (60% to 80%) as medications (*Harvard Mental Health Letter*, 1995). This is based on empirical findings that "feelings follow thoughts." Usually psychotherapy is prescribed along with medications for the best outcomes.

Anxiety Disorders

Anxiety disorders can immobilize a person and dominate his or her life with a pervasive sense of impending doom. Anxiety seems to occur in response to a threat to the ego and is normally handled with the use of ego defense mechanisms. Antianxiety tranquilizers such as the benzodiazepines diazepam (Valium) and alprazolam (Xanax) can bring quick relief in short-term situations, but because they can be addictive, they should not be used on a regular, long-term basis. Buspirone (BuSpar) is an antianxiety drug that does not seem to be addictive.

Stress management techniques such as progressive muscle relaxation, meditation, and guided imagery, if practiced daily, can reduce anxiety. Regular active exercise is helpful for most people. Talking out problems in psychotherapy or with friends can help tremendously, as can prayer and other spiritual rituals. Some people with unyielding, intense anxiety profit from cognitive-behavioral therapy to learn to counter the irrational thoughts that provoke anxiety. Display 15-1 lists some relaxation exercises.

Millions of people (1.5% to 3.5% of the population) suffer panic attacks repeatedly and unexpectedly. Feelings of intense fear occur along with dizziness, nausea, sweating, palpitations, chest pain, and a sense of losing all control. Panic attacks are usually treated with alprazolam. Benzodiazepines prove effective and relatively safe in treating situational intense anxiety for up to 4 to 8 weeks. Antidepressant medications help control and prevent the long-term occurrence of panic attacks. Sometimes the anticonvulsant clonazepam (Klonopin) or the beta-adrenergic blocker propranolol (Inderal) is effective, particularly in post-traumatic stress disorder. Appendix D gives a clinical path for panic disorder.

Strong, irrational fears called phobias affect many American adults. Some people fear animals, insects, or snakes. Others suffer from social phobias and are intensely fearful of situations involving other people. Some people suffer agoraphobia, a fear of crowded places or open spaces. Panic disorder can result in agoraphobia. The most popular treatment of a phobia is desensitization, a type of behavioral therapy. Recently a method of treatment called guided mastery was introduced that expands on desensitization. Treatments try to alter maladaptive thinking and confirm the client's coping capacity (*Harvard Mental Health Letter*, May 1997). Frequently, antidepressant drugs are used along with therapy to prevent panic as the fear is confronted. After becoming very relaxed with the use of progressive relaxation exercises, gradual desensitization is begun by imagining the least fearsome situation. Gradually and systematically, the client moves along to more frightening things, finally imagining and then confronting the chief cause of the phobia.

Flooding approaches the phobia from the other direction by immediately immersing the client in the feared object or situation for a specific length of time until the anxiety subsides. This approach is less popular because of the risk of stimulating panic attacks.

Personality Disorders

SSRIs have been used with some success to treat personality disorders, but these pervasive disorders, previously called "character disorders," generally do not respond well to treatment. They represent a style of maladaptive behavior developed over a long period. Antisocial and borderline personality disorders are the most common.

Compulsive Disorders

Obsessive-compulsive disorder (OCD) is disruptive and is often associated with the disorders listed above. The client becomes dominated by continuous, intrusive thoughts and the need to carry out certain rituals to control his or her anxiety and avoid a panic attack. Frequent handwashing and obsession with microorganisms is an example. Sometimes people with OCD wash their hands so frequently that their hands begin to look like raw meat. Psychotherapy has not been effective in treating this disorder. Some antidepressant drugs, such as clomipramine (Anafranil) and fluoxetine (Prozac), have proved successful. It is not useful to tell clients with OCD that their rituals are irrational; they are well aware of this and want to give them up. Preventing a client from performing rituals may bring on a panic attack. Brain mapping has identified certain areas of the brain that show excess activity in persons with obsessions.

Addiction is also a compulsion and is classified as a mental disorder or disease, although many people refuse to think of it that way. Dual diagnosis (comorbidity) of addiction along with other mental disorders is described later in this chapter. Addiction in the general population without other mental disorders is also discussed later.

Schizophrenia

This diagnostic label applies only to a person who has been psychotic (out of touch with reality) for at least 6 months. This disorder involves gross disruptions in perception, cognition, emotion, and behavior. Bizarre, confused thoughts are a primary feature. Several distinct types of schizophrenia have been noted, and schizophrenia is now thought to be a group of disorders. It affects almost 1% of the population. Autism, or extreme withdrawal from others, is the major symptom and one of the reasons why some homeless people with schizophrenia refuse to go to shelters or group homes.

There is considerable social and occupational dysfunction in schizophrenia, which usually begins around age 20. If the person continues to suffer delusions, hallucinations, and disorganized behavior over a 2-year period, he or she is considered chronic. Sometimes chronic schizophrenics go into remission, especially when they are compliant with their medications. Then they seem normal, exhibiting symptoms only during exacerbations of the disease.

People with schizophrenia react differently to different antipsychotic medications. All these neuroleptic medications have serious side effects. The most serious are agranulocytosis, which can be fatal, and tardive dyskinesia, which is irreversible. Newer medications such as clozapine (Clozaril) and risperidone (Risperdal) are effective for some clients who do not respond well to other antipsychotic medications.

Bipolar Disorder

Previously called manic-depressive disorder, this condition manifests itself in extreme moods, which can be cyclic or predominantly manic or depressive. In both extremes of mood, clients can experience psychosis. Lithium stabilizes the disease in most people and enables them to live fairly normal lives if compliant with the medication regimen. This regimen includes monthly blood tests to monitor the blood level of lithium and to prevent toxic buildup. Another effective drug is carbamazepine. Extreme impulsivity, hyperactivity, and grandiose thinking characterize the manic episodes. See the true case study in ''The Nurse Speaks'' near the end of this chapter.

Community Support Programs

Community mental health services have been successful in primary and secondary prevention but cannot provide all the tertiary prevention services needed by the severely and persistently mentally ill coming out of large state hospitals. Persons with chronic, severe mental illness sometimes decompensate and relapse in the community for a wide variety of reasons and require rehospitalization. Relapses can be caused by the disease process, failure to take prescribed psychotropic medications, or the stressors of life in the community. Rehospitalization compounds their lifestyle stressors: a client fortunate enough to find a decent, affordable apartment may lose it during hospitalization. A vicious cycle occurs when the client is discharged and must adjust to a different community dwelling; he or she may end up homeless in the process. All the stressors of homelessness can lead to another relapse, requiring another period of hospitalization.

In recognition of these problems, in 1977 the National Institute of Mental Health established community support programs targeted at the severely and persistently mentally ill. Case management is provided for consistent support and coordination of needed services. Those who are frequently hospitalized, dually diagnosed, or homeless are the focus of case management because they need intensive and skillful guidance. Psychiatric nurses are best equipped to function as case managers because of their holistic orientation and the fact that these clients have multiple physical needs. Social workers are used as case managers in some communities. Many facilities hire mental health lay workers for these case management roles because they are less expensive than professionals. In addition to case management, other community support programs include social and life skills training, vocational rehabilitation, day hospitals, outpatient clinics, and socialization and support clubs for clients who have been discharged from mental hospitals.

High-Risk Clients Needing Case Management

Recidivism

Frequent relapse to psychotic and threatening symptoms requiring rehospitalization places mentally ill clients in a high-risk category requiring case management. More than two hospitalizations per year is not considered normal, even for severe mental illness. Good case management usually prevents relapses and frequent rehospitalization.

Elderly

There are 2 million chronically mentally ill elderly people in the United States. Many are frail elderly who need case management so they can stay in the community instead of being placed in extended-care facilities. Those who are homebound often need the services of home care nurses who are especially knowledgeable about mental illness. More about the home care nursing needs of these people is found in Chapter 15. Criteria for psychiatric-mental health home care services are found in Display 15-5 and a short mental status examination for dementia is found in Display 11-3.

Mental Retardation

The Mental Retardation Facilities and Community Mental Health Centers Construction Act led to the discharge of many mentally retarded persons to the community. A mentally retarded person is one with an IQ below 75; about 2% to 3% of the population is considered mentally retarded (Harris, 1995). By standard definition, mental retardation means that clients have intellectual limitations associated with seriously impaired adaptive behavior so they cannot attain a level of social responsibility and personal independence appropriate to their age either as children or adults. The same pattern of resistance to the establishment of community residences or neighborhood group homes exists for mentally retarded persons as it does for psychiatric clients. Occasionally there is overlap: persons who are mentally retarded can also suffer from mental illness, as shown in the case study in "The Nurse

Speaks." Emotional disturbances occur in up to 40% of mentally retarded adults (Drapo, 1993). This is referred to as dual diagnosis.

Substance Abuse and HIV Infection

Perhaps because of the drug-ridden neighborhoods where they are forced to live, or perhaps in efforts to self-medicate against the unpleasant feelings of mental illness, many clients with mental illness drift into substance abuse and become addicted (Fig. 10-2). When they come to the health system for treatment, they are said to have a dual diagnosis. Mentally ill clients who become infected with AIDS because they have used infected needles are said to carry a triple diagnosis. Mentally ill clients tend to engage in unsafe sexual practices, putting them at risk for HIV infection. In one study of clients with schizophrenia (Cournos et al, 1994), nearly 50% had been sexually active during the preceding 6 months in ways that placed them at high risk for HIV infection. In another study (Kalichman et al, 1994), high-risk behaviors for HIV infection among mentally ill persons were identified as

- Multiple sex partners
- No or inconsistent condom use

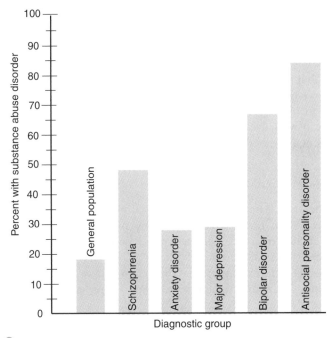

FIGURE 10-2
Lifetime prevalence rates for substance abuse disorder. (Based on data from NIMH-ECA [1990]. Epidemiologic Catchment Area Study. Washington DC: NIMH.)

- Alcohol and drug use in conjunction with sex
- Sex partners who are injection drug users
- Infection with other sexually transmitted infections.

HIV-Related Dementia

HIV infection of the central nervous system resulting in dementia is an increasingly common neuropsychiatric disorder. It results in a progressive loss of cognitive and motor function along with behavioral changes. HIV-related dementia is not limited to the vulnerable clients with chronic mental illness. In the later stages of AIDS, HIV-related dementia is seen more and more frequently. Early symptoms include headaches and seizures. Common behavioral changes include dysphoric mood, apathy, and withdrawal, often misinterpreted as clinical depression. Psychosis and regressive, childlike behaviors occur. Forgetfulness, confusion, psychomotor retardation, muscle weakness, and loss of balance are other indications of HIV-related dementia. Symptoms of forgetfulness and confusion make clients more vulnerable to opportunistic infections because they cannot take adequate care of themselves. These neuropsychiatric symptoms also present enormous challenges to caregivers of persons with AIDS. Home care and hospice nurses see many cases of HIV-related dementia.

Dual Diagnosis: Mental Illness and Substance Abuse

The complex situation caused by the interrelated problems of mental illness and alcohol or other drug abuse is called dual diagnosis or comorbidity. Persons with serious mental illnesses such as antisocial or borderline personality disorder, schizophrenia, or bipolar mood disorder often become addicted to chemicals or misuse them in unhealthy ways. These chemicals can further complicate their psychiatric symptoms. For example, alcohol, a central nervous system depressant, intensifies and prolongs depression. Cocaine, a central nervous system stimulant, increases psychotic symptoms, including acute paranoia, frightening hallucinations, and delusions. Combining street drugs with prescribed psychotropic drugs reduces or complicates the effectiveness of the latter and causes toxic effects such as increased tardive dyskinesia (Olivera et al, 1990). Disorganized behavior is another interaction effect that puts these vulnerable people at extreme risk for HIV infection, for example.

One of the problems in treating persons with dual diagnosis is that another artificial division exists between treatment facilities and programs for serious mental illnesses and treatment programs for substance abuse. Even if they coexist on the same community mental health campus, they are physically separated and treatment is administered by a different staff. This makes integrated treatment for severely mentally ill persons challenging and confusing to the clients. The reason for this division seems to be the effort to distance addiction and substance abuse treatment from other mental illnesses. By not labeling addictions as mental disorders, clients are less stigmatized and more apt to come for treatment.

Addictions in the General Population

Nicotine, Alcohol, and Street Drugs

Alcohol and nicotine are still the most widely abused substances in the United States. In recent years, nicotine has been recognized as a highly addictive and dangerous chemical. One in five deaths is attributed to cigarette smoking in the United States, according to the Institute for Health Policy (Brandeis University, 1993). This includes 90% of deaths from lung cancer, 90% of deaths from chronic pulmonary disease, and 30% of deaths from heart disease (Fiore, 1993). In 1993, the Centers for Disease Control and Prevention (CDC) estimated the medical costs of smoking to be $50 billion dollars (*MMWR*, 1994). Published data in 1989 attributed more than 40% of the total annual medical care expenditures to smoking (USDHHS, 1989) (Fig. 10-3).

Severe liver, pancreatic, brain, and gastrointestinal disease commonly occurs secondary to heavy alcohol use. The addiction rate of alcohol is 10%—that is, out of every 10 persons who drink alcohol from time to time, one person becomes addicted to alcohol. Together, addictions to alcohol and nicotine cause or contribute to a large number of physical disorders. The premature deaths of millions of people are caused by these substances. They rank among the highest of all risk factors in the United States. Alcoholism by itself is the third leading cause of illness and disability in the United States and accounts for 10% of all deaths (National Advisory Mental Health Council, 1993a).

Most people when surveyed reported that they were not screened for alcohol use when seeing their physicians for check-ups (National Institute on Alcohol Abuse

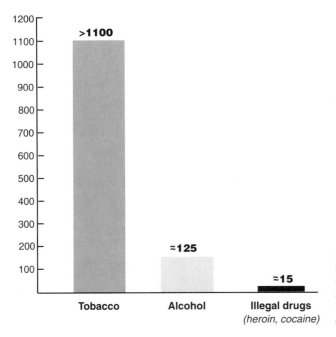

FIGURE 10-3
Drug-related deaths per day. (Reprinted with permission. Stanhope M, Lancaster J, [1996] *Community Health Nursing.* 4th ed. St. Louis: Mosby.)

and Alcoholism, 1994; Substance Abuse Letter, 1994; NIAAA, 1994). The CAGE question-naire is a brief, effective, easy-to-use screening tool:

C: Have you ever felt you should *Cut down* on your drinking?

A: Have people *Annoyed* you by criticizing your drinking?

G: Have you ever felt bad or *Guilty* about drinking?

E: Have your ever taken a drink first thing in the morning to steady your nerves or get rid of a hangover (*Eye-opener*)?

The questionnaire reliably identifies early alcohol abuse. A positive CAGE is defined as one or more affirmative answers. As a screening tool, both its sensitivity (85%) and specificity (89%) are impressive (Bush et al, 1987).

It is estimated that drug and alcohol abuse contributes to more than $163.6 billion dollars in health-care costs, lost productivity, and crime. Estimates of general hospital beds occupied by patients whose physical condition is caused or complicated by alcohol and drug problems range from 25% to 50% (National Advisory Mental Health Council, 1993a). Street drugs such as heroin, crack cocaine, and lysergic acid diethylamide (LSD) are the most widely feared, perhaps because of the deterioration in personality that occurs with their abuse. Alcohol use has become such an intimate part of American culture that we tend to deny or overlook the personality deterioration that can occur with alcoholism. Many people refuse to think of alcohol as a serious drug and still find intoxication somewhat amusing.

Treatment of Addictions

Private treatment centers for drug and alcohol addiction have become a big business. An optimal program for success is an expensive 28-day residential program that includes the 12-step program of Alcoholics Anonymous. The first several days are spent in detoxification, and an educational and counseling program follows. Family members are included in the therapy, usually during a family weekend toward the end of the 28 days. Some studies show residential rehabilitation to be the most effective treatment mode. However, inpatient programs are losing popularity because of their expense, and sources of insurance coverage are drying up. Several recent studies show outpatient and day hospital treatment programs to be equally effective for alcoholics (*Harvard Mental Health Letter*, 1995). Outpatient detoxification can be a problem for addictions to alcohol, barbiturates, and benzodiazepines if done abruptly. Close monitoring by home care or clinic nurses is important for those substances because of the delirium and other effects that can occur.

The Council on Alcoholism has developed a successful strategy to break down the strong denial of persons addicted to chemicals. The strategy is known as "intervention" and was made famous by the Ford family in their efforts to force the former first lady, Betty Ford, to recognize her addictions and enter a treatment program. The Council on Alcoholism offers assistance in planning and training for interventions. If done properly, they are about 96% successful. The "Clinical Application" in this chapter is based on a true account regarding a family's intervention to combat alcoholism in a loved one.

Most treatment centers today treat polyaddiction, addiction to more than one drug. A common combination is cocaine and alcohol. Most addicts under age 45 are polyaddicted. Although alcohol is still the dominant addiction, persons often cite cocaine as their drug of choice.

The recent rise in the number of teenagers using drugs is distressing, especially because that rate had been falling (Fig. 10-4). Marijuana and alcohol are the "entry-level drugs" widely used by teenagers. Some of the marijuana available today is potent or contaminated and potentially harmful. The National Federation of Drug-Free Youth states the dangers of marijuana as follows:

- Smoking just two joints of marijuana can reduce lung capacity more than smoking one pack of tobacco cigarettes.
- Marijuana smoke has 50% more tar than regular cigarettes and produces greater cellular changes in the lungs than does tobacco smoke.
- Marijuana can cause emphysema 20 times faster than tobacco, and marijuana smoke increases airway resistance 25%.
- Marijuana appears to lower testosterone levels in boys and may accumulate in the ovaries of girls.
- Brain wave tests show that teenagers who get high twice a week or more have evidence of diffuse brain impairment for up to 2 months.

All nurses should practice primary prevention in teaching teenage friends and family the facts about the effects of marijuana. The myth among teenagers is that marijuana is basically harmless.

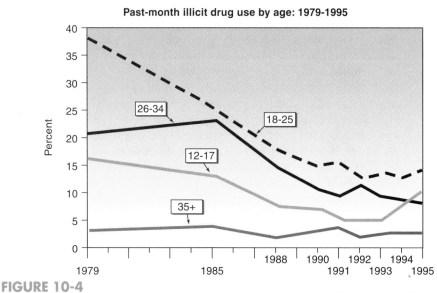

FIGURE 10-4
Surveys show U.S. drug use stays the same; increases among youth. (Source: Advance Report Number 17, Preliminary Estimates from the Drug Abuse Warning Network, Office of Applied Studies, Substance Abuse and Mental Health Services Administration.)

Ambulatory Drug Treatment Programs

Many managed-care programs do not pay for residential treatment programs. Ambulatory drug treatment programs are becoming more prevalent and more successful. Often "detox" day hospital programs are separate from "rehab" programs. Most community mental health centers sponsor drug and alcoholism treatment programs, as do many government and private agencies. To date, the most successful programs in the treatment of addictions are the least expensive: 12-step programs based on the original format of Alcoholics Anonymous established in 1935 by Bill Wilson (Display 10-4). Other 12-step programs include Narcotics Anonymous, Overeaters Anonymous, Emotions Anonymous, and Gamblers Anonymous. One problem with these programs is the high dropout rate, estimated to be as high as 60–75% by 3 months and 88% by 1 year. However, many alcoholics return later to try again. By 5 years, 35% are successful at attaining sobriety

---

DISPLAY 10-4
The Twelve Steps of Alcoholics Anonymous

1. We admitted we were powerless over alcohol—that our lives had become unmanageable.
2. Came to believe that a Power greater than ourselves could restore us to sanity.
3. Made a decision to turn our will and our lives over to the care of God, as we understood Him.
4. Made a searching and fearless moral inventory of ourselves.
5. Admitted to God, to ourselves, and to another human being the exact nature of our wrongs.
6. Were entirely ready to have God remove all these defects of character.
7. Humbly asked Him to remove our shortcomings.
8. Made a list of all people we had harmed, and became willing to make amends to them all.
9. Made direct amends to such people wherever possible, except when to do so would injure them or others.
10. Continued to take personal inventory and when we were wrong, promptly admitted it.
11. Sought through prayer and meditation to improve our conscious contact with God, as we understood Him, praying only for knowledge of His will for us and the power to carry that out.
12. Having had a spiritual awakening as the result of these steps, we tried to carry this message to alcoholics, and to practice these principles in all our affairs.

(The Twelve Steps from Twelve Steps and Twelve Traditions *are reprinted with permission of Alcoholics Anonymous World Services, Inc. Permission to reprint the Twelve Steps does not mean that AA has reviewed or approved the contents of this publication, nor that AA agrees with the views expressed herein. AA is a program of recovery from alcoholism only—use of the Twelve Steps in connection with programs and activities which are patterned after AA, but which address other problems, or in any other non-AA context, does not imply otherwise.)*

(Brownell, et al, 1986). Participants always refer to themselves as recovering, not recovered, from their addiction. The 12 steps have proved so valuable, both for treatment and as a successful way to live life, that they are now included in almost all treatment programs.

Methadone maintenance programs for the treatment of heroin addiction are sponsored by most community mental health centers but are controversial. Methadone is a synthetic narcotic given free to addicts as a substitute drug, paid for by taxpayers. Critics charge that addicts use these programs to reduce the cost of maintaining their habit on the street. Methadone is administered in lower and lower doses and reduces tolerance to narcotics. The goal is that the dose eventually becomes so low that the client is no longer physiologically addicted to the narcotic. According to the *Harvard Mental Health Letter* (1995), methadone maintenance stands out as particularly cost-effective among addiction treatments. These programs have a relatively low dropout rate and when well managed are successful in curing the addiction. Most research suggests that methadone programs work better when they also supply counseling, medical care, and psychiatric services.

Is Addiction a Disease?

Debate continues about whether addiction is a disease associated with chemical dependency. Some people insist that addiction is a learned habit, a character weakness, or a life problem. Professionals who adhere to this model advocate behavioral and cognitive therapy to correct counterproductive actions and attitudes. They say that thinking of addiction as a disease promotes moral irresponsibility, helps explain away and ignore underlying problems, and reduces the client's confidence in his or her ability to master the habit.

However, most professionals who work in the field of addictions advocate the disease model, which regards drug dependence as a chronic brain malfunction. The addiction is a chemically induced disorder that greatly stimulates the brain's reward or pleasure center and may cause lasting physiologic changes associated with alterations in neurotransmitter functioning. Viewing addiction as a disease removes some of the stigma and guilt and makes it easier for clients to seek and accept help. The disease of addiction endangers both physical and mental health and causes huge secondary problems for families and communities.

A spiritual crisis or a required behavioral modification has been known to lead to sudden recovery. This fact, and the estimated 50% or more alcoholics who eventually free themselves from their addiction, are difficult to understand if one adheres only to the disease theory. In one study, a group of self-treated alcoholics was interviewed, with the following results (*Harvard Mental Health Letter*, 1995):

> Fifty-seven percent simply said they decided that alcohol was bad for them. Twenty-nine percent said health problems, frightening experiences, accidents, or blackouts persuaded them to quit. Others used such phrases as "Things were building up" or "I was sick and tired of it." Support from a husband or wife was important in sustaining the resolution.

It appears that addiction is a complex condition that is both physiologically and psychologically driven.

THE NURSE SPEAKS . . .

About Conducting an Intervention

For a long time I was in denial about Tom's drinking. He was always a very social person who enjoyed people and loved to party. It was probably one of the things that made me fall in love with him and marry him. At some time over the past few years, though, things began to get out of hand. Although his drinking never seemed to interfere with his work, it became his regular pattern to stop after work "to relax with the boys over a drink or two," as he used to put it. He always had a beer in his hand around the house, which he claimed that he "nursed" all day. His personality changed at home, and he began to yell at the kids or at me for the least little thing. Once when our youngest son talked back, Tom lost control and hit him. That's when my denial broke down and I started looking for help.

I called the Council on Alcoholism and they helped a great deal, first to confirm that Tom was indeed an alcoholic, based on my description of his behavior. They helped me see that I too had become affected by the disease of alcoholism and needed personal help. They gave me information about Al-Anon and Alateen for my sons. They told me that I couldn't change Tom by harping at him or begging him to change, as I had been doing. They suggested that if and when I felt ready, they would give me guidance on holding an intervention to lovingly but firmly confront Tom with his alcoholism and to break down his strong denial. They explained that such interventions have a 96% success rate when conducted correctly, with guidance.

It took me a while to realize that we could not go on as a family unless Tom sought help, and whatever it took, financially or otherwise, we should try. I went back to the Council for intervention training for two or three sessions, and our sons agreed to do the same. I asked Tom's brother and sister and close friends (nonalcoholics and recovering alcoholics) to participate. They were all concerned about his drinking and agreed to help and go for training. We learned to describe, in a caring way, Tom's behavior that we had observed and how it affected us. I made reservations at a residential 28-day treatment center in the next county for the night of the intervention. I had his suitcase packed and friends ready to drive him there right from the intervention. In my own mind, I was ready to tell him that night that if he did not go into treatment, I would leave him. We made up some ruse about the meeting, and when Tom and I walked in, everyone was waiting.

Tom's denial was incredible. Finally, he admitted that maybe he did have a little problem and would go to some AA meetings, but there was no way he could afford to take off work for a month. I told him that I had already spoken with the occupational health nurse where he works. He would be given the time and considerable help with the expenses, and everything would be handled confidentially. Finally, he agreed to go, but he was very, very angry at me, and I was grateful that a couple of his friends were driving him to the treatment center. During the next 3 or 4 days, he refused to speak with me on the telephone. Then, he started to change.

Since treatment, Tom has been a different person. It's wonderful to have our family working together again. Tom has become an enthusiastic participant in AA and is even instrumental in helping other people attain sobriety. Alcoholics always say they are recovering, not recovered, but Tom has maintained sobriety for many years now. Best of all, AA has helped him discover his own spirituality and source of strength.

Pat
HOME CARE NURSE

CLINICAL APPLICATION

A Critical Thinking Case Study Involving a Client With Bipolar Disorder

On a very cold, windy winter day, Irene comes to the mental health clinic where you work. She wears a thin jacket and no hat or gloves, and is heavily made up. She finds it difficult to sit during the interview and keeps standing up and pacing every few minutes. Her speech is rapid and pressured.

"I only came because the people where I live said I couldn't stay there anymore if I didn't come to the clinic. They say I've been acting crazy, just because I can't sleep at night. They drive *me* crazy! So bossy! I can't do this and I can't do that! I can't go out with guys just because I'm retarded. They're the ones who are retarded!"

 and Think!

- What defense mechanism is Irene using?
- She says she is retarded, but her referral form says she has bipolar disorder. What do you think could be the reason for this discrepancy?
- What are the symptoms of each condition?
- Which symptoms does Irene manifest?
- Irene did not want to come to the clinic and seems angry. What can you say or do to begin to establish a therapeutic relationship with her?

"It must be very hard for you," you reflect sincerely. You note her use of projection and denial and her manic behaviors. Probably she has a dual diagnosis. Let your body language communicate your empathy.

"Tell me about what's been happening," you suggest.

"I moved here from upstate this summer because I heard there were good jobs here. Then my lithium ran out and I didn't know how to get more. Anyway, I was feeling okay. Lately I've been jumpy and I can't sleep."

She gets up from the chair and paces back and forth again.

"You take lithium but it ran out, so you haven't taken it lately and are feeling hyper," you restate. "Tell me more. When did all this start?"

"Years ago. Sometimes I get so high and do bad things, like sleep around with guys and stuff. Then sometimes I get so low I can hardly move. Lithium helps, but it ran out this summer. I don't have any to take now," she says, finally making eye contact.

"That's a tough disease! It sounds like you think you need some lithium. I bet the doctor will agree with you and you'll get some lithium today to make you start feeling better. Did lithium ever bother you in any way? Cause you any problems?"

and Think!

- What is the purpose of your last question?
- What was the main reason you said that the doctor would probably agree with her?
- What is the significance of her eye contact?
- What important instructions need to be taught every client who takes lithium?
- What will you say if she interrupts to say she already knows all about it and doesn't need further instruction?
- How will you evaluate whether learning has taken place without making Irene feel like a child?
- What else do you need to know about Irene?

You need to know if Irene has had any adverse effects from lithium; if so, a different medication, such as carbamazepine, might be ordered. Everything you say to clients like Irene should be respectful and honest, while constantly working to build self-esteem—an example is your comment that the doctor is apt to agree with her. Her eye contact may mean she is beginning to relate to you and trust you. It is crucial to reinforce what Irene already knows about lithium, especially coming back to the clinic for monitoring and monthly blood level tests, and continuing to take the drug as ordered. She needs to remember to drink plenty of fluids (2 to 3 liters a day) and to eat a diet containing 2 to 4 g of salt daily. If she is defensive about the instructions, ask her to summarize with you the important points to teach a patient with bipolar disorder. This is a good way to evaluate her learning as well.

You need to determine if Irene has developed a support system, because she is new to the community. You might tell her about community resources that would be of interest to her. You need to learn about her job and place of residence and any important relationships she has elsewhere. You should also clarify the reason she said she was retarded when she first arrived.

Chapter SUMMARY

Our increasing knowledge of the brain shows that mental disorders have more of a biologic basis than was previously thought. The efficacy of psychotropic medications was a major factor in the emptying of large state psychiatric hospitals and the advent of community mental health programs. These programs include outpatient clinics, community support programs, and community mental health centers. To qualify for federal assistance, the latter must provide emergency services, hospitalization, partial hospitalization, outpatient service, and consultation and education.

Common disorders such as depression, anxiety, panic attacks, and phobias are generally treated on an outpatient basis. More serious disorders such as the schizophrenias and bipolar and borderline disorders may require periods of hospitalization from time to time. High-risk categories needing close case management include dual and triple diagnoses that include mental illness, mental retardation, substance abuse, and HIV infection. Other high-risk clients are those with HIV-related dementia or mental retardation, the mentally ill elderly, and clients who relapse frequently.

Addictions in the general population are common and exact a heavy toll on the health and finances of all Americans. Nicotine and alcohol abuse seriously endanger health. The CDC attributes 40% of the total annual medical care expenses to the effects of smoking! Alcoholism is the third leading cause of illness and disability in the United States, according to the National Advisory Mental Health Council. Personal physicians and other primary care providers generally fail to screen for early alcohol abuse. The CAGE questionnaire is a good, quick screening tool. Drug and alcohol treatment programs are increasingly conducted on an outpatient basis, mainly for financial reasons. The 12-step program of Alcoholics Anonymous is included in most treatment plans. Methadone maintenance programs for heroin addicts have proved to be both successful and cost-effective, despite the controversy that surrounds them in some communities. Most professionals working in the field of addictions consider alcoholism and other addictions to be a disease.

A list of references and additional readings for this chapter appears at the end of Part 3.

11

The Elderly and the Disabled: Major Consumers of Health Care

Key Terms

Americans With Disabilities
   Act of 1990
assisted living facilities
competitive employment
dementia
donepezil (Aricept)
extended-care facilities

integrity vs. despair
long-term care facilities
mental status examination
nursing homes
optimal functioning
physically compromised
polypharmacy

respite
Supplemental Security Income
   (SSI)
skilled nursing facilities
stereotype
unconscionable

Learning Objectives

1. Describe three categories of the elderly population.
2. Identify common health problems of the elderly.
3. Name 15 *Healthy People 2000* objectives for the elderly population.
4. Describe four levels of disability.
5. Explain the common areas of concern of disabled people.
6. Explain the effect of the Americans With Disabilities Act of 1990.
7. Describe the functional limitations of millions of disabled people.
8. Identify factors that result in the abuse of elderly or disabled persons.

The Elderly Population

Erikson's theories about human developmental stages and tasks are well known to nurses. His eighth and last stage, integrity vs. despair, applies to the elderly. Erikson called integrity *wisdom*, or the state of successful integration of all of life's developmental tasks. According to Erikson, success in integrating personal life experiences, both suffering and gladness, results in wisdom rather than despair. We all know people who master that eighth task and attain a measure of wisdom and serenity despite the many losses of aging. We also know people who seem haunted by bitterness and despair about their many losses and disappointments. The incidence of suicide is greater among the elderly than any age group, including adolescents. There are many myths about elderly people; Display 11-1 will test your knowledge about the elderly.

We cannot stereotype the aging population. It is true that the elderly consume more health services than any other age group, but that does not accurately reflect the diversity in physical and mental health among the elderly. Attend a 50th high school reunion to

---

DISPLAY 11-1
What's Your Aging IQ?

	True	False
1. Baby boomers are the fastest-growing segment of the population.	☐	☐
2. Families don't bother with their older relatives.	☐	☐
3. Everyone becomes confused or forgetful if they live long enough.	☐	☐
4. HIV/AIDS does not exist among the elderly.	☐	☐
5. Heart disease is a much bigger problem for older men than for older women.	☐	☐
6. Old age begins at age 65.	☐	☐
7. People should watch their weight as they age.	☐	☐
8. Most older people are depressed. Why shouldn't they be?	☐	☐
9. There's no point in screening older people for cancer because they can't be treated.	☐	☐
10. The elderly prefer to be with people their own age.	☐	☐
11. People begin to lose interest in sex around age 60.	☐	☐
12. If your parents had Alzheimer's disease, you will inevitably get it.	☐	☐
13. Diet and exercise reduce the risk for osteoporosis.	☐	☐
14. As your body changes with age, so does your personality.	☐	☐
15. Older people might as well accept urinary accidents as a fact of life.	☐	☐
16. Suicide is mainly a problem for teenagers.	☐	☐
17. Falls and injuries are inevitable for older people.	☐	☐
18. Everybody gets cataracts.	☐	☐
19. Older people become stubborn and irritable.	☐	☐
20. "You can't teach an old dog new tricks."	☐	☐

Only #7 and #13 are true.

(Adapted from the National Institute on Aging.)

see the astounding differences in the way people age. It is difficult to believe that everyone is the same chronological age: some people look like they are in their 50s, and others appear to be in their 80s or 90s.

According to Dr. Ken Minaker, chief of geriatric medicine at Massachusetts General Hospital, ''Today's elderly are pioneers of a new kind of aging. The next century will be dominated by the concerns of the elderly'' (Lauerman, 1996). The U.S. population is aging. The elderly population increased 20% during the past decade, and each day 3,000 people become 65 years of age. Only 2,000 people above the age of 65 die each day, leaving 1,000 additional people joining the elderly population every day (Fig. 11-1). By the year 2020, that growth rate increase will be 73%, more than twice the growth rate of the general population. The current life expectancy is 78.8 years for women and 72.2 years for men (1996, p. 58). The rate of growth of the oldest old—those over 85—is the most rapid. It is no longer rare to live to be more than 100. A woman in southern France, Jeanne Calment, celebrated her 122nd birthday in February 1997; on her birthday she said, ''I've only ever had one wrinkle, and I'm sitting on it.'' She died in the summer of 1997.

What about the quality of life for the aging? Are people surviving longer just to become dependent, confused, and incontinent, to live in pain and in poverty? Although elderly people do slow down as a rule and are more susceptible to disease (by age 65, most people have at least one chronic disease), there is also evidence that many people in retirement are living lives of quality. A long time ago, the esteemed Dr. William Osler of Canada said that the way to have a long, full life is to develop a chronic disease and learn to take good care of yourself. Advances in modern medicine and public health measures in primary prevention such as immunizations, good hygiene, and nutrition have expanded the years of healthy life. The *Healthy People 2000* objectives include goals applicable to the elderly (Display 11-2).

Polypharmacy—multiple medications prescribed for concurrent conditions—can put elderly and disabled people at risk for dangerous interactions. Medication effects need to be constantly monitored and excellent teaching provided to these people by nurses in all health-care settings.

Active senior citizens (ages 65 to 75) tend to live independently and be involved in many community activities. Many are employed or work as volunteers. Financially, this group is doing fairly well; travel is big business among senior citizens. Senior citizen discounts, Social Security, Medicare, pensions, and the profits from selling a home all contribute greatly to the improved economic status of the elderly population. The elderly in this age group are big consumers of ambulatory care (Fig. 11-2). Preventive education has taught them to take care of themselves and to seek care early, before conditions become complicated. Of course, there are still some seniors living in abject poverty, but as a whole, elderly people are doing better financially and physically than at any time in our nation's history.

Old senior citizens (ages 75 to 85) tend to move in with, or close to, their children or into retirement communities in preparation for increased frailty. Only 5% of America's elderly live in nursing homes (AARP, 1993). Many old seniors are still very active and continue to drive and be active in senior citizen clubs and volunteer and church activities. Contrary to the view that people in other countries have about American children

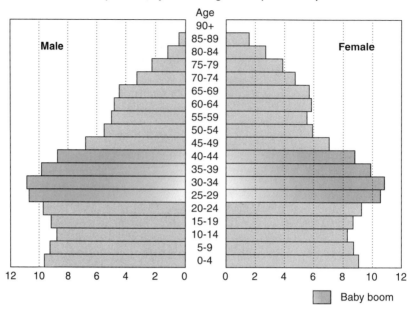

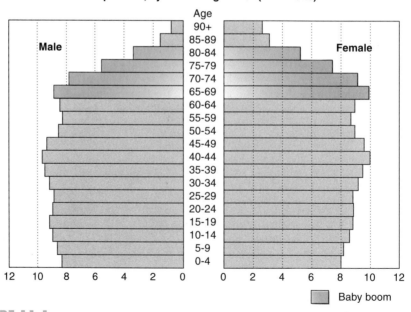

FIGURE 11-1

Population characteristics by age and sex, United States: 1990 and 2030. (From U.S. Bureau of the Census. [1992]. *Sixty-Five Plus in America.* Washington DC: U.S. Government Printing Office.)

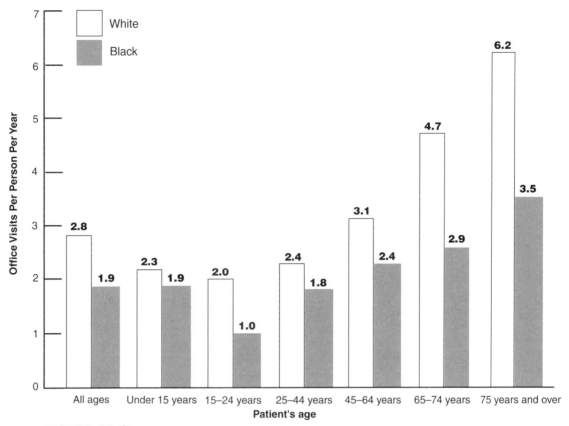

FIGURE 11-2
Annual rate of visits to office-based physicians by patient's age and race: United States, 1991. (From U.S. Department of Health and Human Services, Public Health Service [1994]. *National Ambulatory Medical Care Survey: 1991 Summary,* DHHS Pub No (PHS) 94-1777. Washington DC: U.S. Government Printing Office.)

abandoning their elderly parents, most elderly people hear from their children at least once a week on average. Elderly persons with no close ties to family, friends, or community are three times more likely to die early.

Health problems are generally high in this age group. Heavy losses occur as friends and loved ones die or move away, and these losses are often the catalyst for episodes of depression. Arthritis and diabetes are common afflictions. Cardiovascular disease takes a heavy toll, as does cancer. Elderly women now outnumber men three to two. People prefer to remain at home when they are ill and become heavy users of home care at this age, in addition to ambulatory care.

Dementia is caused by Alzheimer's disease, various other neurologic disorders, or a lack of oxygen to the brain from cerebrovascular disease. Dementia begins more frequently during this age, but it is not a normal, inevitable part of aging, even among

DISPLAY 11-2
Healthy People 2000 Selected National Health Objectives Related to Older Adults

1.5a   Reduce the proportion of people over age 65 who engage in no leisure time physical activity to less than 22%.

2.18   Increase receipt of home food services to those in need to at least 80%.

6.1c   Reduce suicide incidence among white men aged 65 and older to less than 39.2 per 100,000 population.

9.3c   Reduce motor vehicle deaths among those aged 70 and older to less than 20 per 100,000 population.

9.4a   Reduce fall-related deaths and injuries to less than 14.4 per 100,000 people aged 65 to 84 years.

16.12b   Increase the proportion of women over age 70 who have ever had a Pap smear to at least 95%.

17.1   Increase years of healthy life by at least 14 years in those 65 years and over.

17.3   Reduce the proportion of people over age 65 who have difficulty with two or more personal care activities to less than 90 per 1,000.

17.6a   Reduce significant hearing impairment in people over age 45 to less than 180 per 1,000 population.

17.7a   Reduce significant visual impairment in people over age 65 to less than 70 per 1,000 population.

17.18   Increase the proportion of perimenopausal women who have been counseled regarding the benefits of estrogen replacement therapy to at least 90%.

20.11   Increase pneumonia and influenza immunization levels among chronically ill or older people to at least 60%.

(Source: U.S. Department of Health and Human Services.)

those with a family history of dementia. The disease process varies in its rate of progression. Display 11-3 is a short mental status questionnaire. Forgetfulness can make it impossible for an elderly person to live alone safely without caregiver assistance, because he or she may wander off and become lost. In the latter stages of dementia, there is a complete reversal of capabilities so that near death, the person is infantlike and needs total care. The demands on the caregivers of dementia clients are enormous, and more respite services are needed for them.

The "old old" are those with strong genetic constitutions, or they may be people who have avoided smoking, unhealthy diets, lack of exercise, substance abuse, obesity, and social isolation. Meaningful interests and being surrounded by a strong, loving support group is almost essential for a long, healthy life. It seems axiomatic that the longer a person lives, the longer he or she is apt to live. There appears to be a demographic "survival of the fittest" phenomenon. A Mayo Clinic publication (1996) describes a study showing that maintaining mental fitness may delay the onset of dementia. Researchers believe that lifelong mental exercise and learning may promote the growth

DISPLAY 11-3
Short Mental Status Questionnaire

Instructions: Ask questions 1–10 in this list and record all answers. Ask question 4a only if patient does not have a telephone. Record total number of errors based on ten questions.

+   −

_____   **1.**   What day of the week is it? _____

_____   **2.**   What is the date today (month/day/year)? _____

_____   **3.**   What is the name of this place? _____

_____   **4.**   What is your telephone number? _____

_____   **4a.**   What is your street address? _____

_____   **5.**   How old are you? _____

_____   **6.**   When were you born? _____

_____   **7.**   Who is the president of the U.S. now? _____

_____   **8.**   Who was the president before him? _____

_____   **9.**   What was your mother's maiden name? _____

_____   **10.**   Subtract 3 from 30 and keep subtracting 3 from each new number, all the way down. _____

_____   **Total Errors**

To be completed by interviewer

Client Name _____

Sex: 1. Male   2. Female   Primary Language: _____

Years of Education: _____
1. Grade School   2. High School   3. Beyond High School

Interviewer's Name: _____

The total number of errors constitutes the score in the SPMSQ. The test is sensitive to educational attainment.

0–1 Errors: Intact intellectual functioning
3–4 Errors: Mild intellectual impairment
5–7 Errors: Moderate intellectual impairment
8–10 Errors: Severe intellectual impairment

For persons with 8 or fewer years of education, one additional error is allowed for each scoring category. For persons with more than 12 years of education, one less error is allowed for each category.

(Adapted from Pfeiffer E. [1975]. A portable mental status questionnaire for the assessment of organic brain deficit in elderly patients. J of Amer Geriatric Soc 23(10) 433–441.)

of additional synapses between neurons and delay the onset of dementia. This is important: the Alzheimer's Association says that whereas only 6% of people at age 65 suffer dementia, by age 85 that percentage is 49.5%, or almost half of that population. Alzheimer's disease affects an estimated 4 million Americans, according to this group, and places a heavy burden on caregivers.

The Disabled Population

A disability is a physical or mental impairment that substantially limits one or more major life activities, according to the Americans With Disabilities Act of 1990. Disabling conditions with the highest risk of disability are mental retardation, bilateral leg amputations, cancer of the respiratory system, cerebral palsy, multiple sclerosis, blindness, paralysis, rheumatoid arthritis, degenerative disk disorders, severe heart disease, gastrointestinal cancer, emphysema, loss of arms or hands, and cerebrovascular disease (*Disability Stat Bulletin*, 1989). Display 11-4 lists conditions related to disability in persons 15 years old or older.

The level of disability includes activity of daily living (ADL) functioning and employment ability. Four levels have been identified:

- Level I: Partial disability manifested by slight limitation in at least one major life activity. Independent in ADLs. Full-time competitive employment.
- Level II: Partial disability manifested by moderate limitation in one or more major life areas. May need some help with ADLs. Modified employment.
- Level III: Partial disability manifested by severe limitation in one or more major life areas. Unable to work or attend school regularly. Needs ADL assistance.
- Level IV: Total disability manifested by complete dependency on others for ADLs. Unable to work.

Areas of concern for people who are disabled are shown in Display 11-5. Variables affecting a person's adaptation to a disability are listed in Display 11-6.

Economic Considerations

A person who is substantially limited is usually eligible for Social Security disability benefits and Supplemental Security Income (SSI). SSI payments are for aged, blind, or disabled people with very low incomes. Many disabled persons can work and seek employment according to their ability. "Competitive employment" is when a disabled person can work among the general workforce. Sheltered workshops have been established to provide employment for disabled persons who cannot perform competitive employment (eg, Goodwill Industries).

The Americans With Disabilities Act of 1990

The purpose of this law was to allow the disabled to enter the mainstream of life and to lead as normal a life as possible. Employers are prohibited from discriminating against any person with a disability who is qualified to do the work. Ramps, wide aisles and

DISPLAY 11-4
Conditions Related to Disability in Persons 15 Years Old or Older

AIDS or AIDS-related condition
Alcohol- or drug-related problem or disorder
Arthritis or rheumatism
Back or spine problems (including chronic stiffness or deformity of the back or spine)
Blindness or other visual impairment (difficulty seeing well enough, even with glasses, to read a newspaper)
Broken bone/fracture
Cancer
Cerebral palsy
Deafness or serious trouble hearing
Diabetes
Epilepsy
Head or spinal cord injury
Heart trouble (including coronary heart disease and arteriosclerosis)
Hernia or rupture
High blood pressure (hypertension)
Kidney stones or chronic kidney trouble
Learning disability
Lung or respiratory trouble (asthma, bronchitis, emphysema, respiratory allergies, tuberculosis, or other lung trouble)
Mental retardation
Missing legs, feet, arms, hands, or fingers
Paralysis of any kind
Senility/Dementia/Alzheimer's disease
Speech disorder
Stiffness or deformity of the foot, leg, arm, or hand
Stomach trouble (including ulcers and gall bladder or liver conditions)
Stroke
Thyroid trouble or goiter
Tumor, cyst, or growth
Other

(Centers for Disease Control and Prevention [1994]. Prevalence of Disabilities and Associated Health Conditions, United States, 1991-1992. MMRW 43(40):730-731, 737-739.)

doors, and elevators have been installed in public places to ensure access for disabled people. This law focuses on public services, activities, and programs as well as public accommodations. Employment opportunities are mandated by this law, which covers mental as well as physical disabilities. Previous laws ensured access to education for the disabled. Although much headway has been made in public transportation, such as the modified vans that help transport wheelchair-bound persons, facilities are still inadequate for the physically disabled in many parts of the country.

DISPLAY 11-5
Some Areas of Concern for People Who Are Disabled

- Education
- Financial stability
- Employment
- Access to services
- Health care
- Social and recreational opportunities
- Sexuality
- Guardianship
- Community residential opportunities
- Attendant services
- Respite care

Some people who are disabled use homebound instruction to learn a skill or gain education for a career. The U.S. Department of Education recognizes the National Home Study Council (1601 Eighteenth Street, N.W., Washington, D.C. 20009; phone 202-234-5100) and its *Directory of Accredited Home Study Schools* as a resource for locating quality schools of home study.

(Clemen-Stone S, Eigsti D, McGuire S. [1995]. Comprehensive Community Health Nursing, *4th ed. St. Louis: Mosby-Year Book.)*

DISPLAY 11-6
Variables Affecting Adaptation to a Disability

- The stage of grief and mourning
- Age at which the handicapping condition occurred
- Age-appropriateness of the disability
- Rapidity of onset of the disability
- Level of disability caused by the disability
- Visibility of the disability
- Value of the disabled area
- Attitudes regarding self
- Attitudes of significant others
- Community resources available and used
- Coping mechanism used
- Prognosis or expected duration of the disability

(Clemen-Stone S, Eigsti D, McGuire S [1995]. Comprehensive Community Health Nursing, *4th ed. St. Louis: Mosby-Year Book.)*

This act was long overdue and is a major step forward. Disabilities themselves impose enough pain; the unnecessary suffering caused by discrimination and abuse is unconscionable. We must strive to remove the physical, social, and economic barriers to optimal functioning and well-being for the disabled.

Health Care and Personal Assistance

Until the past few years, most ambulatory care health facilities and physicians' offices had no ramps and were inaccessible to the disabled. Disabled persons on Medicaid still have difficulty finding a physician who will accept Medicaid. Some disabled persons claim that health-care personnel are insensitive to their special needs. There is sometimes an attitude of "We can't do much for you" toward clients with a permanent disability. Actually, there is much that can be done to improve their health status and well-being, regardless of whether the disability can be corrected.

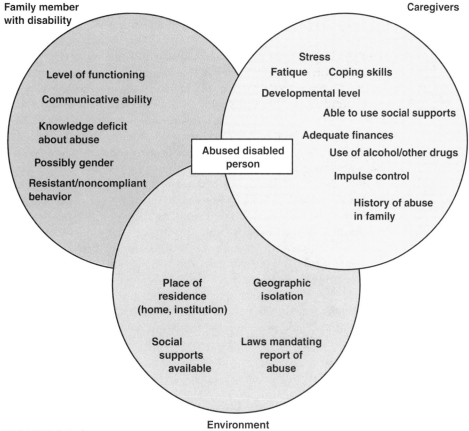

FIGURE 11-3
Factors influencing the abuse of those who are physically compromised. (Stanhope M, Lancaster J [1996]. *Community Health Nursing*. St. Louis: Mosby.)

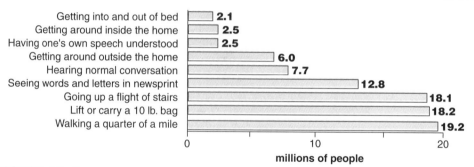

FIGURE 11-4

Functional limitation of adults with disabilities. (Kraus LE, Stoddard S [1989]. *Chartbook on Disability in the United States, an InfoUse Report.* Washington DC: National Institute on Disability and Rehabilitation Research.)

It is disgraceful that 700,000 to 1 million of the elderly population are abused each year (Fulmer, 1995). Some disabled people even suffer abuse at the hands of their caregivers. Figure 11-3 shows the factors influencing the abuse of physically compromised persons.

Many disabled people require assistance with some ADLs (Fig. 11-4). If they are not living with families who can provide this assistance, they need a personal care aide to help them. Medicaid will pay for this service if a physician certifies that it is needed. Some severely disabled persons who do not have adequate assistance from a personal care aide must enter long-term care institutions. There is a serious lack of home care assistance for both the disabled and the frail elderly. This custodial care is said to be too costly, but the alternative, institutional care, seems as expensive, if not more so. A person's quality of life is better if he or she can continue to live independently in the community. New York has developed a long-term care program called "a nursing home without walls." Medicaid clients whose care costs do not exceed 75% of nursing home costs are provided needed care and supplies at home.

When Christopher Reeve became quadriplegic as a result of his horseback riding accident in 1995, greater attention was focused on the plight of people with all disabilities. The actor who played Superman in the movies has become a superhero to the American people because of his courageous coping with his disability and his determination to raise funds for research to help the estimated 250,000 others who are paralyzed. To pursue his dream of finding the means for spinal regeneration in his lifetime, he has established the Christopher Reeve Foundation, which is raising funds for research.

THE NURSE SPEAKS . . .
About Senior Adult Day Care

I work as a registered nurse in a community senior day-care center sponsored by a church. My job is to keep everyone safe around here. Most of the clients have some degree of dementia. I teach the staff how to work safely, and I monitor the clients' activities for safety. I am always assessing and evaluating, especially medication effects. I help plan appropriate activities, and my interventions include involvement with the families.

See that big fellow over there painting birdhouses with that other guy? Bob is a good case in point. His frail, little wife brought him to us about 3 months ago. He comes 2 days a week, and they pay a small amount based on our sliding fee schedule. She doesn't look so frazzled and exhausted since she's been having 2 days a week respite. When Bob first came, he was very withdrawn and quiet—almost mute, in fact. He seemed confused and was often incontinent because he forgot the restroom location or didn't recognize the signal to void. He's a big man to dress and undress. I reviewed body mechanics with the staff and taught them and his wife some helpful techniques for moving and assisting him. He has Parkinson's disease and becomes rigid, in a frozen state at times. I have to constantly remind the staff to allow him plenty of time to do anything because of his bradykinesia and tremors.

As I assessed Bob, I began to suspect that much of his mutism and withdrawal might be due to depression. It's hard to be sure, because the masklike facies and monotone voice of Parkinson's looks like depression. I thought it was worth discussing with Bob's doctor anyway. When I approached Bob's wife about contacting the doctor, she explained that they had just been switched to a new prospective-payment managed-care company by their pension plan, and their old doctor was not included in the system. The thought of finding a new doctor seemed overwhelming to her.

We looked over the list of providers in their new managed-care company together and found a couple of familiar names who do a good job treating other people who come to this center. I called the doctor she selected and discussed Bob's possible depression. I also told the doctor that Bob takes Tagamet, and that we notice more confusion in our clients here when they take Tagamet. The MD agreed that confusion is a common side effect of Tagamet in the elderly. He later put Bob on Zoloft on a trial basis. Within a month, Bob had improved greatly and is no longer confused or mute. See how he is interacting with that other fellow now? Of course, his wife is thrilled. I feel really good about this. The quality of their life is so much better. No wonder I love this work!

Steve
ELDERCARE DAY PROGRAM NURSE

CLINICAL APPLICATION

A Critical Thinking Study About a Confused Woman Who Charges Abuse

You are a community mental health nurse working for Geriatric Evaluation Services. Mrs. Connor, a 90-year-old woman, has been calling the police in the middle of the night, claiming that her granddaughter is trying to kill her. The police notified adult protective services, which called you to do an evaluation because the woman sounds confused. You plan a home visit and find that Mrs. Connor lives alone in her home of over 50 years. About 6 weeks ago, her granddaughter began staying there at night because Mrs. Connor had been wandering around at night.

and Think!

- On what basis will you determine that Mrs. Connor is confused?
- What are the components of a mental status examination?
- How will you evaluate long-term vs. short-term memory loss and concrete vs. abstract thinking?
- How can you evaluate sound judgment?
- Which parameter is most significant when you test to see if Mrs. Connor is oriented to time, place, and persons?
- List conditions that can cause temporary confusion. Explain the difference between dementia, delirium, and depression.
- How would you differentiate between these three conditions, and why is that important to do?

You assess Mrs. Connor's medications and learn that she is taking none. Medication effects are one of the most common causes of confusion in the elderly; all medications should be ordered "low and slow" for this age group. You take her vital signs and ask about urinary frequency and burning to rule out infection, another cause of confusion in the elderly. You note that Mrs. Connor is very thin, but she does not seem to be dehydrated. These are reversible causes of confusion, as is depression when it is treated.

Mrs. Connor's daughter arrives during her lunch hour from work to check on her mother, as she does every day. She tells you that her mother's confusion has developed gradually and consistently with progressive memory loss. You already noted impaired capacity for abstract thought, as evidenced by her concrete interpretation of common proverbs. Her responses to questions such as, "What would you do if you found a newly written letter, stamped and addressed, lying on the sidewalk?" indicate confusion and some lack of judgment ("I wouldn't read it. Maybe I'd just throw it away.").

The daughter adds that Mrs. Connor has become increasingly suspicious and irritable lately. She has been having trouble sleeping at night and tends to wander around the house. She adamantly refuses to leave her home, so the granddaughter has been staying there the past few weeks to make sure the doors stay locked and Mrs. Connor doesn't wander away. This makes Mrs. Connor very angry, and she charges the granddaughter with locking her up so that she can kill her. She also says the granddaughter is stealing her things. The granddaughter has been discarding the large piles of newspapers, empty boxes, bottles, and plastic containers stacked everywhere in the house.

 and Think!

- Is there any way that Mrs. Connor can remain safely in her house?
- Does she belong in an institution?
- What can be done to help her?

- She refuses to live with her family or to see a doctor. Are your assessments complete?
- What did you forget?

To rule out her charges about her granddaughter's abuse, Mrs. Connor requires a good physical assessment. She is very vague about where and how she has been hurt and shows no signs of pain anywhere. There are no lacerations, abrasions, or bruises. She keeps repeating, "She's locking me up so she can kill me!"

On examination, you do not think Mrs. Connor has been abused. However, you believe she should have medical attention, a diagnosis, and probably some medication to treat her paranoia, confusion, and sleep problems. With treatment, her condition may improve enough to enable her to remain safely in her own home. This will require considerable community support services and assistance from her willing family, but will be much more cost-effective than institutionalization. She should have a home health aide with her at night, because the granddaughter cannot leave her own family to stay there permanently. She should have Meals On Wheels during the day to ensure that she eats properly. The knobs can be removed from her gas stove to prevent her from turning on the stove and forgetting she did so. The family will check on her during the day and will spend time with her each evening.

Medicare will not pay for the home health aide custodial care she needs. However, you suspect that once Mrs. Connor's savings have been used up, she will become eligible for Medicaid, which indeed turns out to be the case. But the first step is to persuade Mrs. Connor to see a physician. Her familiar doctor has retired and moved out of state, but she speaks fondly of his nurse, who still lives in the community. "She's a real nurse—wears a white uniform and a cap, you know!" Mrs. Connor says. With Mrs. Connor's permission, you ask that nurse to call her, and she persuades Mrs. Connor to go to a doctor she recommended for a check-up. He diagnoses Alzheimer's disease and prescribes the new drug donepezil (Aricept), 5 mg at bedtime. Mrs. Connor becomes much calmer and less delusional. She sleeps better at night with the help of Tylenol PM, which contains diphenhydramine (Benadryl). She stops calling the police and complaining of abuse. She accepts the plan of care, including the home health aide.

 and Think!

- Has your work been completed?
- Is there anything more you can do to improve this situation?

You guide and teach the family and aides about various strategies to help preserve and maximize Mrs. Connor's functioning. You urge them to use consistent routines, because familiarity and structure prolong optimal functioning. This is why Alzheimer's patients generally do much better in their own homes. You advise them not to argue when Mrs. Connor becomes upset or stubborn. They should talk calmly and soothingly, hold hands, hug or rock her, and use distraction. Frustration can be avoided by not offering Mrs. Connor difficult choices or asking complex questions. They should speak slowly and simply, reinforcing their message with gestures and presenting just one idea at a time. Useful memory aids include lists of daily activities, telephone numbers, and step-by-step instructions for tasks such as dressing. Verbal cues should be provided. Sing old songs and reminisce together to use her intact long-term memory. Mrs. Connor should wear an identification bracelet with a telephone number to call, should she wander and get lost. For safety, extension cords and scatter rugs should be put away and household clutter reduced. Doors should be locked securely at night so she cannot wander outside. Often, a good daytime walk reduces nighttime wandering. A calming bedtime ritual can also reduce nighttime activity. Have her void at bedtime and avoid extra fluids and caffeine late in the day. These strategies should lengthen the moderate stage of Mrs. Connor's Alzheimer's disease and preserve her functioning as long as possible.

Family caregivers will receive valuable support from the Alzheimer's Association. You encourage the granddaughter to attend the support group jointly sponsored by Geriatric Evaluation Services and the local chapter of the association. Support groups give caregivers an opportunity to meet others with similar problems, ventilate their feelings, and plan ahead. Techniques such as validation of the client's feelings are discussed. Support groups are extremely helpful, and they reportedly delay institutional placement by at least a year because caregivers are getting strength and reassurance too.

In the future, Mrs. Connor may need a day-care program as she becomes less able to be alone during the day. She will need more and more home health aide time, eventually requiring a 24-hour live-in aide as her abilities decline. Eventually, she is apt to revert to an infantlike state of total dependency and will require complete care. This will require very heavy care from both the family and the aides. It might be best to place Mrs. Connor in a long-term care facility during her last months, when she is totally confused, helpless, and in an infantile state. You plan to reevaluate the situation at various steps along the way and give guidance regarding the appropriate care.

Chapter SUMMARY

There are many myths about the elderly. People age at different rates, so elderly people vary greatly. Three general categories of the elderly are the active elderly, the old elderly, and the "old old" or frail elderly. Dementia affects about 50% of the latter group. The "old old" are the fastest-growing population group in the United States, although the entire elderly population is growing because of longer life spans.

Disability can result from physical or mental impairment. The highest prevalence of disability occurs among persons who are mentally retarded. There are four levels of disability based on functional and employment capability. The first level describes slight limitation but independence in performing activities of daily living and full-time competitive employment capability. The next two levels describe increasing levels of disability and dependence. The fourth level is defined as total disability and total dependence on others. Social Security and supplemental security income assists disabled people who cannot work to support themselves.

In 1990, the Americans With Disabilities Act was passed to allow the disabled to enter the mainstream of life. Ramps and other facilities became mandatory to make public places accessible. Disabled people can no longer be denied jobs or education if their disability allows them to pursue these things. Disabled persons in level four still have difficulty finding adequate custodial care at home, so many must resort to long-term care facilities. It is tragic that some disabled and elderly persons are victims of abuse by caregivers and others. Risk factors for abuse include caregiver burnout, alcohol and drug abuse, and others.

A list of references and additional readings for this chapter appears at the end of Part 3.

12

Expanding Roles in Nursing Practice

Key Terms

across the continuum
acupuncture
advanced practice
alternative care modalities
ayurvedic techniques
birthing centers
capitation
case management
charting by exception
Civilian Health and Medical Programs (CHAMPUS)
clinical paths
collaborative practice
consultants
consultation liaison psychiatric nurse

cost containment
direct reimbursement
discharge planners
durable medical equipment
entrepreneurs
fax machines
generic
healing touch
integrated system
marketing
massage therapy
multidisciplinary providers
neuropsychiatric disorders
nursing centers
outcomes-driven
prepaid basis

prescriptive authority
primary care
private-duty registry
psychobiologic
quality assurance
reflexology
regulatory issues
scope of benefits
self-insurance contracts
service providers
start-up funding
third-party reimbursements
underserved
utilization review nurse
voice mail

Learning Objectives

1. Describe nursing centers.
2. Identify at least three types of nursing centers.
3. Explain why the Carondelet system is called a health maintenance organization (HMO).
4. Define the term "nurse entrepreneur."
5. Compare the value of direct vs. indirect reimbursement.

6. List the states where nurse practitioners have full prescriptive authority.
7. Describe at least six models of private practice.
8. Explain the role of a nurse consultant.
9. Identify five levels of case managers.
10. Explain the pros and cons of working as a case manager.
11. Describe the advantages of using clinical paths.

Various roles have opened for nurses in recent years. Some of them require advanced practice education, but some do not. Many associate degree and diploma school graduates working in community health feel the need to gain further formal education in baccalaureate add-on programs. Because of the complex problems and multiple variables dealt with in community health nursing, at least a baccalaureate degree is needed. This is particularly true of registered nurses involved in contemporary roles of nursing practice. These roles include work in nursing centers, private practice, consultation, case management, and entrepreneurial activities.

Many people think of these expanding roles as new areas of nursing practice. Actually, none of these roles are really new to nursing. Lillian Wald, Margaret Sanger, and Mary Breckinridge all established nursing centers early in the 20th century. Private practice has had a long tradition in private-duty nursing. Nurses have always done some form of consulting and case management. For many years, creative, courageous nurses have opened new businesses as entrepreneurs.

Then why are these called expanding roles in nursing practice? Perhaps the difference is the *number* of nurses who are involved in primary care today, or perhaps it is the degree of independence and autonomy they exhibit.

Nursing Centers

Nursing centers and nurse-managed clinics that deliver primary care began to appear in the 1970s and 1980s for a variety of reasons. Like other community health centers, many nursing centers were established to serve underserved populations. Several clinics around the country are owned by schools of nursing and operated by their faculty. For example, faculty members of the College of Nursing of the University of Kentucky run a clinic for the homeless. The University of California at Los Angeles School of Nursing Health Center provides primary care for the homeless at the large Union Rescue Mission. Columbia University School of Nursing's Center for Advanced Practice in New York City is run by nurses who have full admitting privileges at the Presbyterian Hospital of Columbia-Presbyterian Medical Center. Such centers serve as a base for faculty research as well as practice. These clinics help correct an unfortunate division in the profession between nursing education and nursing practice. These facilities also provide valuable clinical experience for nursing students. Primary care is done by nursing faculty in advanced practice roles such as nurse practitioners or nurse clinical specialists with prescriptive authority.

Nurse-managed clinics in nonacademic centers are very effective also. The Mercy Mobile Health Program of Atlanta provides care to the underserved from a fully equipped van. HIV testing, substance abuse counseling, and primary care are some of their services. In Tampa, women and children can receive such care at the large Genesis/Tampa Health Center, which has an annual budget of $40 million. Comprehensive family-focused care is provided by the nurse-managed Community Health Clinic of Lafayette, Indiana. In Natchez, adolescents and families of rural Mississippi are served in nursing centers in which nurses are the primary caregivers. These are just a few examples of nurse-managed clinics. Registered nurses assist the advanced practice nurses in most of these clinics.

Figure 12-1 shows a contemporary community nursing center model. A survey of nurse-managed centers conducted by the National League for Nurses (NLN) in 1993

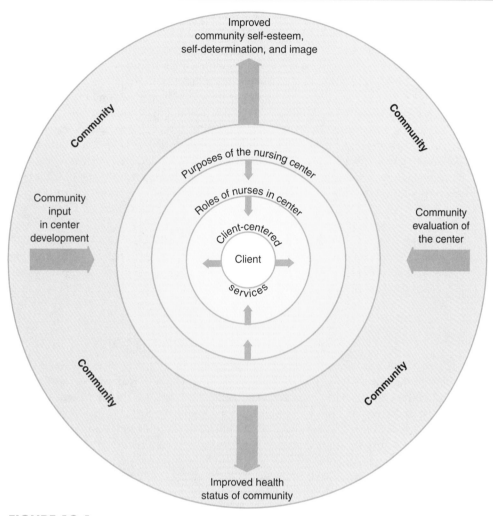

FIGURE 12-1
Contemporary nursing center model. (Stanhope M, Lancaster J [1996]. *Community Health Nursing,* 4th ed. St. Louis: Mosby.)

(Barger & Rosenfeld, 1993) revealed that 30% of clients paid for themselves (some on a sliding fee scale), 20% paid nothing, 14% were covered by Medicaid, 10% were covered by Medicare, and 11% were undisclosed. Some managed-care programs are including nursing centers in their networks of primary care providers because these centers almost always offer cost savings along with high-quality, comprehensive, holistic care.

A Nursing HMO

The Carondelet nursing model in southern Arizona, sponsored by the Sisters of St. Joseph's of Carondelet, is a nationally known integrated system of health services. The system provides a full spectrum of health services across the continuum. Community nursing centers exist at 18 sites, and there are three hospitals (Carondelet St. Mary's Hospital and St. Joseph's Hospital in Tucson and Carondelet Holy Cross Hospital in Nogales, 65 miles to the south). Each city has a licensed home health agency as part of the system. The system also sponsors a skilled nursing facility, Carondelet Holy Family. Finally, the system contains a hospice that provides both inpatient and home-based care.

This comprehensive HMO system has been involved in several creative research and demonstration projects. For example, the Carondelet Community Nursing Organization is one of four national Medicare demonstration projects in which a registered nurse is linked with a specific client to coordinate primary care services. As in other HMOs, this is done on a capitated, prepaid basis to Medicare beneficiaries. The goal is to maximize consumer participation, continuity, and care coordination. A wellness plan is established that includes health screenings at 6-month intervals. Consultation with physicians and families is included. Intermittent skilled nursing services, personal care, and durable medical equipment are provided as needed.

Carondelet's case management program was well designed and is a national model. It serves a population of high-risk persons with exceptional physical and emotional needs and little or no caregiver support. The elderly, newborn, pregnant women, and persons with chronic illness, such as multiple sclerosis, are included. Case management is discussed further later in this chapter.

Birthing Centers

Specialized nursing centers are very successful. Birthing centers established and run by certified nurse-midwives have been operating for many years, serving both middle-class clients and underserved populations. Display 12-1 lists the core interventions of certified nurse-midwives. Lonnie C. Morris founded the Childbirth Center in Englewood, New Jersey, more than 20 years ago. It has a staff of three certified nurse-midwives and 10 registered nurses. She is affiliated with two obstetricians and two pediatricians if there is an abnormal obstetric history or pediatric disorder. She also has privileges at two hospitals if a woman prefers a hospital delivery or a midwife–physician team approach. At the Childbirth Center, total gynecologic and reproductive care is provided for well women through the reproductive years and into menopause. In the following account, Lonnie describes the care provided to one of her earliest clients.

> Sarah first came to me over 20 years ago because she could not consummate her marriage. I worked with her using vaginal dilators, counseling, and teaching. The couple were then able to have pleasurable intercourse, but Sarah was still unable to conceive for more than a year. Then I worked with the couple about their infertility and taught them about ovulation and optimal timing of intercourse. A short while later, Sarah became pregnant, but to our disappointment, she miscarried near the end of her third trimester. A few months later she returned to say that she thought she was pregnant again.
>
> All my prenatal health teaching was followed carefully and she delivered a healthy baby boy. Sarah had some difficulty initiating breastfeeding—98% of our clients successfully breastfeed. With use of our lactation consultant, she was able to pass that hurdle successfully. The couple refused contraception because of Sarah's difficulty in becoming pregnant earlier. Within 6 months, Sarah was pregnant again. The couple were overjoyed!
>
> Now Sarah is 44 years old, and I am currently providing prenatal care for her sixth baby! But she says that after this birth, she will come to me only for contraception and menopausal care. They feel their family will be complete with this baby.

DISPLAY 12-1

Core Nursing Interventions Identified by the American College of Nurse-Midwives

Abuse protection	Health education
Active listening	Health screening
Admission care	Intrapartal care
Anticipatory guidance	Medication management
Attachment promotion	Medication prescribing
Birthing	Newborn care
Breastfeeding assistance	Nutrition counseling
Childbirth preparation	Pain management
Decision-making support	Parent education: Childbearing family
Delegation	Physician support
Discharge planning	Postpartal care
Documentation	Referral
Emotional support	Risk identification: Childbearing family
Environmental management	Sexual counseling
Family integrity promotion: Childbearing family	Suturing
Family planning: Contraception	Teaching: Individual
Family planning: Unplanned pregnancy	Telephone consultation
Fertility preservation	

(Reprinted from Iowa Intervention Project. Core Interventions by Specialty. *Iowa City, Center for Nursing Classification, College of Nursing, University of Iowa, 1996, p. 29. Reprinted with permission.)*

The philosophy of birthing centers is that childbirth is a normal, healthy process, and should be a celebration. Families are involved and clients take an active role in their own health care. Extensive education and support is provided both prenatally and postnatally. Special programs are sometimes offered such as vaginal birth after cesarean section and water labor, which reduces stress on the mother and baby.

Wellness Centers

Nursing wellness centers are being established across the nation. Some specialize in care of the elderly, but most focus on the general population. In northern Minnesota, Karen Woehler's Northwoods Wellness Center seeks to integrate the mind, body, and spirit holistically. Karen is an experienced psychiatric-mental health nurse, parish nurse, and certified massage therapist. She begins with a physical, spiritual, psychosocial, and mental assessment, attempting to understand the client's perceptions of his or her world. Karen's goal is to promote hope, self-esteem, and self-empowerment. She provides comfort through massage, Therapeutic Touch, prayer, and nonpharmacologic pain control measures. She does a great deal of therapeutic communication, health counseling, and teaching, and offers stress management training. She helps clients to identify and use their own strengths, promoting a sense of control and responsibility, and to define their life mission.

Alternative Care Nursing Centers

Another popular type of specialty nursing center emphasizes alternative approaches to health care, such as Healing Touch, massage therapy, herbal interventions, acupuncture, and ayurvedic techniques. For example, the New Mexico Center for Nursing Therapeutics was founded and is owned by Pamela Potter Hughes, a certified Healing Touch practitioner and instructor. She offers a holistic approach to mental health counseling and physical wellness and helps clients with stress and burnout, grief and loss, and life transitions. She helps to identify emotional energy blocks affecting physical health and well-being. Other registered nurses in her center are also licensed massage therapists and nutritionists. There are nurse practitioners, pastoral counselors, acupuncturists, and clinical specialists. Individual and family therapy and stress management training is offered. There is strong emphasis on learning self-care and management of one's own health using a holistic, mind–body approach.

Nurse Entrepreneurs

The three nurses mentioned so far in this chapter—Lonnie, Karen, and Pamela—are good examples of nurse entrepreneurs. Nurses who start a business must assess the needs of the community and the legal and regulatory issues involved in providing care. They must plan how the services will be delivered, how patients will be referred to them, and how they will market the business. Obtaining start-up funding can be especially challenging. Funds will be needed to pay for office supplies and forms for recordkeeping, employee salaries, benefits, and continuing education. About 20,000 nurses have established their own businesses, and that number is growing. "The Nurse Speaks" near the end of this chapter gives an account by a nurse who established a home care agency.

Entrepreneurs must first develop a sound business plan. *Entrepreneuring: A Nurse's Guide to Starting a Business* (Vogel & Doleysh, 1994) explains how to formulate such a plan. Start-up funding can be sought from a variety of sources. Grants are available from some foundations and federal, state, and local agencies, but this money is drying up in the current financial climate. Often nurses start off using personal and borrowed funds and then use fee-for-service and third-party reimbursement contracts to finance the business as time goes on. The National Independent Nursing Network, a network of nurse-owned home health agencies and hospices, was established in 1995.

Direct Reimbursement

Direct reimbursement from third-party payers is far preferable to payment through another provider, such as a physician or an agency who then pays the entrepreneur. In 34 states, advanced practice nurses receive direct reimbursement, but some of these states strictly limit what can be reimbursed (Pearson, 1994). Nurses working in underserved rural areas are eligible for direct Medicare reimbursement. Medicaid reimbursement is available for advanced practice nurses in 49 states, but often at a much lower rate than physicians receive. Direct reimbursement to nurse practitioners is provided by the Civilian Health and Medical Programs (CHAMPUS), a federal payment program for medical services for dependents of active or retired military personnel. CHAMPUS outpatient care is reimbursed at 75% to 80% of the allowable funds.

Prescriptive Authority

The right of nurses to write prescriptions varies from state to state. More and more states are granting this right to advanced practice nurses. In 1995, 48 states and the District of Columbia granted prescriptive authority. The ability to write prescriptions has a great impact on a nurse's ability to function as a primary caregiver (Table 12-1).

Self-Employed Nurses

Self-employed nurses function in a variety of ways. A major advantage of independent practice is personal freedom and control over your time. You can choose the days you will work and the days you will go on vacation, for example. A major disadvantage of self-employment is lack of a preset income; knowing what your income will be can help in personal planning and budgeting. Self-employed persons do not receive employee benefits such as health insurance. All self-employed persons must keep careful business records for taxes and other purposes. It is difficult to estimate what the shift toward managed care and other major changes in health care will mean for self-employed nurses.

TABLE 12-1. Who Can Prescribe What?

Authority	State
Nurse practitioners can prescribe (including controlled substances) independent of a physician's involvement.	Alaska, Arizona, Colorado, Delaware, Iowa, Maine, Montana, New Mexico, New Hampshire, Oregon, Vermont, Washington, Washington DC, Wisconsin, Wyoming
Nurse practitioners can prescribe (including controlled substances) with some involvement by the physician.	Arkansas, Connecticut, Georgia, Indiana, Louisiana, Maryland, Massachusetts, Minnesota, Mississippi, Nebraska, New York, North Carolina, North Dakota, Pennsylvania, Rhode Island, South Carolina, South Dakota, Utah, West Virginia
Nurse practitioners can prescribe (excluding controlled substances) with some involvement by the physician.	Alabama, California, Florida, Hawaii, Idaho, Kansas, Kentucky, Michigan, Missouri, Nevada, New Jersey, Ohio, Tennessee, Texas, Virgina
Nurse practitioners have no prescriptive authority.	Illinois, Oklahoma

(Remember, state statutes and regulations are subject to change. Verify the current status of the law in your area.)
(Pearson LJ [1994–95]. How each state stands on legislative issues affecting advanced nursing practice. *Nurse Practitioner* 20:23–38.)

Private Practice

The number of nurses establishing private practices is on the increase. Psychiatric-mental health clinical specialists trained in psychotherapy go into private or group practice fairly often and see clients by appointment. Midwives also have a strong tradition in private or group practice. Some parish nurses work with large congregations or two or three smaller congregations as private practitioners, earning a salary or an hourly rate. Some nurses sign contracts for certain periods of time with camps, private schools, or small businesses. Independent case managers are in private practice but contract with employers to manage complex cases more cost-effectively, with a better quality of care and improved outcomes for clients. Companies and local governments that provide self-insurance contracts are particularly apt to hire independent case managers. Lamaze teachers and La Leche League consultants usually work in private practice.

Collaborative Practice Arrangements

Nurse-midwives, pediatric and family nurse practitioners, and psychiatric nurse clinical specialists sometimes work in physicians' offices, not as employees but in collaborative private practice. The latter diagnose and treat mental health problems in clients with somatic complaints. Depression, anxiety, and substance abuse often compound medical problems; in fact, it is estimated that many persons visit their primary care providers because of anxiety, depression, or other mental health problems.

Private-Duty Nursing

Private-duty nursing also offers freedom and control of working days. A private-duty nurse gives comprehensive, intensive care to one client; a physician supplies primary medical care. Often the client is quite sick and needs a great deal of physical and mental care (eg, severe burns, stroke, spinal injury causing paralysis). Some clients with chronic conditions can afford private nurses and wish to have someone constantly at hand for safety and reassurance. Most private-duty nurses work through a nurses' employment agency or registry. Most registered nurses who do private duty in clients' homes work through contract agencies.

Consultants

Role Characteristics

All competent nurses assist other health professionals by providing information and guidance from time to time. The formal role of nurse consultant is somewhat different, however; it is more than imparting knowledge or giving advice. A consultant collaborates with the seeker of help in solving problems. The help-seeker is generally an agency or group that can afford to hire a consultant. A consultant may add to the seeker's knowledge, but the primary tasks of consultation are to stimulate the seeker to think productively and to promote the seeker's ability to handle a troubling or potentially troubling situation. A consultant has no administrative power or authority over the seeker, nor is the consultant responsible for the outcome. The seeker may accept or reject the consultant's recommendations in part or in entirety. Whatever power the consultant has results from his or her expertise only.

A consultant may be hired to work on an individual case or client problem, a program problem, or an administrative problem. The purpose for which the consultation is requested must be clearly established and communicated at the beginning. If the seeker has unrealistic expectations, the consultant must identify and communicate this up front. Consultation requires close teamwork and equal accountability between the seeker and the consultant. In the contract, everything must be specifically spelled out in advance, including the amount of time the consultant will spend on the project and the amount he or she will be paid. Agreements in writing can help prevent misunderstanding and discord. At the end of the project, the consultant prepares a report with specific recommendations. Whether or not the seeker accepts the recommendations, the agreed-on consultation fee must be paid.

Each nurse consultant has expertise in a certain area or areas of nursing (eg, education, administration, mental health, medical-surgical, pediatric). Many nurse consultants work for the government; some work for nursing organizations. Referrals come from various professional organizations.

Consultation–Liaison Psychiatric Nurses

Several hospitals and home care agencies have consultant–liaison psychiatric nurses on staff. They work indirectly with staff or directly with challenging, difficult clients who are not progressing according to expectations. Ambulatory care agencies, rehabilitation facilities, mental health settings, extended care facilities, schools, and businesses also hire these consultants to work with staff, persons, or families with chronic problems or acute crises. Industries find these consultants to be cost-effective in preventing employee absences and expensive treatment programs. Many serious conditions are due to lifestyle choices such as alcohol and drug abuse, smoking, obesity, unsafe sexual practices, and unhealthy diets. Motivation strategies and psychotherapy, as well as education, are needed to effect change in these difficult and serious problems. The International Society of Psychiatric Consultation Liaison Nurses was established in 1994 as a subspecialty of psychiatric-mental health nursing. Contact information is listed in Appendix B.

Case Management

The term *case manager* can be used to describe several roles and activities. A case manager can be:

1. A primary hospital or home care nurse who coordinates and organizes the daily care of clients
2. A hospital utilization nurse coordinator or discharge planner
3. A social worker or mental health worker who oversees the care needs of chronic psychiatric clients in the community for multidisciplinary providers.

4. An independent practitioner who consults with employers on complex and expensive cases requiring extensive services. Such a case manager may be employed by a case management firm that provides consultation services.

5. An employee of an insurance company or HMO who is assigned to manage complex cases through several episodes of illness; the goals are quality care and cost containment.

The last definition is the one most often used in contemporary literature about managed care. This is a fast-growing field of opportunity for nurses. Today, 80% of case managers are nurses. In the past, the case management field was dominated by social workers, especially in the fields of rehabilitation and chronic mental illness. Today, the depth of clinical knowledge required of a case manager makes nurses much better suited for the role. Even in mental illness cases, in-depth psychobiologic and pharmacologic knowledge is required because of more recent knowledge of the brain and increased understanding of mental illnesses as neuropsychiatric disorders.

Case management is more than a role and a service: it is also a system and a technology, and many forces affect it (Figs. 12-2 and 12-3). It is an outcomes-driven system. The system includes assessment, planning, negotiation for and procurement of appropriate services for clients, delivery and coordination of services, and monitoring and evaluating the multiple services to ensure good client outcomes. Because of the complexity of organizing multiple care providers, case managers use modern technology, including fax machines, beepers, voice mail, portable computers, and cellular telephones. Case managers who work for an HMO try to use service providers within that system, although they may go outside the system if necessary to provide optimal care. Independent case managers negotiate with many different service and equipment providers to find the one that will deliver the best service at the least cost.

Case managers are client advocates, working for good outcomes for their clients. Cost containment and the provision of quality care are their major responsibilities (Display 12-2). Nurses who take case management positions are often shocked by the

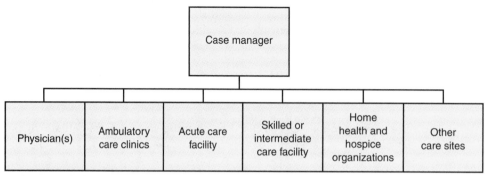

FIGURE 12-2

The community-based case manager continuum. The case manager, working collaboratively with the primary physician, is responsible for monitoring and coordinating all elements of the patient's plan of care along the health-care continuum to include discharge from all formal agencies. This cycle will continue as long as the patient is considered frail and requires case management services. (Marelli TM, Hilliard LS [1996]. *Home Care and Critical Paths*. St. Louis: Mosby.)

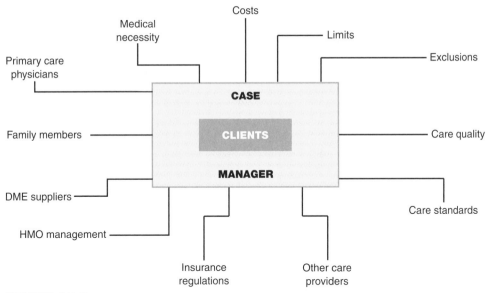

FIGURE 12-3
Forces affecting solutions in the case management process. (Hicks LL, Stallmeyer JM, Coleman JR [1993]. *The Role of the Nurse in Managed Care.* Washington DC: American Nurses Publishing. Reprinted with permission.)

DISPLAY 12-2
Case Management Creed

GOALS

To maintain and promote health

To restore the member to his or her highest level for the long term

To allocate health resources that are available within the health plan and to investigate services within the community

To assist providers and members in navigating the health-care delivery system

To facilitate communication among all health-care providers, health plan administrators, and the member

To secure the best possible economic and clinical outcomes

To advocate for the member

GOALS WILL BE *SMART*

Specific

Measurable

Achievable

Realistic

Timely

OUTCOMES

Outcomes will demonstrate value-added services, such as provision of high-quality, effective medical care, appropriate use of resources, improved quality of life, and patient, payer, and provider satisfaction.

amount of waste they see in the health-care system. Case managers work with hospital utilization and discharge planning nurses to set up appropriate plans of care for clients when they return to the community. Some managed-care companies do both in-hospital and community planning. Within the scope of benefits provided by the plan, case managers work fairly independently. They can approve added services but cannot deny benefits provided by the plan without approval of the medical director.

Case managers must look at the total picture. They must be knowledgeable about the care needed and the resources available in the community to make best use of the funds available for a client. Because case managers usually carry the same clients over time through multiple episodes of illnesses, they come to know these clients' needs. Most case management is generic, but subspecialization is beginning to occur—for example, some case managers specialize in AIDS clients, others in diabetic or hospice clients.

Using Clinical Paths

Planning effective care that provides the best client outcomes for the least cost is complex and challenging. Clinical paths (also known as care maps or critical pathways) are helpful in case management (see Appendix D and Display 12-3). According to Ignatavicius and Hausman (1995), who have written extensively about clinical paths:

> Clinical paths are interdisciplinary plans of care with timelines. They provide an outline of the optimal timing and sequencing of interventions for clients with a particular diagnosis, symptom, or procedure. Paths are designed to minimize use of resources and time while maximizing the quality of patient care, serving as guides for care of clients with a predictable course of illness. Clinical paths are developed for high-volume, high-risk or high-cost diagnoses, procedures, or symptoms. Individual differences are recorded under "variances." Regardless of individual differences, clinical paths usually have four major features:
>
> - *Client outcomes.* They are based on expected client outcomes. Some include daily outcomes.
> - *Timeline.* Specific timelines are given for sequencing interventions, hour by hour in emergency rooms, day by day or week by week in home or rehabilitation settings.
> - *Collaboration.* Clinical paths are jointly developed by multiple health-care professionals and reflect interdisciplinary interventions.
> - *Comprehensive aspects of care.* Paths track various aspects of care, such as diagnostic tests, treatments, medications, nutrition, mobility, client teaching, and discharge planning.
>
> Benefits of clinical paths may be standardized, organized care; increased patient and staff satisfaction; decreased length of stay and decreased costs; and availability of data for evaluating care (Adapted from Ignatavicius DD, Hausman KA, 1995.

The Carondelet HMO described earlier in this chapter uses clinical paths in its integrated system that provides health care across the continuum from ambulatory care center to acute hospital care to extended care facility to home care to hospice. High-risk clients with long-term chronic or catastrophic health problems are managed across the continuum of care (see Chap. 14).

Clinical paths are a system of "charting by exception." Variance codes help individualize the clinical paths. If a client's expected outcomes are not met within the designated

DISPLAY 12-3
Why Use Clinical Paths to Improve Patient Care?

ADMINISTRATIVE GOALS
- Provide a defined clinical budget for care
- Demand data collection and management
- Allow for examination and comparison of similar care (eg, benchmarking)
- Assist in effective orientation for new staff by designating expectations related to patient care
- Provide the basis for determining patient care variances (as the core framework for CQI)
- Decrease or streamline documentation (reducing duplicative paperwork)
- Reduce limited resource utilization
- Focus on systems, not individual practice patterns

CLINICAL GOALS
- Initiate discharge planning on admission
- Encourage ongoing staff education
- Provide clinical standardization of care (including definitions of patient care terms)
- Encourage the patient and family to be equal partners in care
- Support improved care coordination and communication
- Provide the basis for continuity among caregivers
- Support holistic and multidisciplinary care
- Clarify patient expectations regarding care
- Create a visual overview of care for the planning team
- Solidify a structure for collaborative care planning

(Marrelli T, Hilliard L [1996]. Home Care and Critical Paths. *St. Louis: Mosby.)*

time frame or not achieved at all, the variance code is designated as patient-related, situation-related, or systems-related.

Clinical paths are formulated for certain client populations and are based on assessments of client needs. Agencies often create their own clinical paths to suit the aggregates they serve. There is not one correct clinical path for every client, every diagnosis, every problem, or every community. However, clinical paths serve as effective tools to assist with case management and reduce excess paperwork.

THE NURSE SPEAKS . . .
About Being an Entrepreneur

Thirteen years ago, another nurse and I established a home care agency. Today we have over 500 employees, more than 300 of them full-time. We have four area offices and will soon be opening a fifth. Our agency has a reputation for delivering high-quality care, and we offer diverse services such as infusion therapy, ventilator care, and high-tech pediatric care.

Running a business requires a great deal of hard work, especially at the beginning. At first, we both had to continue working nights at our hospital jobs while running the business during the day. We needed start-up capital to cover expenses because insurance companies are very slow in paying agencies. At first we did everything ourselves: all the clerical work, marketing, and nursing care. I had a background in sales before becoming a nurse, and that helped. We also had an excellent network of coworkers, nurses, and aides to call on as the business grew.

Our first contract was with a rehabilitation hospital; we supplied the extra staff they needed for in-hospital care. When the patients were discharged, they were referred to us. The two of us did a careful assessment while the patients were still in the hospital and never took a case unless we felt we could provide excellent care at home. This led us gradually into high-technology home care—that is, by spending time with the patient in the hospital before discharge, we could become thoroughly aware of and familiar with all aspects of the care that would be required at home. It was a natural progression.

When we began, proprietary agencies were not licensed. This seemed strange to us because we believed that home care agencies should be carefully regulated and monitored. We sought licensure as soon as our state's department of health opened it up, about 10 years ago. Then we began our own training program so that our home health aides could become certified. This assures us that they are well trained. All our employees must pass our examination; we have high standards. We are also certified by the Joint Commission, which is a mark of excellence. We have a director of quality management and regular continuing education programs for our staff. Good people stay with us for years because we offer benefits such as a 401(k) retirement plan and health insurance. This costs a lot of money, but we think it is worth it to keep good people.

We try to keep up on trends and are always looking for ways to improve our efficiency. We now have a computerized management information system for all our scheduling, billing, and other clerical work. The system we use has a clinical module available, and we are looking ahead to providing laptop computers for the nurses to use in the homes and then download to our main system. We have contracts with many managed care companies. We do the assessments for their case managers to determine the amount of care needed. We use clinical paths to help establish a sound plan of care. We like working with case managers, most of whom are nurses, understand nursing care, and are willing to negotiate what is best for the patients. They are trying to control waste, not necessary care.

As you can see, our agency has become quite an enterprise! It keeps us very busy, but it makes us proud also.

Kathleen
HOME CARE ADMINISTRATOR

CLINICAL APPLICATION

A Critical Thinking Case Study About Case Management

You are a nurse case manager for a large HMO. Your goal is to provide quality care to clients at the minimum cost. This means avoiding waste, duplication, and unnecessary care.

Mrs. Forenski was hospitalized for uncontrolled diabetes and staphylococcal septicemia secondary to cellulitis from a wound in her right foot. The wound was debrided, with removal of osteophytes from bone. Irrigation and deep packing was started in the hospital. Mrs. Forenski's 82-year-old husband watched this procedure several times. Mrs. Forenski was happy to be discharged after 4 days. However, because it was not certain whether Mr. Forenski could manage her wound care at home, it was decided that he would bring her to the HMO clinic every day for the wound to be packed there.

 and Think!

- Do you foresee any problems with this plan?
- What might they be?
- What are the potential complications of this type of wound?

After 5 days, you receive a call from the clinic nurse saying the plan was not working. Twice the couple had missed their appointment, once because they had car trouble and the other time because Mrs. Forenski did not feel well enough to leave the house. Furthermore, the clinic nurse and doctor thought the wound should be packed twice a day. She said that the funnel-shaped wound was 1.5 cm deep, going right to the bone.

You phone the visiting nurse service with which your firm contracts for service. Your home care referral allows four nursing visits to teach the husband the procedure.

 and Think!

- Do four home care nursing visits seem adequate to teach Mr. Forenski this procedure?
- Why is strict aseptic technique essential in this situation?

On Monday morning, you receive a call from the home care nurse, Nancy, who was quite irritated. She had made her first visit on Sunday, per your referral, and found the elderly couple utterly exhausted and anxious. The lengthy trip to the HMO clinic in heavy traffic had been too much for both of them. They were told at the clinic that the wound was not healing well and in fact looked worse than when Mrs. Forenski left the hospital.

One of Nancy's biggest complaints is that neither the clinic nor the hospital had sent the couple home with any supplies. The wound protocol required a 4% acetic acid solution, among other things, and Nancy had to phone and drive all around the city on a Sunday afternoon trying to find supplies. Although Nancy carries routine dressing supplies in her nursing bag and in the trunk of her car, she does not carry special supplies and solutions. Discharged hospital patients are supposed to be sent home with needed supplies. Laurie added that trying to teach Mr. Forenski yesterday was impossible and that she would probably need more nursing visits, especially because the clinic physician wanted wound care done twice a day. You agree to approve payment for three more nursing visits.

Three days later, Nancy calls again. She had just completed the allowed number of nursing visits and insists that more were needed to ensure that Mr. Forenski can perform the procedure without contamination. She reminds you of the depth of the wound and that bone was exposed, so there is a real risk of osteomyelitis developing. She also reminds you that Mrs. Forenski is diabetic and therefore more open to risk and delayed healing. She insists that more nursing visits are needed.

 and Think!

- What do you think a case manager's reaction is apt to be to an insistent nurse like this?
- Did Nancy overstep her bounds?

You thank Nancy for her opinion and explain that your job is to minimize costs. However, your job is also to see that quality care is delivered to your clients. You express great appreciation for the fact that Nancy did not just complain, but she backed up her complaints with a sound rationale for additional services. With these sound reasons, you can and do approve increased services. You ask Nancy to estimate the number of additional visits needed; she says that would be difficult to do until improvements are observed. You agree that Nancy will visit twice a day for another 4 days and then report back if further visits might be needed.

Chapter SUMMARY

Many nurses are seeking new models of nursing practice. Nursing centers and nursing clinics are developing all across the United States. Birthing centers, founded by nurse-midwives, have been in existence for some time. Wellness centers are increasing in number, as are alternative therapy centers. Nurse entrepreneurs have founded home care agencies and other businesses that provide nursing services. Direct reimbursement and prescriptive privileges are available to advanced practice nurses in most states. Nursing consultants work in a wide range of roles. Some nurses work as independent, self-employed case managers and are hired on a contract basis by agencies and institutions. Case management is demanding but is a rapidly growing field for nurses. Clinical paths are excellent tools used by case managers to plan client care across a continuum of health-care settings.

A list of references and additional readings for this chapter appears at the end of Part 3.

PART 3

References and Additional Readings

Adler J (1994). A dose of virtual Prozac. *Newsweek*, February 7:43.

Advanced Practice Nursing (1993). New age in health care. *Nursing Facts*. Washington DC: American Nurses Association, August.

Ahn H et al (1994). Architectural barriers to persons with disabilities in businesses in an urban community. *J Burn Care Rehab* 15(2):176-180.

Alcoholics Anonymous (1939). The Twelve Steps. In *Twelve Steps and Twelve Traditions*. Alcoholics Anonymous World Services, Inc.

American Nurses Association (1994). *A Statement on Psychiatric-Mental Health Clinical Nursing Practice and Standards of Psychiatric-Mental Health Clinical Nursing Practice*. Washington DC: American Nurses Association.

American Association of Retired Persons (1996). AIDS and the Elderly: Facing facts. *Perspectives* 11(1):1-12.

American Association of Retired Persons (1995). *Alcohol, Medications and Older Adults: How to Help*. Washington DC: AARP.

American Association of Retired Persons (1993). *A Profile of Older Americans*. Washington DC: AARP.

American Academy of Nursing (1993). *Managed Care and National Health Care Reform: Nurses Can Make It Work*. American Academy of Nursing.

American Psychiatric Association (1994). *Diagnostic and Statistical Manual of Mental Disorders*, 4th ed. Washington DC: American Psychiatric Association.

American Nurses Association (1993). *Nursing Case Management*. Kansas City, MO: The Association.

American Nurses Association (1993). *Nurse Practitioners and Certified Nurse Midwives: Meta-Analysis of Process of Care, Clinical Outcomes, and Cost-Effectiveness of Nurses In Primary Care Roles*. Washington DC: The Association.

American Nurses Association (1993). Consumers willing to see a nurse for routine doctoring, according to Gallup poll. News release, Sept. 7.

American Nurses Association (1993). *Innovation at the Work Site: Delivery of Nurse-Managed Primary Health Care Services*. Washington DC: The Association.

American Nurses Association (1994). *Credentializing Center Certification Catalog*. Washington DC: The Association.

Anderson G (1995). *Caring for People With Alzheimer's Disease*. Baltimore: Health Professions Press.

Anderson A et al (1995). Unsung heros. *Home Healthcare Nurse* 13(6):9-15.

Anthony W et al (1989). Research on community support services: What we have learned. *Psychosoc Rehabil J* 12:55.

Bahr R (1995). Sleep disturbances. In Stanley, Beare, eds. *Gerontological Nursing*. Philadelphia: FA Davis.

Baker LC, Baker LS (1994). Excess cost of emergency department visits for nonurgent care. *Health Affairs* 13(5):162-171.

Banez-Car M, McCoy N (1994). Training for the transition to case management. *Caring* 5(3):37-40.

Barer B (1994). Men and women aging differently. *Int J Aging Hum Dev* 38(1):29-40.

Barger SE (1996). The nursing center: A model of community health nursing practice. In Stanhope M, Lancaster J, eds. *Community Health Nursing*. St. Louis: Mosby.

Barger S, Rosenfeld P (1993). Models in community healthcare: Findings from a study of community nursing centers. *Nursing and Health Care* 14(8):402-431.

Barnes L (1993). Residential care operators: Perspectives on mental illness and caregiving roles. *New Directions for Mental Health Services* 58:33-42.

Barnett A, Mayer G (1992). *Ambulatory Care Management and Practice*. Frederick, MD: Aspen.

Bartels S et al (1993). Substance abuse in schizophrenia. *J Nervous Mental Disease* 81(4):227–232.

Bartling AC (1995). Trends in managed care. *Healthcare Exec* 10(2):6–11.

Bauer T, Barron C (1995). Nursing interventions for spiritual care: Preferences of community-based elderly. *J Holistic Nurs* 13(3):268–279.

Beck J (1994). Geriatric assessment: Focus on function. *Patient Care* Feb. 28.

Begley S (1994). Beyond Prozac: Personality in a pill. *Newsweek* Feb. 7, pp. 37–40.

Benson E, McDevitt J (1994). When third-party payment determines service. *Holistic Nurs Pract* 8(2):28–36.

Berggren-Thomas P, Griggs M (1995). Spirituality in aging: Spiritual need or spiritual journey? *J Gerontological Nurs* 21:5–10.

Berkowitz C (1997). Conscious sedation. *RN* 60(2):32–35.

(1997). Best ways to stop hearing loss. *Johns Hopkins Medical Letter* 8(12):4–9.

Bielenson P et al (1995). Politics and practice: Introducing Norplant into a school-based health center in Baltimore. *Am J Pub Health* 85(3):309–311.

Birchfield P (1996). Elder health. In Stanhope B, Lancaster J, eds. *Community Health Nursing*. St. Louis: Mosby

Borthwick-Duffy, Eyman R (1994). Who are the dually diagnosed? *Am J Ment Retard* May:586–596.

Boyle P (1995). *What Price Mental Health? The Ethics and Politics of Setting Priorities*. Baltimore, MD: Georgetown University Press.

Brady R (1993). Mental health of the aging. In Johnson B. *Adaptation and Growth—Psychiatric-Mental Health Nursing*, 3rd ed. Philadelphia: JB Lippincott.

Brandeis University (1993). Effects of smoking. *Institute for Health Policy Report*.

Brooks C (1995). Health care organizations. In Yoder-Wise, ed. *Leading and Managing Nursing Care*. St. Louis: Mosby.

Broussard M, Pitre S (1996). Medication problems in the elderly: A home healthcare nurse's perception. *Home Healthcare Nurse* 14(6):441–443.

Brown SA, Grimes DE (1993). *Nurse Practitioners and Certified Nurse-Midwives*. Washington DC: American Nurses Publishing.

Brownell K, et al (1986). Understanding and preventing relapse. *American Psychology* 41:765–782.

Brubakken KM et al (1994). Roles in implementation of a differentiated case management model: Primm's model of differentiated case management. *Clin Nurs Spec* 8:69–73.

Bruce M et al (1994). The impact of depressive symptomatology on physical disability: McArthur studies of successful aging. *Am J Pub Health* 84(11):1796–1799.

Burrell LO et al (1997). *Adult Nursing: Acute and Community Care*, 2d ed. Stamford, CT: Appleton & Lange.

Busch P (1996). Panic disorder. *Home Healthcare Nurse* 14(2):111–116.

Bush B et al (1987). Screening for alcohol abuse using the CAGE questionnaire. *Am J of Medicine* 82:231–235.

Bushy A (1994). Women in rural environments: Considerations for holistic nurses. *Holistic Nurs Pract* 8:67–73.

Callahan C et al (1994). Depression in late life: The use of clinical characteristics to focus screening efforts. *J Gerontology* 49(1):m9–m14.

Callahan D et al (1995). *The World Growing Old: The Coming Healthcare Challenge*. Baltimore, MD: Georgetown University Press.

Campbell JC et al (1993). Violence as a nursing priority: Policy implications. *Nursing Outlook* 41(2):83–92.

Canobbio M (1996). *Mosby's Handbook of Patient Teaching*. St. Louis: Mosby.

Capuano TA (1995). Clinical pathways: Practical approaches, positive outcomes. *Nurs Mgmt* 26(1):34.

Carpenito LJ, Neal MC (1994). Nurse entrepreneurs. In McCloskey J, Grace HK, eds. *Current Issues in Nursing*, 4th ed. St. Louis: Mosby.

Carroll J (1997). *Measuring and Managing Ambulatory Care Outcomes*. Frederick, MD: Aspen.

Carroll P (1997). Pulse oximetry at your fingertips. *RN* 60(2):22–26.

Cary A (1996). Case management. In Stanhope M, Lancaster J, eds. *Community Health Nursing*. St. Louis: Mosby.

Case C, Seigal N (1996). A community-based long-term care alternative: A case study. *Home Health Care Management & Practice* 8(2):59–64.

Centers for Disease Control & Prevention (1993). Prevalence of Work Disability—U.S., 1990. *MMWR* 42(39):757–759.

Centers for Disease Control & Prevention (1994). Prevalence of disabilities and associated health condition, U.S. 1991–92. *MMWR* 43(40):730–739.

Cerrato P, Amara A, (1997). Alternative complementary therapies: Use research to weigh the alternatives. *RN* 60(2):53–56.

Cesta T et al (1997). *The Case Manager's Survival Guide*. St. Louis: Mosby-Year Book.

Chafetz L (1996). The severely and persistently mentally ill in the community. In Wilson H, Kneisl C, eds. *Psychiatric Nursing*. Menlo Park, CA: Addison-Wesley.

Chen H (1994). Hearing in the elderly: Relationship of hearing loss, loneliness, and self-esteem. *J Gerontol Nurs* 20(6):22–28.

Christopher M et al (1993). Neighborhood nursing: Community as partner. *Caring* 12:44–47.

Chubon S et al (1994). Too little money, too little medication: How do patients cope? *Public Health Nursing* 11(6):412–415.

Clearly A (1994). A better place to be: Integrated/capitated care gives frail elderly a choice over nursing homes. *Hosp Health Netw* 68:58–60.

Clemen-Stone S et al (1995). *Comprehensive Community Health Nursing*, 4th ed. St. Louis: Mosby-Year Book.

Coleman J (1993). Medical case management and managed care. *Case Manager* 4(1):39.

Considine C (1996). Measurement of outcomes: What does it really mean? *Home Healthcare Nurse* 14(6):417–418.

Consumers Union (1995). Who pays how much? How to choose a plan. *Consumer Reports* 60(11):735.

Consumers Union (1995). Does mental health therapy help? A survey. *Consumer Reports* 60(11):734–739.

Consumer Union (1996). Can HMOs help solve the health care crisis? Medicare HMOs luring the elderly. *Consumer Reports* 61(10):28–37.

Consumer Union (1996). How good is your health plan: Ratings of 51 plans. *Consumer Reports* 61(8):28–42.

Corbett DF, Androwich IM (1994). Critical paths: Implications for improving practice. *Home Health Care Nurse* 12:6.

Corley NC et al (1994). The clinical ladder: Impact on nurse satisfaction and turnover. *J Nurs Admin* 24:42–48.

Cournos F et al (1994). Sexual activity and risk of HIV infection among patients with schizophrenia. *Am J Psychiatry* 151(2):228–232.

Cramer C (1996). Saving the unseen patient. *AJN* 96(9):80.

Dalton J, Busch K (1995). Depression: The missing diagnosis in the elderly. *Home Healthcare Nurse* 13(5):31–35.

Davis JE (1993). Ambulatory surgery . . . How far can we go? *Med Clin North Am* 77:365–375.

DeGroot-Kosolcharoen J (1996). Solving the infection puzzle with culture and sensitivity testing. *Nursing '96* 26(9):33–40.

(1997). Depression that won't quit. *Johns Hopkins Medical Letter* February, p. 3.

(1989). Disability risks of chronic illnesses and impairments. *Disability Stat Bull* 2(Fall):1–4.

Donnelly G et al (1994). A faculty-practice program: Three perspectives. *Holistic Nurs Pract* 8:71–80.

Dossey B (1996). Help your patient break free of anxiety. *Nursing '96* 26(10):52–54.

Drapo P (1993). Mental retardation. In Johnson B, ed. *Psychiatric–Mental Health Nursing*. Philadelphia: JB Lippincott.

Dunham-Taylor et al (1996). Surviving capitation. *AJN* 96(3):26–29.

Ebersole P (1994). *Toward Healthy Aging: Human Needs and Nursing Response*, 4th ed. St. Louis: Mosby.

Editors (1996). What you should know about chlamydia. *Nursing '96* 26(9):24f–24h.

Editors (1994). A star-spangled career. *Am J Nursing Career Guide*, pp. 238–242.

Editors (1994). Medical-care expenditures attributable to cigarette smoking—US 1993. *MMWR* 43(26):469–472.

Ernst RL, Hay JW (1994). The U.S. economic and social costs of Alzheimer's disease revisited. *Am J Public Health* 84:1261–1263.

Ethridge P, Lerma D (1996). The Carondelet model. In Marrelli T, Hilliard S, eds. *Home Care and Clinical Paths*. St. Louis: Mosby.

Feil N (1993). Communicating with the confused elderly patient. *Geriatrics* 39:131.

Feingold E (1994). Health care reform—more than cost containment and universal access. *Am J Public Health* 84(5):727–728.

Fiore M (1993). Treatment options for smoking in the 90s. *J Clin Pharmacol* 34(3):195–199.

Fisher L, Lieberman M (1994). Alzheimer's disease: The impact on spouses, offspring, and in-laws. *Fam Process* 33:305–325.

Fisher P (1995). *More Than Movement for Fit to Frail Older Adults*. Baltimore: Health Professions Press.

Fitzpatrick J, Shinners M (1996). How to make assessing as easy as ABC. *Nursing '96* 26(8):51.

Flanagan L (1993). *Self-Employment in Nursing*. Washington DC: American Nurses Publishing.

Florian V, Dangoor N (1994). Personal and familial adaptation of women with severe physical disabilities. *J Marriage Fam* 56(3):735-746.

Foreman M, Zane D (1996). Nursing strategies for acute confusion in elders. *AJN* 96(4).

Fortinash K et al (1995). *Psychiatric Nursing Care Plans*. St. Louis: Mosby.

Francis S (1995). Disability and chronic illness. In Johnson B, ed. *Child, Adolescent and Family Psychiatric Nursing*. Philadelphia: JB Lippincott.

Frawley K (1994). Confidentiality in the computer age. *RN* 57:59-60.

Fulmer I (1995). Elder mistreatment. In Stanley, Beare, eds. *Gerontological Nursing*. Philadelphia: FA Davis.

Galanter M, Kleber H (1994). *Textbook of Substance Abuse Treatment*. Washington DC: American Psychiatric Association Press.

Gelfand D (1994). *Aging and Ethnicity*. New York: Springer.

Glass LK (1989). The historic origins of nursing centers. In *Nursing Centers: Meeting the Demand for Quality Health Care*, Pub. No. 21-2311. New York: NLN.

Goldenberg G (1996). Aches and pains? Call your primary care nurse. *Columbia* Winter:34.

Goodwin DR (1994). Nursing case management activities. *JONA* 24(2):29.

Gorman M (1996). Culture clash: Working with a difficult patient. *AJN* 96(11):58.

Gorrie et al (1994). *Maternal-Newborn Nursing*. Philadelphia: WB Saunders.

Grace HK, ed. (1994). *Current Issues in Nursing*. St. Louis: Mosby.

Gray J (1996). Meeting psychosocial needs. *RN* 59(8):23-28.

Griffiths D, Unger D (1994). Views about planning for the future among parents and siblings of adults with mental retardation. *Family Relations* 43(2):221-227.

Haber D (1994). *Health Promotion and Aging*, 2nd ed. New York: Springer.

Hall J et al (1995). Standardized care plan: Managing Alzheimer's patients at home. *Gerontological Nursing* 211(1):37-47.

Harris M (1996). Medicare managed care. *Home Healthcare Nurse* 14(2):185-187.

Harris MD (1995). Caring for individuals in the community who are mentally retarded/developmentally disabled. *Home Healthcare Nurse* Nov-Dec. p. 27.

Harvard Medical School (1995). Treatment of drug abuse and addiction. *Harvard Mental Health Letter* 12(4):1-4.

Harvard Medical School (1997). Brain imaging and psychiatry. *Harvard Mental Health Letter* 13(8):1-4.

Harvard Medical School (1997). Self-Efficacy. *Harvard Mental Health Letter* 13(9):4-6.

(1994). Healthcare consulting boom fuels cutbacks in RN staff. *AJN* 94:75-80.

Heerkens Y et al (1994). Impairments and disabilities-the difference. *Phys Ther* 74(5):430-442.

Hicks L et al (1992). Nursing challenges in managed care. *Nursing Economics* 10:265.

Hicks LL et al (1993). *The Role of the Nurse in Managed Care*. Washington DC: American Nurses Publishing.

Hoff L (1993). Health policy and the plight of the mentally ill. *Psychiatry* 56:400-419.

Hoge M et al (1994). Defining managed care in public sector psychiatry. *Hosp Commun Psychiatry* 45:1085-1089.

Howe R (1996). *Clinical Pathways for Ambulatory Care Case Management*. Frederick, MD: Aspen.

(1996). *How to Avoid Pitfalls When Trying to Choose an HMO*. Associated Press.

Huggins M (1993). Community support and rehabilitation. In Johnson B, ed. *Psychiatric-Mental Health Nursing*. Philadelphia: JB Lippincott.

Hurley ML (1994). The push for specialty certification. *RN* 36-44.

Hurley PM, Ungvarshi M (1994). Mental health needs of adults with HIV/AIDS referral for home care. *Psychosoc Rehabilitation J* 17:117-126.

Ignatavicius DD, Hausman KA (1995). *Clinical Pathways for Collaborative Practice*. Philadelphia: WB Saunders.

Iowa Intervention Project (1996). *Core Interventions by Specialty*. Iowa City: Center for Nursing Classification, University of Iowa, p. 29.

Irvine J (1995). *Sexuality Education Across Cultures: Working With Differences*. San Francisco: Jossey-Bass.

Jenkins M, Sullivan-Marx E (1994). Nurse practitioners and community health nurses: Clinical partnerships and future vision. *Nursing Clin North Am* 29(3):459-470.

Kalichman SC et al (1994). Factors associated with risk for HIV infection among chronic mentally ill adults. *Am J Psychiatry* 151(2):221-227.

Kalisch PA, Kalisch BJ (1995). *The Advance of American Nursing*, 3rd ed. Philadelphia: JB Lippincott.

Kane R et al (1994). *Essentials of Clinical Geriatrics*, 3rd ed. New York: McGraw-Hill.

Kassirer JP (1994). What role for nurse practitioners in primary care? *N Engl J Med* 330:204-205.

Kasten B (1996). The client with a dual diagnosis. In Wilson H, Kneisl C, eds. *Psychiatric Nursing*. Menlo Park, CA: Addison-Wesley.

Kaufman R (1996). Profiles in caregiving. *Take Care* 5(3):1-6.

Kelly L, Joel L (1995). *Dimensions of Professional Nursing*. New York: McGraw-Hill.

Kennedy G (1995). The geriatric syndrome of late-life depression. *Psychiatr Services* 46(1):43-43.

Killien M (1993). Returning to work after childbirth: Considerations for health policy. *Nursing Outlook* 41(2):73-78.

King E, Cheatham D (1995). Health teaching for people with disabilities. *Home Healthcare Nurse* 13(6):52-58.

Kneisl C (1994). On the brink of healthcare reform: Vital issues for psychiatric nursing. *Psychiatric Nursing* 1(2):4-17.

Kneisl C (1996). HIV/AIDS in vulnerable psychiatric populations. In Wilson H, Kneisl C, eds. *Psychiatric Nursing*, 5th Ed. Menlo Park, CA: Addison-Wesley.

Krach P (1993). Nursing implications: Functional status of older persons with schizophrenia. *Gerontological Nurs* 19(8):21-27.

Kraus E, Stoddard S (1989). *Chartbook on Disability in the United States*. Washington DC: National Institute on Disability & Rehabilitation Research.

Kreiger N (1993). Analyzing socioeconomic and racial/ethnic patterns in health and health care. *Am J Public Health* 83:1086-1087.

Kuhlman G (1996). Applying the nursing process with the elderly. In Wilson H, Kneisl C. *Psychiatric Nursing*, 5th ed. Menlo Park, CA: Addison-Wesley.

Lauerman J (1996). Toward a natural history of aging. *Harvard Magazine* 99(1):57-65.

Lavin J, Enright B (1996). Charting with managed care in mind. *RN* 59(8):47-48.

LeClere F, Kowalewski B (1994). Disability in the family: Effects on children's well-being. *J Marriage Fam* 56(5):457-468.

Lehman F (1995). Consultation liaison psychiatric nursing care. In Stuart G, Sundeen S. *Psychiatric Nursing*. St. Louis: Mosby.

Lewis P (1996). A review of prayer within the role of the holistic nurse. *J Holistic Nursing* 14(4):308-315.

Lilley L, Guanci R (1996). Polypharmacy in Elders. *AJN* 96(11):12-14.

Lindbloom E (1993). America's aging population: Changing the face of health care. *JAMA* 269(5):674-676.

Lipman TH, Deatrick JA (1994). Enhancing specialist preparation for the next century. *J Nurs Educ* 33:53-58.

Long C et al (1995). The elderly and pneumonia: Prevention and management. *Home Healthcare Nurse* 13(5):43-47.

Lubic R (1993). Birthing centers: Delivering more for less. *AJN* 83:1053-1056.

Lundeen SP (1994). Community nursing centers: Implications for reform. In McCloskey et al. *Current Issues in Nursing*, 4th ed. St. Louis: Mosby.

Luquire R (1994). Focusing on outcomes. *RN* May, p. 57.

Lutz B (1996). Total parenteral nutrition in the older patient. *Home Healthcare Nurse* 14(2):123-125.

Mackel C et al (1994). The challenge of detection and management of alcohol abuse among elders. *Clinical Nurse Specialist* 8(3):129-135.

Madden MJ, Ponte PR (1994). Advanced practice roles in the managed care environment. *J Nurs Admin* 24:56-62.

Marrelli T, Hilliard L (1996). *Home Care and Critical Paths: Effective Care Planning Across the Continuum*. St. Louis: Mosby.

Mathre M (1996). Substance abuse in the community. In Stanhope B, Lancaster J, eds. *Community Health Nursing*, 4th ed. St. Louis: Mosby.

Mayo Clinic (1996). *Alzheimer's Disease*. Rochester, MN: Mayo Foundation for Medical Education and Research.

McClellan M (1996). The physically compromised. In Stanhope B, Lancaster J, eds. *Community Health Nursing*, 4th ed. St. Louis: Mosby.

McGurrin M, Worley N (1993). Evaluation of intensive case management for seriously and persistently mentally ill persons. *J Case Manage* 2:59.

McIntosh J (1993). *The Suicide of Older Men and Women: How You Can Help Prevent a Tragedy*. Washington DC: AARP.

Mechanic D (1991). Strategies for integrating public mental health services. *Hosp Commun Psychiatry* 42:797.

Metler M, Kemper D (1996). *Healthwise for Life.* Boise, ID: Healthwise.

Michaels C (1991). A nursing HMO: 10 Months with Carondelet St. Mary's Hospital-based nurse-case management. *Aspen Adv Nurse Exec* 6:3-4.

Middlestadt PC (1994). Federal reimbursement of advanced practice nurses' services empowers the profession. In Harrington C, Estes CL, eds. *Health Policy and Nursing.* Boston: Jones & Bartlett.

Mihaly LK (1991). *Homeless Families: Failed Policies and Young Families.* Washington, DC: The Children's Defense Fund.

Miller N (1994). An interview with Phyllis Ethridge: Challenges for nursing executives. *Nursing Econ* 12(2):65-70.

Miller C (1995). *Nursing Care of Older Adults*, 2nd ed. Philadelphia: JB Lippincott.

Milone-Nuzzo R (1996). The emergency department and home care: Strange bedfellows. *Home Healthcare Nurse* 14(6):451-452.

Mion L et al (1994). Nutritional assessment in the ambulatory care setting. *Nurs Pract Forum* 5(1):46-51.

Molloy SP (1994). Defining case management. *Home Health Nurse* 12(3):51-54.

Montessoro A, Bixen C (1996). Public policy and adolescent pregnancy: A reexamination of the issues. *Nursing Outlook* 44(1):31-36.

Moskowitz E, Jennings B (1996). *Coerced Contraception? Moral and Policy Changes of Long-Acting Birth Control.* Baltimore: Georgetown University Press.

Mullin M (1994). Where in the world are the new grad jobs? *Imprint* 41:6-8.

Mundinger M (1994). Community-based care: Who will be the case managers? *Nurs Outlook* 32(6): 294-95.

National Advisory Mental Health Council (1993). Health care reform for Americans with severe mental illness. *Am J Psychiatry* 150(10):1447-1463.

National Advisory Mental Health Council (1993). Key facts about mental illness. *Am J Psychiatry* 150:1447.

Neal L (1996). The home care client With Alzheimer's disease. *Home Healthcare Nurse* 14(3):175-178.

Newman S (1994). The housing and neighborhood conditions of persons with severe mental illness. *Hosp Commun Psychiatry* 45(4):338-342.

NIAAA (1994). *Alcohol Health and Research World.* Vol. 18, no. 2.

NIMH-ECA (1990). *Proportions of U.S. Population Affected By Selected Mental Disorders: Epidemiologic Catchment Area Study.* Washington DC: National Institute of Mental Health.

Oermann M (1994). Professional nursing education in the future: Changes and challenges. *JOGNN* 23:153-159.

Olivera AA et al (1990). Tardive dyskinesia in psychiatric patients with substance use disorders. *Am J Drug Alcohol Abuse* 16(1):57-66.

Olson L (1994). *The Graying of the World: Who Will Care for the Frail Elderly?* New York: Haworth Press.

Pappas G (1994). Elucidating the relationship between race, socioeconomic status and health. *Am J Public Health* 84:892-893.

Pearson LJ (1994-95). Update: How each state stands on legislative issues affecting advanced nursing practice. *Nurse Pract* 20:23-38.

Perkel R, Wender R, eds. (1996). *Primary Care Models of Ambulatory Care.* Philadelphia: WB Saunders.

Petit J (1994). Continuing care retirement communities and the role of the wellness nurse. *Geriatric Nursing* 15:28-31.

Pfeiffer E (1975). A portable mental status questionnaire for assessment of organic brain deficit in elderly patients. *J Am Geriatric Soc* 23(10):433-441.

Phelps G (1994). Adaptability or extinction: Trends in generalist and subspecialty medicine. *Am Fam Physician* 49:1055-1058.

Phillips DL, Steel JE (1994). Factors influencing scope of practice in nursing centers. *J Prof Nurs* 10:84-90.

Pica-Furey W (1993). Ambulatory surgery-Hospital-based versus freestanding. *AORN J* 57:1119-1127.

Planned Parenthood of America (1994) *Fact Sheet.*

Porter S et al (1995). A comparison of the eyewitness accounts of deaf and hearing children. *Child Abuse Negl* 19(1):51-61.

Price J, Everett S (1994). Perceptions of lung cancer and smoking in an economically disadvantaged population. *J Community Health* 19(5):361-375.

Proehl J, Jones L (1997). *Mosby's Emergency Department Patient Teaching Guides.* St. Louis: Mosby.

(1993). Profile of the rural U.S. *Aging* 365:10-11.

Ragland G (1997). *Instant Teaching Treasures for Patient Education.* St. Louis: Mosby.

Rector C (1997). Innovative practice models in community health nursing. In Spradley B, Allender J. *Readings in Community Health Nursing.* Philadelphia: Lippincott-Raven.

Rheaume A et al (1994). Case management and nursing practice. *J Nursing Admin* 24(3):30–36.

Rhodes A (1996). Update on advanced practice. *MCN* 21(4):257.

Roemer M (1988). Resistance to innovations: The case of the community health center. *Am J Pub Health* 78:1234–1239.

Romaine D (1995). Case management challenges present and future. *Cont Care* 14(1):24–31.

Rooks JP et al (1989). Outcomes of care in birth centers: The National Birth Center Study. *N Engl J Med* 321:1804–1811.

Rosella JD (1994). The need for multicultural diversity among health professionals. *Nurs Health Care* 15:242–246.

Saba V et al (1994). *Computers in Nursing Management*. Washington DC: American Nurses Publishing.

Santos A et al (1993). Providing assertive community treatment for severely mentally ill patients in a rural area. *Hosp Commun Psychiatry* 44:34.

Schoenfelf D et al (1994). Self-rated health and mortality in the high-functioning elderly. *J Gerontol Med Sci* 49(3):109–115.

Schreter R (1994). *Allies and Adversaries: The Impact of Managed Care on Mental Health Services*. Washington DC: American Psychiatric Press.

Seligman M (1995). *What You Can Change and What You Can't*. New York: Balantine Books.

Shames K (1996). Harnessing the Power of Guided Imagery. *RN* 59(8):49–50.

Sharp N (1992). Community nursing centers coming of age. *Nurs Manage* 23:18–20.

Sherwen L, Scoloveno M, Weingarten C (1995). *Nursing Care of the Childbearing Family*. Norwalk, CT: Appleton & Lange.

Simmons-Alling S (1996). Psychobiology. In Wilson, Kneisl, eds. *Psychiatric Nursing* 5th ed. Menlo Park, CA: Addison-Wesley.

Smeltzer S, Bare B (1996). *Brunner and Suddarth's Textbook of Medical-Surgical Nursing*, 8th ed. Philadelphia: Lippincott-Raven.

Smith S et al (1995). Assessing and treating anxiety in elder persons. *Psychiatr Services* 46(1):36–42.

Smith C, Mauer F (1995). *Community Health Nursing*. Philadelphia: WB Saunders.

Solomon J (1995). Retirement living equals jobs for nurses. *RN* 58:52.

Solomon R, Peterson M (1994). Successful aging: How to help your patients cope with change. *Geriatrics* 49(4):41–47.

Sowell R, Meadows T (1994). An integrated case management model: Developing standards evaluation and outcome criteria. *Nurs Admin Q* 18(2):52–64.

Spath PL (1994). *Clinical Paths-Tools for Outcome Management*. Chicago: American Hospital Publishing.

Spear H (1996). Anxiety: When to worry, what to do. *RN* 59(7):40–46.

Spragins E (1996). America's best HMOs. *Newsweek* June 24:56–64.

Stackhouse J (1997). Facilitative verbal responses. In Leasia S, Monahan F. *A Practical Guide for Health Assessment*. Philadelphia: WB Saunders.

Stanhope M, Knollmueller R (1996). *Handbook of Community and Home Health Nursing*. St. Louis: Mosby.

Stocker S (1996). Six tips for caring for aging parents. *AJN* 96(9):32–33.

Stroul B (1988). *Community Support Systems for Persons With Long-Term Mental Illness: Questions and Answers*. Rockville, MD: National Institute of Mental Health.

Substance Abuse Letter (1994). Physicians said not to screen routinely for alcohol use. *PACECom, Inc.*

Sullivan E (1995). *Nursing Care of Clients With Substance Abuse*. St. Louis: Mosby.

Sullivan P et al (1993). Characteristics of repeat users of a psychiatric emergency service. *Hosp Commun Psychiatry* 44(4):376–380.

Taguay P (1994). Successful information system implementation. *Remington Report* 11.

Talley C, Caverly S (1994). Nursing update: Advanced-practice nursing and health care reform. *Hosp Commun Psychiatry* 45:545–557.

Torrey E et al (1992). Criminalizing the seriously mentally ill: The abuse of jails as hospitals. Arlington, VA: U.S. Govt. Printing Office.

Turner-Hensen A, Holaday B (1995). Daily experiences for the chronically ill: A life-span perspective. *Fam Community Health* 17(4):1–11.

Turnock BJ et al (1994). Implementing and assessing organizational practices in local health departments. *Public Health Rep* 109:478–484.

Ugarriza DN, Fallon T (1994). Nurses' attitudes towards homeless women: A barrier to change. *Nurse Outlook* 42:26–29.

USDHHS (1991). *Healthy People 2000*. Washington DC: U.S. Govt. Printing Office.

USDHHS (1996). *Healthy People 2000: Midcourse Review and 1995 Revisions*. Washington DC: U.S. Govt. Printing Office.

USDHHS PHS (1994). *National Ambulatory Medical Care Survey*. Pub. No. 94-1777. Washington DC: U.S. Govt. Printing Office.

USDHHS PHS (1996). Substance Abuse and Mental Health Services Administration helps states manage managed care. *SAMHSA Newsletter* 4(4):4–8.

USDHHS PHS (1996). Substance Abuse and Mental Health Services Administration releases study of co-occurrence between mental syndromes and substance abuse. *SAMHSA Newsletter* 4(4):8–9.

USDHHS PHS (1996). New study shows treatment reduces drug use *SAMHSA Newsletter* 4(4):21–23.

USDHHS PHS (1996). Study shows two-parent family lowers teen drug use. *SAMHSA Newsletter* 4(4):25–26.

U.S. Department of Justice (1991). *Americans With Disabilities Act Handbook*. Washington DC: U.S. Govt. Printing Office.

Vahldieck R et al (1993). A framework for planning public health nursing services for families. In Wegner, Alexander, eds. *Readings in Family Nursing*. Philadelphia: JB Lippincott.

Vogel G, Doleysh N (1994). *Entrepreneuring: A Nurse's Guide to Starting a Business*, 2nd ed. New York: National League for Nursing.

Wagner J (1996). Wandering and fall prevention: New solutions to a perennial problem. *Nursing '96* 26(8):24s–24t.

Walker M, Doherty A. Healthy cities: Empowering vulnerable populations for health through partnerships. *Fam Community Health* 17(2):77–79.

Walker PH (1994). Comprehensive community nursing center model: Maximizing practice income—A challenge to educators. *J Prof Nurs* 10:131–139.

Washington Consulting Group (1994). *Survey of Certified Nurse Practitioners and Clinical Nurse Specialists* (December 1992, Final Report). Rockville, MD: Division of Nursing.

Weiden P, Havens L (1994). Psychotherapeutic management techniques in treatment of outpatients with schizophrenia. *Hosp Commun Psychiatry* 45(6):549–555.

Wheeler L (1996). Managed mental health care. In Wilson H, Kneisl C. *Psychiatric Nursing*, 5th ed. Menlo Park, CA: Addison-Wesley.

Wills E (1996). Nurse–client alliance. *Home Healthcare Nurse* 14(6):455–459.

Wilson HD (1993). Family caregiving for a relative with Alzheimer's dementia: Coping with negative choices. In Wegner, Alexander, eds. *Readings in Family Nursing*. Philadelphia: JB Lippincott.

Wilson H, Kneisl C (1996). *Psychiatric Nursing*, 5th ed. Menlo Park, CA: Addison-Wesley.

Worley N, Lowery B (1988). Deinstitutionalization: Could the process have been better for patients? *Arch Psychiatric Nursing* 2:126.

Worley N (1995). Community psychiatric nursing care. In Stuart J, Sundeen S, eds. *Psychiatric Nursing*, 5th ed. St. Louis: Mosby.

Yale R (1995). *Developing Support Groups for Individuals With Early-Stage Alzheimer's Disease*. Baltimore: Health Professions Press.

Yates S (1994). The practice of school nursing: Integration with new models of health delivery. *J School Nurs* 10(1):10–19.

Zander K (1995). *Managing Outcomes Through Collaborative Care*. Chicago: AHA.

Zweig R, Hinrichsen G (1993). Factors associated with suicide attempts by depressed older adults. *J Psychiatry* 150:1687–1692.

Part 4

Nursing Practice in Home Care

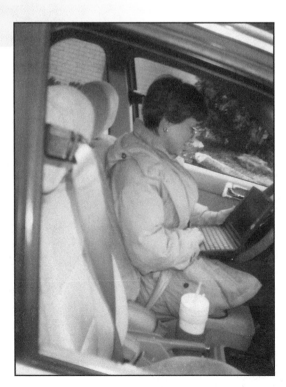

A home care nurse using her computer.

13

The Home Care System

Key Terms

capitation

case coordination

case managers

certified home care agencies

combination agencies

Community Health Accreditation Program (CHAP)

conditions of participation

continuity of care

discharge planning

durable medical equipment

freestanding agencies

Health Care Financing Administration (HCFA)

home care surveys

hospices

hospital-based home care

informal caregivers

Joint Commission on Accreditation of Healthcare Organizations (JCAHO)

medically indigent

National Home Caring Council

official public agencies

Outcomes Assessment Information Set (OASIS)

proprietary home care agencies

referrals

reimbursement payments

shared-risk system

subsidized care

United Way contributions

visiting nurse associations

Learning Objectives

1. Describe the growth of home care.

2. Differentiate between the types of home care agencies.

3. Explain the licensing, certification, and accreditation system for home care agencies.

4. Define eight home care reimbursement systems.

5. Trace the history of discharge planning.

6. Contrast Medicare and Medicaid.

7. Explain the characteristics of good discharge planning.

8. List referral sources for home care services.

9. Identify three levels of case coordination.

10. Compare the case coordination roles of the discharge planner, the primary nurse, and the managed-care company's case manager.

11. Describe recent and proposed changes in Medicare.

Six million Americans currently receive health care at home. The home care system continues to grow dramatically, as does the need for registered nurses to work in home care (Fig. 13-1). In the 5 years between 1989 and 1994, the number of certified home care agencies grew from 11,097 to 15,027, a 26% increase. The number of hospices grew even more during the same period, from 597 to 1,459 (National Association for Home Care [NAHC], 1995a). The largest number of clients needed care for diseases of the circulatory system (25.6%); endocrine, nutritional, and metabolic diseases and immunity disorders ranked second (9.8%); and diseases of the musculoskeletal system and connective tissue ranked third (9.3%) (NAHC, 1995a). Diabetes mellitus has recently become the number-one diagnosis of home care clients (*Home Health Digest,* December 1996).

Most home care is provided informally by unpaid caregivers, usually family members. Three quarters of informal caregivers are female; nearly a third are over age 65. The total number of family caregivers is estimated to be 18 million (National Family Caregivers Association, 1994). Family caregivers provide assistance in three areas: housework and transportation (66%); emotional support and guardianship (57%); and health care and assistance with activities of daily living (43%). These patterns of caregiving are correlated with the nature of the client's illness or disability (National Family Caregivers Association, 1994).

Types of Home Care Agencies

The home care system comprises several types of agencies. Modern home care began in England in 1859 when William Rathbone, with the help of Florence Nightingale, started a school to train visiting nurses. The main purpose was to care for poor, sick people in their homes. In the United States during the late 1800s, the waves of poor immigrants with health problems induced philanthropists to help establish visiting nurse agencies in Boston, Buffalo, New York, and Philadelphia. Because of the high quality of care given by these agencies, middle-class people sought and received home care services, first in Philadelphia. As visiting nurse agencies spread to other areas, sliding-scale fees were developed, based on the client's ability to pay.

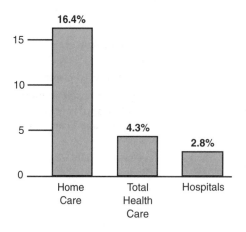

FIGURE 13-1

Annual employment growth rate. (Source: Bureau of Labor Statistics)

Visiting nurse associations (VNAs) grew across the United States in cities, small towns, and rural areas. In places where no public health nursing service was available, they incorporated preventive services such as school nursing and maternal-child care. VNAs are freestanding agencies—that is, they are not owned by hospitals or other institutions but are governed by a board of directors and are not-for-profit. VNAs are voluntary organizations that do not depend on state and local tax revenues. Much of their income is from third-party payment reimbursements from Medicare, Medicaid, and private insurance, including managed-care organizations. Private endowments, donations, United Way contributions, and private payment of fees also help support them. The Visiting Nurse Association of America represents more than 500 local agencies across the United States.

Official public agencies such as local health departments traditionally provide public health nursing services in health promotion and disease prevention. This includes home visits for potential problems in maternal-child health and other situations of a preventive measure. In 1965, when Medicare was signed into law, funding was provided for home care for sick people. In locations where no VNA existed to offer home care services, local health departments began to provide these services as part of their mission to fill gaps in community health services. These home care services were then organized and certified as Medicare-approved home health agencies. Traditional public health nursing services were continued along with the home care visits to the sick, so these agencies also came to be called "combination agencies." These agencies receive third-party reimbursements for the home care visits to the sick. As the number of referrals from hospitals, physicians, and other sources increased, many of the traditional preventive services have been pushed aside because they have less immediacy than the care of the sick. Thus, in some areas, the old pattern of ignoring prevention to serve people who are already sick is repeated because of a shortage of home health agencies.

Hospital-based home care agencies began to develop across the United States because of this need and because of economic factors. In the retrospective, fee-for-service system, hospitals set their own fees for services and could include some of the expensive hospital costs in those fees. Thus, it became cost-effective for hospitals to establish their own home care departments rather than refer clients to VNAs or health department home care agencies. With today's trend toward managed-care prospective-payment systems, all agencies face fierce competition over the fees they charge, resulting in lower fees and less profit.

Proprietary home care agencies are freestanding, for-profit agencies that provide home health services. Persons, groups, or corporations may own proprietary agencies. These agencies are growing most rapidly. Not all proprietary agencies are licensed, certified, or accredited, so their quality varies. There are several national chains of proprietary agencies that are administered through corporate offices. Some proprietary agencies are owned and operated by nurses experienced in home care. Some proprietary agencies are certified to participate in the Medicare program; some are not. Revenues are generated by private payments or managed-care or other insurance reimbursements. Many of these agencies act as private-duty nursing registries. Some proprietary agencies specialize in a particular aspect of care such as pediatric home care, oncology home care, or high-technology home care. Some agencies specialize in just one aspect of care, such as infusion therapy. Others specialize in home health aide and homemaker personnel only and may contract with other home health agencies to provide these services.

Durable medical equipment agencies, often referred to as home care agencies, supply equipment needed in the home such as hospital beds, commodes, ventilators and other oxygen equipment, wheelchairs, and walkers. These agencies are more product-oriented than service-oriented, although they do set up and teach the use of their equipment in the home and will return if problems arise with the use of their products. These agencies are for-profit businesses.

Agency Licensing, Certification, and Accreditation

Thirty-nine states require licensure for home care agencies (Humphrey & Milone-Nuzzo, 1996). An agency must be licensed by the state in which it is located before it can become a Medicare-certified agency and receive direct Medicare reimbursements. The conditions of participation are the federal regulations that certify home care agencies to participate in Medicare. These conditions were developed by the Health Care Financing Administration (HCFA), which administers Medicare and sets rules and standards for Medicare participating agencies.

Surveys of licensed home care agencies must be conducted at least every 15 months. In some states, the HCFA has contracts with state health departments to conduct a survey for Medicare certification. The state then surveys the agency for both licensure and certification at the same time. If the agency meets the state's licensing law criteria, it receives a license. If it is deficient, it may be given a certain period of time to attain compliance. Sometimes seriously deficient agencies are closed by the state until the deficiencies are corrected.

Accreditation is a different matter. It is a voluntary process, but it demonstrates that an agency meets high standards and delivers quality care. Managed-care organizations are increasingly demanding that agencies to which they award contracts be accredited. There are three important accrediting organizations in the United States.

The Joint Commission on Accreditation of Healthcare Organizations (JCAHO), which surveys hospitals and provides highly valued voluntary accreditation status, began in 1988 to accredit home care agencies as well. Depending on the size of the agency, the survey visit may last 1 or more days. Charts are audited, staff members are interviewed, and home visits are made as part of the survey. Standards to be met are provided in the *Accreditation Manual for Home Care*. The survey team reviews and scores the findings and the agency is assigned to one of five categories:

1. Accreditation with commendation
2. Accreditation with or without recommendations
3. Conditional accreditation
4. Provisional accreditation
5. Not accredited

Even when highly accredited, agencies are subject to unannounced surveys about midpoint between the scheduled accreditation visits each 3 years. Roughly 5% of accredited agencies are randomly selected for unannounced visits, which can change the accreditation status if standards have not been maintained. Display 13-1 lists the issues the JCAHO would look at in a home care agency's orientation program for new nurses.

The second major accrediting program is called the Community Health Accreditation Program (CHAP). CHAP is related to the National League for Nursing (NLN) and has been accrediting home care agencies since 1965. CHAP accreditation involves four steps:

1. An application is filed with CHAP.
2. A contract is written by CHAP with the home care agency.
3. The agency compares itself to CHAP standards.
4. A survey visit of several days is made to the agency. A board of review then looks at both the self-study and the survey results and, if satisfied, awards a 3-year accreditation.

DISPLAY 13-1
JCAHO Topics Surveyed for Orientation of Home Care Nurses

- An understanding of the types of care or services to be delivered in the client's environment
- Confidentiality of client information
- Appropriate policies and procedures
- Appropriate actions in unsafe situations
- Emergency preparedness
- Home safety issues, including bathroom, fire, environmental, and electrical safety
- Identification, handling, and disposal of hazardous or infectious materials and wastes in a safe and sanitary manner and in accordance with law and regulation
- Principles of infection control, including personal hygiene, precautions, aseptic procedures, communicable infections, and appropriate cleaning, disinfection, or sterilization of equipment and supplies
- Storage, handling, and access to supplies, medical gases, and drugs appropriate to the care or service provided
- Equipment management, including safe and appropriate use of equipment as applicable to the care or service provided
- Any specific tests or procedures to be performed by the staff
- Screening for abuse and neglect, appropriate to the staff
- Information regarding care or service provided by other members of the staff to better coordinate care and appropriately refer the client
- Guidelines for appropriate referrals, which include timeliness
- Policies and procedures regarding advance directives
- Organizational policies and procedures regarding death and dying
- Any other client care responsibilities

(Adapted from Joint Commission on Accreditation of Healthcare Organizations [1995]. "Management of Human Resources." In Accreditation Manual for Home Care, Volume II: Scoring Guidelines.*)*

The National Home Caring Council is the third major accrediting body for home care agencies. This program focuses on home health aide services. A self-study and a survey visit are conducted; if successful, a 3-year accreditation is granted.

Benchmarking is the process of developing criteria or standards of comparison with other similar agencies or measuring progress within an agency.

Reimbursement Systems for Payment of Home Care Services

Medicare (Title XVIII)

The federal government provides national health insurance to persons over 65 and persons who have been declared disabled for 2 years or more. Persons with end-stage renal disease are also included. More home care payments come from Medicare than any other source of reimbursement. Most Medicare benefits go to hospitals; about 25% goes to reimburse physicians, 8% pays for home care benefits, and only 1% pays for hospice programs (Humphrey & Milone-Nuzzo, 1996). Medicare consumes 20 cents out of every federal tax dollar. For the nation's financial health, this extremely costly system must be reformed. A federal budget reduction act agreed on by Congress and the president reduces Medicare spending by $115 billion over 5 years. Medicare Part B premiums, paid by clients, will increase by about $2 per month, with wealthier clients paying more. Gradually, Part B will cover 25% of home care, which will make Part A more solvent in the future.

The HCFA, a branch of the U.S. Department of Health and Human Services, governs the Medicare program and each year produces the *Medicare Handbook,* which describes Medicare benefits. In various areas of the nation, appointed fiscal intermediaries (usually insurance companies such as Blue Cross and Blue Shield) handle the payments, although program regulations and policies are still governed by the HCFA. A special HCFA form must be used as a generic plan of care (Display 13-2). For the agency to receive reimbursement, this form must be filled out carefully and accurately for each client. The nurse and the physician must sign the form, and the latter must certify that the client is essentially homebound, under medical care, and in need of reasonable and necessary skilled home care services. The plan of care is in force for 60 days, after which the client must be recertified.

The HCFA is revising Medicare conditions of participation for home care agencies. This includes mandated use of the Outcomes Assessment Information Set (OASIS), a group of 89 questions used to assess clients' health and functional status. Each client must have an OASIS on admission and at least every 62 days. The new conditions will be the most thorough revamping of Medicare regulations since 1973, when they were established. They switch the focus to outcomes instead of process.

Before long, prospective payments and a capitation system similar to the diagnostic related groups imposed on hospitals will be used for home care agencies. This means that the HCFA will strictly limit the frequency and duration of home visits based on the diagnosis. This ignores the multifaceted nature of many home care situations and the multiple diagnoses of most elderly people. It will require nurses to be extremely efficient. Some experts are estimating a 15% cut in Medicare reimbursements for home care in 1998 (Moore, 1997).

DISPLAY 13-2

Department of Health and Human Services Health Care Financing Administration

Department of Health and Human Services Health Care Financing Administration	FORM APPROVED OMB No. 0938-0357

Home Health Certification and Plan of Treatment

1. Patient's Name and Address	2. Patient's HI Claim Number
	3. Medical Record Number
4. Dates: Start of care and verbal order for SOC	5. Certification Period: From: To:
6. Home Health Agency Name and Address	7. Principal Diagnosis: Narrative, Dates of Onset/Exacerbation, ICD-9-CM Code □□□.□□
	8. Surgical Procedure(s) Revelant to Care: Narrative, Date, ICD-9-CM Code □□□.□□

9. Other Pertinent Diagnosis–Narrative, Dates of Onset/Exacerbation, ICD-9-CM Code(s)

□□□.□□   □□□.□□
□□□.□□   □□□.□□

10.

Functional Limitations		Activities Permitted	
□ Amputation	□ Ambulation	□ Bedrest	□ Crutches
□ Bowel/Bladder	□ Mental	□ Complete	□ Cane
(incontinence)	□ Speech	□ BRP	□ Wheelchair
□ Contracture	□ Vision	□ Up as Tolerated	□ Walker
□ Hearing	□ Respiratory	□ Transfer Bed/Chair	□ No Restrictions
□ Paralysis	□ Other(Specify)	□ Exercises Prescribed	□ Other (Specify)
□ Endurance		□ Partial Weight Bearing	
		□ Independent at Home	

11. Safety Measures:

12. Orders for Services and Treatments (Specify Modality, amt/freq/dura)	13. Medications: Dose/Frequency/Route (N) New (C) Changed

14. Mental Status: □ Oriented   □ Forgetful   □ Disoriented   □ Agitated
    □ Comatose   □ Depressed   □ Lethargic   □ Other

15. Nutritional Requirements:

16. Medical Supplies & DME Ordered	17. Allergies

DISPLAY 13-2 (*Continued*)

18. Goals/Rehabilitation Potential/Discharge Plans	19. Significant Clinical Findings/Summary from each discipline

20. Prognosis: ☐Poor ☐Guarded ☐Fair ☐Good ☐Excellent

21. Attending Physician's Name and Address	22. Physician Certification: I ☐certify ☐recertify that the above home health services are required and are authorized by me with a written plan for treatment which will be periodically reviewed by me. This patient is under my care, is confined to his home, and is in need of intermittent skilled nursing care and/or physical or speech therapy or has been furnished home health services based on such a need and no longer has a need for such care or therapy, but continues to need occupational therapy.
23. Attending Physician's Signature and Date	

Form HCFA-485(U4)(4-85)	PROVIDER

Private insurance companies generally adhere to Medicare policies and regulations for clinical and reimbursement matters (Harris, 1994). In recent years, Medicare and Medicaid Health Maintenance Organizations (HMOs) have been developed by private companies (Display 13-3). Some people purchase Medigap insurance from a private company. Medigap provides coverage for some of the several gaps in Medicare coverage.

Consumers Union recently compared the overall value of Medicare HMOs versus regular fee-for-service Medicare with Medigap insurance and reported that people are generally better off with the latter, even if it costs a few dollars more a month (Consumers Union, October 1996). Many home care nurses complain that many Medicare HMO plans provide inadequate home care services. These plans advertise benefits such as free eyeglasses that regular Medicare does not provide, and many elderly people who sign up for Medicare HMO plans do not realize that some of these plans are deficient in needed services when serious illness strikes. HMOs vary a great deal in the quality of care provided.

The criteria for regular Medicare services are considered conservative. Medicare does not provide care when the client's condition is stable; an acute, changing situation must exist. The word "stable" should never be used to describe a client's status, because reimbursements are then likely to be denied. Medicare offers short-term assistance and will not pay for long-term custodial care. Medicare reimburses up to 80% of the cost of needed rented durable medical equipment. To receive Medicare reimbursement, clients must be sick enough to be essentially homebound. Medicare pays for home health care when five basic conditions are met:

1. The client requires intermittent skilled nursing care, physical therapy, or speech therapy.

DISPLAY 13-3
How Do Medicare HMOs Work?

- HMOs provide all Medicare benefits and sometimes more.
- There is little or no paperwork for clients.
- Clients must continue to pay Medicare Part B premiums.
- Some HMOs require additional small monthly premiums and copayments that can change yearly.
- Clients do not pay Medicare deductibles and copayments.
- Some plans promote preventive health and include extras such as routine physicals and immunizations.
- Some plans include prescription drugs, hearing aids, and eyeglasses for little or no extra fees.
- Clients must receive all health care from the HMO network providers or the plan will not pay.
- Clients select or are assigned a primary doctor who is their gatekeeper for specialists.
- Emergency care outside the plan's network will be paid; Medicare will not pay otherwise.
- Point-of-service riders may be bought, allowing clients to use some outside services.
- To enroll, clients
    - Must live in the HMO service area
    - Must not be receiving care in a Medicare-certified hospice
    - Must not have permanent kidney failure
    - Must continue to have Medicare Part B

(Adapted from Health Care Financing Administration [1996]. The Medicare Handbook.)

2. The client is confined to home.
3. The client's physician determines that home health care is needed and sets up a plan.
4. The home health agency providing the care participates in Medicare.
5. The services must be reasonable and necessary.

Medicare's definition of skilled nursing care is given in Display 13-4.

Medicaid (Title XIX)

Medicaid, which is paid out of shared federal and state funds, was developed to help the medically indigent. About 25% of all home care sources of payment come from Medicaid reimbursement. Medicaid, unlike Medicare, pays for custodial care for chronic conditions. Many frail, elderly persons can remain in their own homes with the assistance of a home health aide several hours a day. Often this is the only service they need. If their income is low enough to be Medicaid-eligible, the aide will be paid by Medicaid. It is estimated that reduced federal benefit spending requirements will decrease Medicaid spending by $60 billion over the next 10 years (*USA Today*, 1997, p. 8A). This means that some valuable Medicaid services must be reduced or eliminated.

DISPLAY 13-4
"Skilled Nursing Care" Reimbursed by Medicare

A registered nurse using professional knowledge and skills, rendering judgments, and evaluating process and outcomes is performing skilled nursing. Specific examples include:

- Assessment and monitoring (eg, cardiovascular, neurologic, mobility, mental status)
- Medication administration and teaching
- Evaluation of effects of medications and treatments
- Wound and sterile dressing care, including decubitus care and teaching
- Teaching and training caregivers and clients
- Recent ostomy and ileostomy care and teaching
- Evaluation of client safety and progress
- Infusion therapy
- Psychiatric assessments, interventions, evaluations
- Ventilator care
- Tracheostomy care and teaching
- Foley catheter insertion
- Bladder instillation
- Teaching bowel and bladder routines
- Nasogastric tube insertion
- Teaching G-tube feedings
- Chest physiotherapy, including postural drainage
- Diabetic teaching
- Inhalation therapy and teaching
- Bowel disimpaction
- Management and evaluation of patient care plan

A particular function is probably not skilled nursing if a nonprofessional can perform it.

Private Insurance Coverage

Private insurance companies differ as to what home care services they reimburse, but most companies follow Medicare guidelines. Insurance plans are also called indemnity plans with retrospective fee-for-service reimbursements. Clients have maximum freedom to select their doctors and other health-care services but must fill out forms and await reimbursement. Long-term health insurance plans are becoming increasingly popular. A daily reimbursement rate is paid for needed care in a skilled nursing facility or for assisted living or home care services. The amount varies with the cost of premiums. Long-term health insurance premiums are expensive but provide older people with a sense of security should they ever need long-term care.

Before establishing a plan of care, a hospital discharge planner or a home care agency must determine exactly what the client's policy will cover. In many cases, it is insurance reimbursement, more than client need, that determines what services the client will receive.

Managed-Care Plans

The two basic types of prospective-payment managed-care plans are preferred provider organizations (PPOs) and HMOs. Some HMOs also allow members to purchase an extra point-of-service rider that allows members to select their own physicians outside the HMO. This permits freedom similar to that of a PPO, where members can go to physicians outside the organization, although they pay slightly more for the privilege. Case managers develop the most cost-effective plans they can for clients while trying to maintain quality of care.

Wide variations exist in the quality of managed-care programs. Some provide very satisfactory care. The not-for-profit plans generally offer the best care, particularly the Kaiser plans, which have been in existence the longest. HMO programs have not been adequately monitored, regulated, and controlled. One criticism is that some for-profit plans pay their administrators enormous salaries and provide good returns to their stockholders at the expense of quality health care. More information about managed care can be found in Chapters 2 and 9.

No-Fault Auto Insurance

Home care for automobile accident victims is often reimbursed by no-fault auto insurance. This is most often seen in high-technology agencies when severe injuries (eg, paraplegia, quadriplegia, severe head injuries resulting in neurologic deficits) require extensive skilled nursing care.

Worker's Compensation Insurance

The worker's compensation insurance paid by employers offers reimbursement if workers become injured on the job. Both no-fault and worker's compensation reimbursement is sought first, before other reimbursement plans.

Free or Subsidized Care

Free or reduced-payment care is provided by many home health agencies that are solvent financially. Some VNAs receive donations or United Way grants for this purpose. Subsidized care is given by home care agencies when it is necessary for a client's well-being but is not covered by his or her insurance policy. A sliding-scale fee schedule is used; some people may be charged only $1 or $2. Some people have no insurance coverage and no resources. However, if a home care agency allows the amount of free care given to exceed its financial resources, its future could be in jeopardy.

Private Payments

Some traditional, basic home care services are paid privately. Extra services not covered by third-party reimbursements are usually paid privately. These include private-duty nurses or extra home health aide time. Some insurance programs pay for private-duty nurses under special circumstances.

Other Payment Sources

Local, state, and national programs have been set up to help needy clients who fall between the cracks of Medicare, Medicaid, or other insurance programs. Of the total amount of money spent for home care across the country, these monies amount to less than 10%. Special gifts, grants, and endowments fund these programs.

There is a great need for custodial care for elderly persons who wish to remain in their homes but have no family caregivers to assist them. Many live alone. Often they refuse to "spend down" their nest egg until they reach the Medicaid level, which would then pay for needed custodial care. Many elderly persons, too thrifty and too proud to apply for Medicaid, exhaust themselves, become sick, and end up in hospitals or extended-care facilities. In the long run, this is an expensive drain on the system. It costs taxpayers much more for institutional care, which is reimbursed by Medicaid or Medicare.

Discharge Planning and Referrals to Home Care

Referrals for home care services come from various sources. The most common sources are hospitals. Hospitals that have their own home care agency usually refer cases to that agency if the client lives in the community. Social service departments of county and state governments tend to make their referrals to health departments if those are combination agencies. Physicians' offices, nurses, mental health inpatient or outpatient agencies, managed-care case managers, families, and self-referrals are generally made to the closest agency with a reputation for providing quality, cost-effective care.

Referrals should be made only if there is a need and if the services are available. Sometimes the need can be better met by family, friends, neighbors, or religious groups than by a health-care agency. Parish nurses are often involved in discharge planning and may use services available from their church or synagogue. Most importantly, the client or the family should agree to a referral before it is made.

Discharge planning facilitates the transfer of a client from one setting to another or one level of care to another. The continuity of care provided by good discharge planning enables the client's gains made in one facility to continue in the new one without regression or complications. In 1965, Medicare and Medicaid legislation mandated discharge planning. In 1982, the prospective-payment system, aimed at reducing the number of days spent in the hospital, was enacted. Nurses or sometimes social workers were designated to begin discharge planning as early as possible in the hospitalization process. Thus, good discharge planning becomes cost-effective to hospitals by reducing the length of stay. The American Hospital Association and the Omnibus Budget Reconciliation Act of 1986 strengthened the role of discharge planners. Medicare mandates a standardized needs assessment process for all Medicare clients. Many hospitals call their discharge planners "case managers." Managed-care case managers look for good discharge plans that facilitate client access to needed care and at the same time make the money for services stretch as far as possible.

Characteristics for good discharge planning include the following:

1. Identifying clients who will need posthospital care as early as possible during their hospitalization, and begin to set the plan in motion.
2. Using assessment, planning, analysis, intervention, and evaluation as systematic problem-solving steps of the discharge plan—in other words, using the nursing process. An accurate in-hospital assessment of the client's physical and functional status and support system is crucial in developing a successful discharge plan.
3. Including the client and the family in the discharge planning process.
4. Always keeping in mind the best environment for the client, and planning according to the setting where the client is going.
5. Applying knowledge of appropriate community resources.
6. Working with other health-care disciplines (eg, social services or physical therapy) as necessary.
7. Ensuring that the physician's orders are complete and are carried out in the discharge plan.
8. Ensuring that the client leaves the hospital with all necessary prescriptions, medications, supplies, and written instructions.
9. Maintaining good follow-up communication with the managed-care case manager, the primary home care nurse, and the client to evaluate the discharge plan.

Case Coordination

Coordination of the client's plan of care takes place on three levels. First, the discharge planner sets in motion the plan of care before the client goes home or enters an intermediate facility (eg, a nursing home or a rehabilitation hospital). Second, when the client goes home, the primary home care nurse is the primary case coordinator. He or she works with other disciplines (physical therapy, social work, speech therapy, occupational therapy) to meet the client's needs. Home health aides may be needed on a part-time basis to assist with bathing and personal care. The nurse must supervise the aide at least every 15 days. If needed, homemaker services, although not covered by most third-party payers, must be included in the plan. The nurse must provide all team members with regular reinforcement of all services and should schedule case conferences with the whole team as needed (at least every 60 days). Good communication with the client, the family, the physician, and other community providers of care is an essential part of the primary nurse's job.

Third, a case manager has a coordination role if the client is enrolled in a managed-care plan and if the situation is complex and requires services from multiple agencies. A managed-care case manager is responsible for maximizing the efficiency of the home care benefits provided by the company. An HMO case manager will make sure that the discharge planner uses the home care or other agencies that are within the HMO system, if needed. However, when that system does not have the needed service, most HMO case managers can go outside the system to provide the needed care. The case manager stays in close touch with the primary home care nurse and may modify the originally approved number of nursing visits based on the primary nurse's recommendations. In fact, most case managers never meet the clients and must assess and make recommendations based on reports and telephone conversations.

If the primary nurse can show that the client needs more care than originally planned, it will be approved by most managed-care plans. However, if client outcomes are not achieved because the nurse wastes time on unimportant matters, the necessary extra visits may not be reimbursed by the managed-care company, and the home care agency will have to absorb the cost of those visits. This is called a shared-risk system because the home care agency shares some of the financial risks of inefficient care with the managed-care or health insurance company. This is a reason why home care nurses must perform with maximum efficiency and productivity. It is important for home care nurses to understand these financial pressures and plan their care efficiently for both their clients' sake and their agency's financial solvency.

THE NURSE SPEAKS . . .
About Caring for a Client With Congestive Heart Failure

I work for a visiting nurse association. About a year ago, I met a client who, herself, was a diligent caregiver. Bertha, a 60-year-old, heavy-set black woman, has become very dear to me, and I will never forget her. She sacrificed her own needs as a loving caregiver during her husband's long illness until he died of lung cancer a year ago. Bertha now lives alone in a ramshackle apartment building. She dresses in second-hand clothing from the Salvation Army. Most of her life, she worked hard as a cleaning woman. She is still hard-working, independent, and motivated to do the right thing. She is a woman of deep religious faith.

Bertha now has end-stage congestive heart failure. During the past year, she has been rushed to the hospital six or eight times with fulminating pulmonary edema. Each time she returned home and again overworked her weak heart. Finally, the hospital discharge planner, at the urging of her parish nurse, referred her to the VNA for a home care program, despite her poor insurance coverage.

My goal has been to improve the quality of her life by enabling her to use her limited energies to do the things she most enjoys. A major goal has been to prevent pulmonary edema and keep her out of the hospital. She needed social work as well as nursing services. She refused a home health aide.

During the first home visit, I noticed that Bertha could hardly see, although she tried hard to cover this up. In fact, Bertha is legally blind. There is so much potential for her to make a medication error by picking up the wrong bottle, and I assume this has happened. I prepared her many medications for several days ahead and later brought her a container with q.i.d. compartments for 1 week. Her niece offered to visit weekly and prepare her medications when I must discharge her from home care services. I taught the niece how to prefill Bertha's syringes and prepour her other medications.

We went to her cupboards. Bertha explained that she is on a low-salt diet and never adds salt to anything. She really thought she had been adhering to a low-salt diet until I read her the salt content of the prepared soups and other foods in her cupboard and freezer! She was horrified. "Let's get these out of here! I'll just give these to my niece!" she exclaimed, as she filled a couple of large brown bags. Bertha insisted on making me a cup of tea. We sat down together and I taught her the early, subtle signs of impending congestive heart failure to report early to her doctor. She agreed that having Meals On Wheels visit would be a good thing when I explained that the meals would be low in sodium. She wasn't sure that she could afford them, but we were able to get her a reduced rate from Meals On Wheels, and her church also helped with the cost. My other purpose in securing Meals On Wheels was to spare her the exertion of shopping and carrying grocery bags up four flights of stairs.

Bertha was less willing to accept the twice-monthly housecleaning services available through a special community fund sponsored by one of the service clubs. "It ain't welfare, is it?" she demanded proudly. When I assured her that it was not, and that it would help spare her heart and keep her out of the hospital, she agreed to it.

Bertha has learned so quickly and so well that I am nearly ready to discharge her. In fact, her insurance benefits have already run out and we are using United Way funds to pay for her care. I'm working on finding a better place for her to live with the help of the agency social worker. The four flights of stairs are just too much for Bertha. The building is cockroach-ridden and the stairs do not look safe. During my last visit, the air was so heavy with insect repellent that even I couldn't breathe, and Bertha and I had to leave the building. That day she said to me, "I just praise the good Lord that He sent you to teach me how to take care of myself."

Diane
VISITING NURSE

CLINICAL APPLICATION

A Critical Thinking Case Study About Caring for a Noncompliant Client

One of the first cases assigned to you after orientation to your hospital's home care agency involves a man named Mr. Edwards. He is staying with his sister, a divorcée, because his house burned down when he was smoking in bed. Your orders indicate three approved visits to teach him to change the sterile burn dressings on his thighs, groin, and chest.

Mr. Edwards greets you at the door dressed in dirty sweat pants and a tee shirt. You notice several brown stains on the tee shirt and the dressing is dislodged. You ask what happened. "Oh, I guess I knocked it against something when I was heating some soup for my lunch," he says. In changing the other dressings, you note that they all seem contaminated. "The tape was pulling or something, so I moved them a little," he admits. "They're so damn uncomfortable!"

 and Think!

- Is there a problem?
- How should you proceed to deal with it?

While changing all the dressings and cleaning the burns, you stress the importance of cleanliness and aseptic technique to prevent infection. Mr. Edwards seems uninterested and complains about the discomfort. You decide it might be better to teach his sister. Mr. Edwards agrees and insists he will inform her. She works part-time, so you schedule a time for your next visit when the sister is at home.

The next day you arrive at the prearranged time only to discover that the sister is not present. "Oh, I forgot to tell her," says Mr. Edwards. He is dressed in the same dirty clothing, with dried blood on his shirt, and he is unshaven. Again, some of the dressings are dislodged, even though you applied them very securely. Using gloves you change the dressings, double bag the soiled dressings for disposal, and bag the blood-stained shirt for soaking in chlorine bleach solution.

 and Think!

- What will you say?
- What will you do?
- What do you think is going on?
- What can you do about it?
- What are the risks?

You strongly remind Mr. Edwards about the importance of cleanliness to avoid infection and leave a note for the sister to call you about the next day's visit. You ask that he wash and be in clean clothes when you arrive. You call the doctor to discuss Mr. Edwards' poor hygiene, dislodged dressings, and need for pain medication before the dressing changes. The physician decides to order daily showers and says he will call Mr. Edwards to reinforce the need for cleanliness and will tell him to take ibuprofen about 30 minutes before the dressing change.

The sister does not call you back, so you call her and discuss her need to learn the dressing technique and to supply her brother with clean clothing daily after his shower. Before setting up an appointment for the next day, you ask the sister if he seems more depressed than usual.

"He's disgusted with himself, and I guess I'm disgusted with him too. He tried for years to quit smoking and was never able to do it. Now he's lost his house because of it and had to move in with me. But he doesn't care what happens to him because of. . . his situation."

You encourage the sister to express her feelings about having him move in with her.

 and Think!

- What can you suggest?
- Is there any help available for Mr. Edwards?
- What if he refuses help for his depression?
- Can he be forced?

You meet the sister the next day and teach her how to change the dressings. You teach Mr. Edwards about showering, and he says the physician already talked to him. You suggest the sister lay out clean clothing and dressing supplies just before Mr. Edwards enters the shower. You urge her to stay nearby the first few days to make sure Mr. Edwards is steady on his feet. He seems embarrassed to have her change his dressings. You feel confident that she can handle the procedure, and she does a return demonstration with good technique. However, you think that Mr. Edwards can and should do his own dressings, and you inform him that on your third and last visit the next day, you expect to watch him do so.

You bring up your observation that Mr. Edwards seems depressed, and you describe the help available to him with medications and psychotherapy. You are not surprised that he adamantly refuses to secure help for his depression. You mention that he might consider doing so for his family, if not for himself, and leave information about the community mental health center and three private psychiatrists.

 and Think!

- Under what conditions can Mr. Edwards be forced to seek help for his depression?
- How else can you help the sister?

You talk with the sister and explain that Mr. Edwards cannot legally be forced to go for help against his will unless he becomes suicidal. If he threatens suicide or makes an attempt, he meets the criteria for treatment against his will—he is a threat to himself. Counseling for the sister would be good primary prevention if she continues to feel so resentful and frustrated about having him live with her, and you provide information for her regarding counseling and a caretakers' support group.

Chapter SUMMARY

The U.S. home care system is growing at a rapid rate, but informal, unpaid caregivers, usually family members, continue to provide the bulk of home care, supplemented by services from home care agencies. There are various types of home care agencies. Quality is evaluated by state licensure, Medicare certification, and voluntary accreditation.

Reimbursement payments for service mainly come from Medicare, which is administered by the federal government. Medicare service is for those over age 65, those with kidney failure, and the disabled. Criteria for care include the need for skilled nursing or physical, occupational, or speech therapy of a restorative, intermittent nature to a homebound client. A physician must sign the plan of care and the agency must participate in Medicare. Medicare conditions of participation are being revised, with emphasis on outcomes rather than process. A major overhaul of Medicare regulations will result in lower reimbursements to agencies.

Medicaid, the second-largest reimburser for home care services, is designed for the medically indigent of all ages. Medicaid, unlike Medicare, covers chronic situations needing custodial care. Free and subsidized care, private payments and special grants, and no-fault and worker's compensation insurance are other types of reimbursement.

Referrals come to a home care agency from various sources. Hospitals and physicians are the largest source of referrals. Self-referral and family referral and community agencies and organizations are other sources. Continuity of care programs prevent complications and regression as clients move from one level of care to another. Characteristics of good hospital discharge plans include early client identification; good use of the nursing process, especially assessment; client and family participation in planning; selection of the best environment for the client; use of community resources as needed; complete physician's orders and an accurate plan of care; all necessary supplies, equipment, instructions, and medications provided at discharge; and good follow-up communication.

Care coordination occurs at three levels: discharge planner, primary home care nurse, and managed-care case manager. The responsibilities and interactions of each are described.

A list of references and additional readings for this chapter appears at the end of Part 4.

14

The Role of the Home Care Nurse

Key Terms

access code
chart audits
care maps
clinical paths
conceptual models
critical pathways
G-tube
integrated information system
litigation
medication clocks

needlefree injections
Omnibus Reconciliation Act of 1990
Patient Bill of Rights
recertification
self-determination
PEG tube
P.E.S. system
personal protective equipment
point-of-care documentation
variance

Learning Objectives

1. Differentiate between hospital and home care nursing practice.

2. Compare the roles of the associate degree, baccalaureate, certified, and advanced practice nurse in home care.

3. Describe how to do a home visit.

4. Explain how to develop a therapeutic relationship.

5. Identify the role of the home health aide.

6. List the equipment commonly used in home care.

7. Describe the nursing responsibilities related to medication management.

8. Explore the value of each step of the nursing process in home care nursing practice.

9. Identify common client problems seen in home care.

10. Describe the important components of infection control in the home.

11. Explain learning barriers for clients and caregivers.

12. Identify legal documentation guidelines in home care nursing.

13. Describe the value of clinical paths.

14. Explain the purpose of a variance.

15. Contrast the terms "point-of-care documentation" and "integrated information system."

How Hospital and Home Care Nursing Differ

As any nurse who has transferred from hospital to home care nursing will say, the role of the nurse in home care is very different from that of the nurse in the hospital. In the hospital, there is a sense that the *nurse owns the environment*. In the home, *the client or family owns the environment*; the nurse is a *guest* in the home. In home care, there is dynamic family involvement in a way that seldom occurs in the hospital. In home care, the nurse's assessment is much more holistic than in the hospital and includes not only the client and the family, but the total environment, including economic and social issues affecting the client. Although home care focuses on the assigned client, in reality the whole family is usually the client.

As mentioned in the previous chapter, the home care primary nurse prepares and coordinates a multidisciplinary plan of care. This means that the home care nurse must have well-developed skills in *clear, complete, concise communication*. Some knowledge of group process is required. The ability to solve problems is essential. In the hospital, the physician and the client are in daily direct contact. In home care, the nurse is the intermediary; the physician depends on the nurse's assessment skills, judgment, and efficiency in timely, concise communication. Teaching clients the best way to communicate with their physicians is a basic intervention for all home care nurses.

If the case is a complex one, there is apt to be a case manager. Collaborating with the case manager about the number and frequency of home visits to achieve the desired client outcomes is essential in the delivery of good care. It is the case manager's job to prevent waste and to minimize the number of visits and services. It is the primary home care nurse's job to determine what care is needed if there is a variance and to inform the case manager. The home care nurse is an advocate for the client.

Nurses must know the criteria of third-party payers and the benefits they will cover. In hospital nursing, all this is done by the billing office. Home care supervisors must know the payment criteria in great detail, but primary care nurses must also develop considerable knowledge so they can be aware of the strengths and weaknesses of clients' third-party coverage. Very few families can afford to pay medical and nursing costs out of pocket, nor can they afford to be faced later with large bills for services they thought would be paid by third-party payers.

Within these economic constraints, the home care nurse operates with a great deal of autonomy, much more so than in hospital nursing. Time management is extremely important. The nurse decides which clients need to be seen, at what time, and for how long each day. The nurse plans an efficient travel route to avoid backtracking. There are professional demands on a nurse's time, such as multidisciplinary case conferences, agency meetings, and staff in-service training sessions. Nurses must make numerous telephone calls before and after each home visit and must fill out extensive paperwork for clients' records and reports. The nurse leaves his or her daily schedule in the office before leaving in the morning and notifies the supervisor if any changes occur so that he or she can be reached if emergencies arise. Emergencies often require an unplanned nursing visit or numerous telephone calls. Such events disrupt the original plan for the day and often require reorganization.

The home care nurse *works alone*. Of course, a home care supervisor is available by telephone, but this is not the same as being surrounded and supported by colleagues, as in the hospital nursing. A home care nurse's assessment and teaching skills must be excellent, because no other nurse is present to assist. Assessment and teaching are high priorities and consume a large proportion of the visits. A primary home care nurse must have an excellent knowledge base (Fig. 14-1) because clients' conditions, diagnoses, and ages vary so much. Although most home care clients are elderly, all ages are included in case loads.

The home care nurse must be *creative and adaptive*. Sometimes needed supplies and equipment are not available in the home, so safe improvisation is required. If the client is poor, the nurse should know how to teach a special diet using low-cost foods. The nurse should also know about the preferred foods of clients of other cultures. Many home care nurses practice in the homes of people of varied cultures and religions; the nurse must incorporate awareness and sensitivity of these differences into the plan of care. Creativity is necessary for good client and family teaching. For instance, in the hospital, where food is served on trays, it is easy to assess the client's food intake. This isn't so easy to do in a client's home. The client may tell the nurse that he or she adheres to a low-salt diet, meaning that no salt is added at the table, but if the nurse is creative and sensitive enough to review food cupboards and the refrigerator (diplomatically), it is not unusual to find them full of high-sodium canned, frozen, and processed foods. (See "The Nurse Speaks" in Chapter 13.)

The home care nurse, unlike the hospital nurse, must be very *knowledgeable about community resources*. The nurse who is not, does clients a disservice. Use of certain resources can bring tremendous improvement to a client's quality of life. Most home care nurses develop a resource file and share the information with colleagues as well as clients and families. It is sometimes difficult to determine reliable resources within a client's family; doing so may require excellent communication skills.

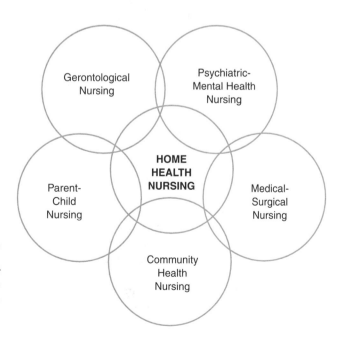

FIGURE 14-1

A conceptual model of home health nursing. (Reprinted with permission from *A Statement on the Scope of Home Health Nursing Practice*, © 1992, American Nurses Association, Washington DC.)

The advocacy role is important in home care. The nurse may discover that a client is living in substandard housing or is being exploited in various ways. The home care nurse must be familiar with resources to effect change in such situations. The nurse must address any unsafe situations in the home, such as clutter or scatter rugs. Some situations may exist in the home that are undesirable from the nurse's perspective; however, if they do not present a safety threat to the client, the nurse must accept those conditions without verbal or nonverbal negative communication. Hospital nurses do not have to work in unsavory environments; home care nurses sometimes do.

Performing Skilled Nursing Care

Some people think of skilled nursing as "hands-on" or "high-tech" nursing care, but skilled nursing is broader than that and includes assessment, teaching, and evaluation skills (see Display 13-4). Medicare will not reimburse for skilled nursing if the client's condition is stable, so home care nurses should strike the word "stable" from their vocabulary if reimbursement is to occur. It takes skill to assess an acute, changing status, whether it is upward or downward. Medicare does not reimburse for preventive care, nor for general health maintenance, nor for nursing visits made to meet the client's and the family's socioeconomic or emotional needs, even though nurses recognize that those visits may require greater skill. Only if the client requires a "skilled service" (nursing, physical therapy, or speech therapy) is the plan of care reimbursable by Medicare. Then social work or home health aide services are also covered if deemed "reasonable and necessary" and if the physician orders them and signs the proper form.

Comparing the Role of the Associate Degree, Baccalaureate, Certified, and Advanced Practice Nurse in Home Care

Most home care agencies require that registered nurses have at least 1 year of hospital experience. That is changing in many places, though; some agencies are hiring nurses right after licensure or with other types of nursing experience. Obviously, the large amount of knowledge and diverse skills of home care nursing require as much advanced education and experience as possible. The more education or other qualifications (eg, job experience or certifications) a nurse has, the better, as the nursing employment market becomes more competitive. In general, a registered nurse with a baccalaureate degree is considered best prepared for the entry-level home care generalist's role. Until very recently, community health nursing courses were not included in any curriculum for associate degree nursing, whereas community health nursing has always been part of baccalaureate programs.

Home care nurses differ a great deal in the personal qualifications they bring to the role. Many associate degree and diploma school graduate nurses work in home care and perform very competently. They would probably be the first to agree about the value of additional education and training to meet the high demands of the role.

In 1993, the first certification examinations from the American Nurses Association were the beginning of national certification in home care nursing. Home care certification is available at two levels: generalist and specialist. Generalists provide care for clients and must have a baccalaureate degree. Specialists manage home care delivery and have graduate degrees. They work in quality management and staff education programs as well as clinical coordination. Large agencies also hire certified nurses such as diabetic education, enterostomal, and psychiatric nurse clinical specialists to serve as consultants to the rest of the staff.

How to Do a Home Visit

A home visit requires more than just the time spent in the home: preparation in the office, travel, the actual visit, and follow-up are required. It is no wonder that each visit is so time-consuming that home care nurses can average only five or six visits a day.

Preparation time includes ascertaining the purpose of the visit. A nurse cannot plan his or her day without knowing how much time a visit will take or if there is a reason to schedule the visit at a particular time of day. For example, if the purpose of the visit is to supervise a home health aide, the visit must be made when the home health aide is present. If the purpose is to teach a procedure that must be done at a specific time, the visit must be scheduled accordingly. The nurse must become familiar with the client's chart or referral form to understand the purpose of the visit.

Making a telephone call to the client to verify the time of the visit and to obtain directions saves a great deal of time. So does a brief inquiry about how the client is feeling and if there have been any significant changes. This prevents surprises when the nurse arrives and allows him or her to make necessary changes in the plan in advance.

Occasionally, additional information is required before visiting. A conference with the supervisor or nurse specialist or even a quick reading about an unfamiliar condition may be part of the preparatory work.

The last thing to be done is to gather the nursing bag and other needed equipment to take along. A daily route schedule is always left for the supervisor so the nurse can be reached during the day.

As a guest in the client's home, the nurse usually enters briefly into small talk after introductions. It is important to ascertain who is the primary caregiver and to assess family dynamics. Some knowledge of family theory is important. Do not talk to the caregiver as if the client were not present, even when the client is very frail. It may be necessary to talk to one or both of them separately at some point during the visit. Staying focused regarding the purpose of the visit is essential despite the many variables that capture the nurse's attention. Do not ignore these variables, but prioritize them so that you can make notes in the car or in the office about them. Assessment, teaching, and some direct care will no doubt be part of your visit. Inform the client about the next visit. Of course, good handwashing at the start and at the end of the visit is basic.

Follow-up care may require some revision to the plan of care. The primary nurse or supervisor should be informed. If a first visit was done, the plan of care needs to be developed; extensive documentation needs to be done and appropriate contacts need

DISPLAY 14-1
Nursing Bag Contents

- Soap, paper towels, hand wipes
- Stethoscope, sphygmomanometer
- Thermometers, oral and rectal
- Airway and resuscitation mask
- Adrenaline (some agencies)
- Sterile and nonsterile gloves
- Scissors, forceps, penlight
- Syringes, needles, alcohol wipes
- Plastic apron, disposable gowns
- OSHA masks, protective eyewear
- Disinfectant, cotton balls
- Tape measure, tongue depressors
- Assorted gauze and nonallergenic tape
- Agency forms, business cards, maps

to be made. Referrals to other community agencies are often needed, as well as reports to the physician and case manager.

Nursing bags are still used in many agencies and should be checked and replenished at the end of the day (Display 14-1). Never put items removed in a client's home back inside the bag, and always set the bag on a paper towel.

In high-crime areas, nurses may not carry the easily recognizable nursing bags because of the risk of robbery; they may substitute a cloth or paper shopping bag for necessary supplies and equipment (Display 14-2). Uniforms are not worn, and home care nurses in these areas seldom carry purses (clothing with pockets is invaluable). Equipment and supplies are kept locked in the car trunk out of sight. In some areas, agencies hire escorts to accompany nurses.

Relating to the Client and the Family

Of all the important things that must be accomplished during a home care visit, the most important is establishing a good relationship, especially on the initial visit. Much depends on that relationship. A helping, supporting relationship must be established with both the caregiver and the client. The caregiver is often on duty 24 hours a day, 7 days a week, and will not appreciate a condescending nurse who whizzes in and out of the home talking about what should be done better! The goal should be a relationship of trust. Trust is built with empathy. Empathy is best communicated by reflecting, with acute observation and sensitivity, what the nurse senses the client and caregiver are feeling.

An attitude of trust is built on consistency and confidentiality as well as empathy (Wendt, 1996). Trust-building begins with the first contact. Testing behaviors by the client or caregiver are common. Guarding the client's privacy is crucial, as is demonstrating reliability. If the nurse perseveres in building the relationship and demonstrates trust, a therapeutic nurse–client relationship is likely to occur. Then the nurse can assess the client's coping mechanisms, support systems, and caregiver stress. Such a relationship enhances the learning process tremendously.

DISPLAY 14-2
Safety Precautions in Home Care

1. Know the phone number of the agency, police, and emergency services.
2. Let the agency know your daily schedules and the phone numbers of your patients so that you can be located if you do not return when expected.
3. Know where the patient lives before leaving to make the visit and carry a map for quick referral.
4. Keep your car in good working order and have sufficient gas in the tank.
5. Park near the patient's home and lock your car during the visit.
6. Do not drive an expensive car or wear expensive jewelry when making visits.
7. Know the routes when using public transportation or walking to the patient's house.
8. Carry agency identification and have enough change to make phone calls in case you get lost or have problems. (Some agencies provide cellular phones for their nurses to enable them to contact the agency in case of an emergency or if unexpected situations arise.)
9. When making visits in high-crime areas, visit with another nurse rather than alone.
10. Schedule visits only during daylight hours.
11. Never walk into a patient's home uninvited.
12. If you do not feel safe entering a patient's home, leave the area.
13. Become familiar with the layout of the house, including exits.
14. If a patient or family member is intoxicated, hostile, or obnoxious, reschedule the visit and leave.
15. If a family is having a serious argument or abusing the patient, reschedule the visit and contact your supervisor and report the abuse to the appropriate authorities.

(Smeltzer S, Bare B [1996]. Brunner and Suddarth's Textbook of Medical-Surgical Nursing. *Philadelphia: Lippincott-Raven)*

Experienced home care nurses were asked to describe their feelings about working in the home setting (Stulginsky, 1993b). They reported:

> Building trust and rapport is essential. Caregiving in the home involves common sense, imagination, improvising, and at times "making do." Priorities need to remain fluid, and setting limits encourages self-care in an atmosphere where professional boundaries are rarely secure. The flexibility and autonomy of home health practice enable nurses to be the nurse they were taught to be while practicing on the cutting edge of health care reform (Stulginsky, 1993b).

Home Health Aide Functions and Supervision

Families and clients are often disappointed to learn how little home health aide time is covered by third-party payers. They read the *Medicare Handbook* and assume that because home health aide service is listed, it will be paid for full time. Actually, Medicare generally provides only 3 or 4 hours of home health aide time a few days a week, and then only when the need can be documented. Rarely is there a need for full-time, 7-days-per-week home health aide care.

Home health aides provide personal care and some basic housekeeping. The goal is to provide a healthy and clean environment, with bathing, grooming, and some meal preparation. There are gradations of home health aide services. In general, a home health aide III is assigned in a medically supervised Medicare plan. These home health aides are state-certified and have completed 65 to 100 hours of approved training and passed an examination. Competency must be evaluated yearly, and 12 hours of in-service training must be completed each year. Regulations about home health aide training vary from state to state. Medicaid-financed aides assigned for custodial care are usually grade I or II aides; in these positions, less training is required and more homemaking duties are part of the role.

A form listing specific home health aide duties is prepared by the primary home care nurse, reviewed with the aide, and posted in the client's home, usually on the refrigerator. The nurse also reviews the aide's assigned duties with the client or caregiver to avoid misunderstandings. Common home health aide functions are listed in Display 14-3. At least every 14 days, the nurse documents the evaluation of the aide's functions and performance.

Equipment Commonly Needed in the Home

Clients vary in their mobility status. Homebound status means that it is a taxing effort for the client to leave, and trips outside the home are infrequent or of very short duration.

Medicare clients can and do leave the home for medical treatment. Walkers or wheelchairs may be required. At home, frail clients who are essentially bedbound usually need a hospital bed with side rails. A commode or raised toilet seat is another commonly

---

DISPLAY 14-3
Home Health Aide Functions

- Performing bedbath or shower, as ordered
- Assisting with toileting
- Assisting with oral care, shampoo, shaving
- Dressing and grooming
- Vital signs, including blood pressure in some cases
- Food preparation, cutting and feeding
- Assisting with transfers (bed to chair)
- Assisting with ambulation
- Accompanying clients to medical care
- Reminding clients to take medication
- Doing light housecleaning

- Changing bed linens as needed
- Doing client's laundry
- Shopping when indicated
- Reporting to the nurse: needed supplies, changes in client's condition
- Measuring intake and output, in some cases
- Applying thromboembolytic disease support (TEDs) hose
- Assisting with prescribed exercises, in some cases
- Preparing special modified diets
- Helping clients relearn household skills

DISPLAY 14-4
Equipment and Supplies for Home Care

- Alternating-pressure mattress
- Apnea monitor
- Blood glucose machine
- Cane, crutches, walker
- Commode, bedpan
- Enteral feeding equipment
- Hospital bed with rails
- Hydraulic lift
- Infusion pump
- Intermittent positive pressure breathing (IPPB) machine
- Lamb's wool pad
- Nebulizer
- Oxygen equipment
- Suction machine
- Traction equipment
- Wheelchair

---

needed piece of equipment; the nurse arranges its rental. A list of covered durable medical equipment is found in Display 14-4. Catheters and dressing and injection supplies are frequently needed, as well as the specialized equipment necessary for high-technology nursing care.

Medication Management

A crucial responsibility of the home care nurse is medication management. While caring for elderly clients who take many medications and often live alone, nurses frequently discover medication mistakes. Display 14-5 outlines nursing responsibilities in medication management.

Using the Nursing Process in Home Care

The nursing process is a highly flexible, convenient, and effective method of problem solving that adapts well to the multiple problems that need to be untangled in home care situations. Nursing care plans based on the nursing process focus on client outcomes. As mentioned previously, managed care and case management are outcome-driven. The nursing process adapts very well to various systems of documentation and aids in the development of Medicare's plan of care or clinical paths. Because the nursing process is a deliberate and systematic approach to client care, it helps to organize care that is specifically related to the client's needs. The steps of the nursing process are as follows.

Assessment

Data are collected from various sources. Referral forms from discharge planners or physicians and the client's previous charts supply valuable information. In most cases, the client is the primary, most important source. Interviews, observations, and a systematic physical examination provide the most valuable data. Demographic information such

---

DISPLAY 14-5
Medication Management Responsibilities of the Home Care Nurse

- Ask that *all* medications be gathered for review, including over-the-counter medications.
- Include the caregiver in all evaluation and teaching sessions, best done in short sessions.
- Have the client identify the medication in each container and tell why it is being given.
- Ask the client to describe dosage, frequency, duration, and side effects of each medication.
- Instruct the client to keep all medications in original containers.
- Examine containers for expiration date and changes in color or consistency of medication.
- Ask client to describe any unusual, untoward effects to any therapy, or any allergy.
- Identify physiologic dysfunction: swallowing, eating, diarrhea, or malabsorption syndromes.
- Ask about use of home remedies, herbs, or traditional medicine practices of the client's culture.
- Evaluate visual and mental acuity and capacity for safe self-administration.
- Verify with physician any discrepancies between orders and medications being taken.
- Check for unfilled prescriptions; determine the reasons and intervene if possible.
- Teach and use adaptive devices to facilitate self-medication management:
  Visual aids: charts, flashcards, medication clocks, pictograms
  Prepour pill boxes with daily q.i.d. containers
  Color-coded containers for liquids
  Magnified insulin syringes, or prefilled syringes stored in refrigerator
  Needlefree injection system
  Automated medication dispenser

(Surrency G [1997]. Medication management in the home. In Zang S, Bailey N, eds. Home Care Manual, Making the Transition. *Philadelphia: Lippincott-Raven.)*

---

as age, ethnic and marital status, children's ages, locations, and occupations, education, occupation, primary caregivers, support systems, and health insurance data are gathered. Clients' perceptions of their health and current problems, psychosocial situations, and current lifestyle patterns must be included in detail. Clients' chief complaints are best stated in their own words. Onset and symptoms are elicited in detail. A thorough assessment of current medications and treatments and the client's knowledge about them is vital. Data on past histories and family histories are important.

Often it is best to have a caregiver or family member present during the interview. Sometimes it is good to follow up later with the client in private if the nurse suspects that the client cannot be candid with someone present. Observation of nonverbal communication and interactions is important. A thorough and systematic physical assessment is performed, and notations are made. Vital signs are always monitored. Patterns of data are noted. The information is organized, and analysis of the data begins in the nurse's mind.

Diagnosis

Diagnosis involves a critical appraisal and analysis of the gathered data to identify the problems, needs, strengths, and weaknesses in a client's situation. Common client problems addressed by nurses have been catalogued and defined by the North American Nursing Diagnosis Association (NANDA). If the PES system is used to describe the client's problem, one of these problem statements usually forms the stem of a nursing diagnosis. The "P" represents the client problem statement, a NANDA-defined problem statement. The "E" represents the etiology or factors related to the problem. The "S" represents the significant symptoms that confirm or validate the problem statement. One defined problem statement is used per need. There may be more than one etiology and symptom. For example, a common nursing diagnosis fully written is as follows:

P: Constipation
E: Related to inadequate fluid intake (E) and lack of roughage in the diet (E)
S: Client has not had a bowel movement for 5 days (S). States she dislikes fluids and seldom drinks (S). Eats mainly pasta (S).

Planning

Planning is based on desired client outcomes. It is not based on what the nurse will do, but on what is expected to happen to the client, and what is desired, as a result of nursing actions. Plans address the problem statement (nursing diagnosis). Together with the client, needs are prioritized during planning, and long- and short-term goals are identified. A specific, realistic time is estimated for the client outcome to be achieved. The Nursing Outcome Classification (NOC) is a standardized list of nursing-sensitive, measurable client outcomes (Johnson & Maas, 1997).

Interventions

Interventions are all the actions that address the causes or factors related or contributing to the problem; the goal is to achieve the expected outcomes for the client. When a nursing care plan is written, the interventions serve as nursing orders for all nurses caring for that client. The interventions are specific and individualized for each client. Assessments that must be done on each visit are listed in detail. All the care that the nurse is to do is specified. Whatever teaching is needed is listed as scheduled. The standardized Nursing Interventions Classification (NIC) system includes 433 specific interventions with numerical codes (McCloskey & Buleckek, 1996).

Evaluations

Expected outcomes are evaluated on the estimated dates set in the planning step. When expected outcomes are not met, or only partially met, the plan must be carefully evaluated to determine the reason and then modified accordingly until the goals are met. In some agencies, the plan of care follows this format. Most agencies follow a modified format. Some agencies use standardized care plans, some use clinical paths, and some use a computerized system of documentation. Some agencies use Medicare forms for the plan of care and the progress or recertification plan.

Whatever form the written care plan takes, the nursing process is a mental framework that should take place in the nurse's mind. The steps of the process do not necessarily occur separately and in exact order, but they do provide a systematic, workable way to attack a problem. The "Standards of Home Health Nursing Practice" of the American Nurses Association are based on the nursing process.

Common Client Problems in Home Care

Diabetes and heart failure are now the most common problems referred for home care. The seven top principal diagnoses of home care clients are shown in Figure 14-2. Most people on home care are elderly and have more than one chronic disease. These people have high-acuity needs: about 80% need help with activities of daily living, and almost 90% have restricted activity or are on bedrest. Many home care clients are taking multiple drugs, sometimes prescribed by different physicians and dispensed by different pharmacies under either generic or brand names. Nurses often discover clients taking double doses of the same medication for this reason.

There are diverse needs for home care. Increasingly, AIDS clients are referred for home care, whether they are young or elderly. The encouraging reports of the effect

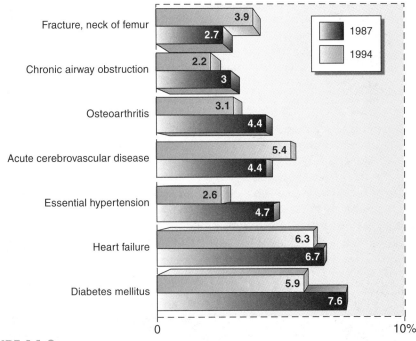

FIGURE 14-2
Medicare home health statistics: percentage of home health patients with top seven principal diagnoses. (Source: Health Care Financing Administration, Bureau of Data Management and Strategy: Data from the Medicare Decision Support System; data development by the Office of Research and Demonstrations. Reported in *Health Care Financing Review*, 1996 Statistical Supplement.)

of combination therapies in controlling AIDS may help stem the increase in the number of AIDS clients on home care. Large numbers of mothers and newborns were referred for home care as a result of the ''drive-by deliveries'' instituted by some managed-care companies. With federal legislation requiring at least 48 hours in the hospital for new mothers, the number of these postpartum visits has dropped. Some home care referrals relate to abuse of children, the elderly, or the disabled. Nurses' records are subpoenaed if cases go to trial; in some instances, nurses are subpoenaed to testify. Hospice clients most often have cancer as their primary diagnosis.

Because people are being discharged earlier from the hospital, more and more clients are receiving complex therapies at home. High-technology and specialized home care nursing is covered in the next chapter.

Infection Control in the Home

There are two aspects of infection control in home care. One is to protect the nurse, family, and community from a client who has an infectious disease; the other is to protect immunodeficient clients from infections from others. Generally, clients have more resistance to the microorganisms in their own homes. However, homes vary in sanitary conditions and in facilities to maintain good hygiene and preventive measures. Families vary in their knowledge of asepsis and hygiene practices and may inadvertently place a client at risk for infection. Clients are increasingly being discharged from the hospital with nosocomial infections of wounds, the urinary tract, or the respiratory system. Clients are referred to home care with communicable diseases such as AIDS, hepatitis, and tuberculosis as their primary problem. Measures must be taken to control the spread of infection in the home.

Standard Precautions and Occupational Safety Health Administration (OSHA) Requirements

The new term ''Standard Precautions'' has been recently adopted by the Centers for Disease Control and Prevention to replace the terms ''Universal Precautions'' and ''body substance isolation'' because of the confusion surrounding those terms (Borton, 1997). Standard precautions are based on the wise assumption than anyone can be infectious, and personal protective equipment (PPE) must be used at all times when handling blood and body fluids. A supply of gloves and other PPE should be kept in the client's home where exposure to blood and body fluids is expected. The home care agency is responsible for supplying necessary PPE to employees and cleaning, repairing, replacing, or disposing of damaged PPE, according to OSHA regulations. Every home care agency must have written procedures for infection control, called the exposure control plan, with specific compliance with OSHA standards.

Handwashing

Washing hands thoroughly with soap and running water for 10 to 15 seconds is the best method of infection control. Hands should be washed at the beginning and end of the visit. Hands also should be washed both before and after applying gloves. Families must be taught this, because many lay people think gloves avoid the need for handwashing. In homes where sinks are nonexistent or so filthy, infested, or full of dirty dishes that access is impossible, nurses use antiseptic hand wipes that they carry with them, along with soap and paper towels. They wash their hands under running water as soon as possible after leaving the home. They do not take their nursing bags inside homes with filthy conditions. A paper towel is used to turn off the water after handwashing in a client's home.

Caring for Contaminated Materials and Equipment

Wearing gloves and other needed PPE, the nurse should flush liquid waste materials down the toilet, never pour them into a sink. If the latter happens inadvertently, the sink should be thoroughly cleansed using a solution of 1 part bleach and 10 parts water. Soaked dressings, catheters, intravenous equipment, saturated menstrual pads, or suction equipment that is semiliquid should be double-bagged to prevent leakage. All other materials containing moist or dried body wastes should be well bagged and disposed of immediately. Biohazard labels should be used. It is said that the hepatitis B virus can survive dry on surfaces for at least a week at room temperature, so avoid contact with dried blood on linens and clothing. HIV seems to be inactivated as soon as it dries.

Disinfection measures in the home vary. The following are frequently found in the home: bleach, 1:10 dilution in water; alcohol, 70% solution; white vinegar, 1:3 in water; and Lysol or Pine-Sol, per directions on the bottle. A 1:10 solution of chlorine bleach is recommended for HIV. Before submerging items in disinfecting solutions to soak them, make certain that all organic matter has been cleansed and removed with soap and water. Generally, items are soaked for 10 minutes for disinfection.

Other methods of disinfection in the home include baking for 1 hour in a flat pan at 350°. Boiling for 15 to 20 minutes is a common method used in the home. The pan should be covered. However, boiling melts some plastics, causes rubber to deteriorate, and promotes rust on some metals. Microwaving hard plastic items such as syringes or self-catheters in a Zip-Lok bag with moisture (a wet paper towel) on a high setting for 10 to 15 minutes is recommended (Doughty, 1991). Some people like to use a pressure cooker at 15 pounds pressure for 10 minutes. These methods render equipment adequately disinfected for use for most procedures in the home. Of course, it is best to use sterile, disposable supplies and equipment in home care, but that is not always possible. If supplies and equipment are not covered by the client's health plan, the client may not be able to afford to use something once and discard it. He or she may reuse it unsterile unless taught these methods. "Clean technique" (not sterile) may be appropriate for intermittent self-catheterization at home.

Care of Used Needles and Sharps

Containers must be waterproof, puncture-proof, and opaque, and must have a secure lid and be labeled, according to OSHA regulations. Most containers are red. They are often supplied by the agency for use in the home. Nurses often carry a container in the trunk of their cars if they have to give an unexpected injection in a home that has no container. Used needles should never be recapped. Syringes should never be carried by themselves unless they are self-sheathing or needleless systems. Containers should be discarded when they are 75% full and should be taped shut. Nurses usually return them to the agency for disposal. Sometimes coffee cans with a lid are used in the home.

Precautions for Immunosuppressed Clients

Immunodeficient clients should be taught the symptoms of early infection that they should report. Display 14-6 lists the symptoms that HIV clients should promptly report. Measures that should be taught to prevent infection include household cleanliness and good, regular personal hygiene and handwashing. Avoidance of crowds and persons with infections needs to be emphasized, and proper food preparation needs to be taught. Display 14-7 contains infection control guidelines for care of AIDS clients at home.

Teaching in Home Care Nursing

Health teaching, which is basic to the role of the home care nurse, is never more important than in regard to controlling the spread of infection. The nurse must demonstrate and consistently model what is taught. A teaching plan should be developed so that no aspect is inadvertently overlooked. Appropriate and creative teaching methods

---

DISPLAY 14-6
Teaching HIV-Positive Clients Symptoms That Require Immediate Medical Evaluation

Instruct the client to seek prompt medical attention for any of the following symptoms:

- New cough with or without sputum production
- Shortness of breath or dyspnea on exertion
- Increased fatigue or malaise
- Fever
- Night sweats
- Headache
- Stiff neck
- Visual changes such as floaters, blurred vision, loss of visual field(s), and sensitivity to light
- Changes in mental status, such as loss of consciousness, loss of memory, forgetfulness, mood swings, and depression
- Development of skin lesions
- Pain
- New or increased diarrhea with or without abdominal cramping
- Sudden, unintended weight loss
- Increased size of or painful lymph node(s)

(Monahan F, Drake T, Neighbors M [1994]. Nursing Care of the Adult. Philadelphia: WB Saunders.)

DISPLAY 14-7
Infection Control Guidelines for Care of AIDS Clients at Home

- Wash hands thoroughly with soap and water before and after giving direct care and preparing foods, and in between preparing different food items.
- Wear latex gloves when handling blood or body fluids. Rubber gloves made for household cleaning should also be used when cleaning up body fluid spills. These can be disinfected and reused.
- Cover any cuts or broken skin that may come into contact with blood or body fluids with Band-Aids.
- When using needles, be very careful to avoid needle sticks. Place used needles in a puncture-proof container such as a coffee can immediately after use. Never recap, bend, or break a needle. A puncture-proof container should be returned to the agency in which needles are used and discarded.
- Wash dishes used by the client in hot soapy water. Clients with HIV infection do not require separate dishes or eating utensils.
- Use usual cleansers for normal household cleaning. Clean the bathroom regularly using a household disinfectant. Clean up blood spills with a diluted bleach solution (1 part bleach mixed with 10 parts water); wear gloves for this task. A new bleach solution should be made every 24 hours because old solutions are less effective.
- Allow the client to prepare food for others provided that he or she does not have any open lesions on the hands or arms and does not have diarrhea.
- Do not share personal items such as toothbrush or razor with the client.
- Wash clothing and linen in the usual manner with soap or detergent in either hot or cold water. It is not necessary to add bleach to kill a virus unless dried blood is on the cloth (hepatitis B virus).
- Prevent exposure of the neutropenic client to people with active infections.
- Protect patients with HIV infection from pathogens found in foods:
  - Avoid use of raw or undercooked meat, poultry, fish, shellfish, or eggs as well as raw (unpasteurized) milk.
  - Wash utensils before reusing with other foods that are being prepared.
  - Do not mix raw foods or their juices with other foods.
  - Use a plastic rather than a wooden cutting board, because plastic ones are easier to clean.
- Wash fruit and vegetables thoroughly.

(Monahan F, Drake T, Neighbors M [1994]. Nursing Care of the Adult. *Philadelphia: WB Saunders.)*

should be used based on the nurse's assessment of the client, the family, and the environment.

Assessing Readiness to Learn

Assessment of the client's and caregiver's motivation and ability to learn must precede formulation of a teaching plan. Nurses, who tend to read a great deal, may mistakenly think that clients can simply read an instruction sheet and learn its contents. This is anything but true. Clients and caregivers are usually elderly, and some have difficulty seeing to read. Some were immigrants and never learned to read English. Also, illiteracy or semiliteracy is a bigger problem than most people realize: one of five Americans reads below the fifth-grade level and is classified as functionally illiterate (Humphrey & Milone-Nuzzo, 1996). Most published health teaching material is written on the eighth-grade level or above. This does not mean that all written material is useless, but it does mean that nurses cannot rely on the written word to teach for them. No piece of health literature should ever be handed to clients or caregivers without the nurse reviewing it with them in detail and highlighting the most important points.

Preparing Supplemental Literature

Most health literature should be modified and simplified, with only one or two major points presented at a time (Display 14-8). Present practical information. Be precise and concise. Use plain language and remove polysyllabic words and technical terminology. Emphasize headings and groupings with good spacing. Use lists rather than narratives.

The advantage of written material is that clients and caregivers can refer to it to refresh their memories when the nurse is no longer present. It is also a useful tool to reinforce verbal teaching. Use written material only as a supplement to verbal teaching and demonstration. Videotapes, if well prepared, make excellent learning supplements because so many people are accustomed to watching television and learning in that way. Use as many senses as possible to enhance the learning process. People learn in different ways and at different rates. Remember that adult learners are pragmatically motivated and are rarely interested in theoretical information.

Learning Objectives

Whether or not the nurse writes out a formal teaching plan, he or she must clearly know the learning objectives. These are based on the assessment data and the analysis and identification of the problem, which is usually some form of knowledge deficit. The client and the caregiver should know the learning objectives also. The content of material to be taught to meet those objectives should be written in the client's chart. For information about the three domains of learning and more about health teaching, review Chapter 5.

Teaching Methods

In teaching, timing is everything. If the client is in pain, the dog is barking, the telephone is ringing, the baby is crying, or the caregiver is anxious, those things must be addressed before teaching and learning can begin in the home. Inform the family in advance that health teaching is a major purpose of the visit so they can prepare the environment as much as possible. Multiple distractions are major barriers to learning, so the nurse may have to decide either to try to modify the environment or to postpone the teaching. Elderly clients need time to absorb and process new information, so do not rush the teaching. Do not teach too much at a time; the average span of attention is about 20 minutes. Allow time for questions and feedback to evaluate what aspects of the teaching

DISPLAY 14-8
A Quick Guide to Good Instructions

Define your readers and assess their background and understanding of the topic.

SIMPLIFY YOUR WRITING

Use short sentences.
Use easy-to-understand words.
Define all medical terms and abbreviations.

INTRODUCE INSTRUCTIONS BY ANSWERING WHO, WHAT, WHERE, WHEN, AND WHY

Who should perform the procedure?
Who can be called for assistance?
What will the reader be doing?
What materials are needed?
Where can these materials be purchased?
When should the procedure be done?
Why should the procedure be done?

INCLUDE WARNINGS OR CAUTIONARY STATEMENTS

Place them in the introduction.
Restate them in the main text immediately before the numbered step to which they pertain.
Highlight them so they are noticeable.

MAKE THE MAIN TEXT READER-FRIENDLY AND CLEAR

Use the imperative.
Organize the text into numbered steps.
Place pictures or diagrams next to the step that describes them.
Use large type and plenty of white space.

CONCLUDE WITH ANSWERS TO "WHAT IF . . ." SITUATIONS

Explain what results the reader should expect.
Provide troubleshooting advice.
Explain when and where to ask for outside help.

(Agee B [1996]. How to write clear instructions. Published in RN 59 [11]: 26—28. Copyright 1996, Medical Economics, Montvale, NJ. Reprinted by permission.)

have been learned and what information needs to be repeated. Offer frequent, sincere encouragement. Do not talk down to learners. The fact that someone is illiterate does not mean that the person is unintelligent. If a major mistake is made in some procedure, say, "Let me show you a better way to do it," not "That's wrong. Try again." Try to relate new learning to something already mastered—for instance, "Preparing this solution is not much different than what you've been doing all your life in the kitchen. Just follow the recipe!''

Teach the smallest amount necessary at a time, and then seek feedback by asking the learner to describe, explain, list, or do whenever possible. Try to make each point as dynamically as possible with pauses, inflections, illustrations, or examples. Perform frequent demonstrations and repeat them as necessary. Summarize every so often. Repeat, review, reinforce, and summarize.

Evaluation of learning is crucial to the process. The teaching may be wonderful, but nothing happens unless learning has taken place. The nurse, the client, and the caregiver all must be sure that learning has been achieved.

Documentation in Home Care Nursing

Different agencies use different documentation formats, but all the formats are comprehensive. The amount of detailed paperwork required in home care is a surprise to many nurses transferring from hospital work. There are several reasons for the amount of paperwork needed. The adage "If it wasn't written, it wasn't done" certainly applies in home care. Legal coverage, third-party reimbursements, Medicare, licensure, and certification all rely on nurses' documentation for chart audits.

Legal Documentation Guidelines

The chart is the place where home care nurses demonstrate whether or not care was given as legally required. Documentation protects the nurse and the agency should litigation occur later, when memory can no longer be relied on. Humphrey and Milone-Nuzzo (1996), in their *Manual of Home Care Nursing Orientation,* list guidelines that can help home care nurses meet practice standards and the legal duty to communicate. The following suggestions are adapted from those guidelines:

1. *Accuracy and completeness*: Unless the record is totally accurate, errors in client care can occur and can be perpetuated by weekend nurses or other caregivers.
2. *Objective, measurable information*: Subjective remarks by health-care providers do not belong in the chart. Subjective remarks by the client or caregiver are appropriate if recorded accurately and in quotes. Vague comments such as, "Appears comfortable" are not measurable and require additional detailed explanation.
3. *Initial and ongoing assessments and interventions should all be documented.* Monitoring for changes in the client's condition, compared with an initial complete assessment, must be demonstrated. Changes in the client's condition must be recorded in detail, including the person notified, date, and time. Notification of essential findings to the physician and anyone else who needs to know is a legal obligation. Some agencies use flow sheets and progress notes that nurses take with them to the home to document data on the spot, lest some detail be forgotten later. All phone calls should be documented.
4. *Include exactly what was taught and the client's or the caregiver's response to teaching.* This documents what the client or caregiver are expected to know,

whether or not learning took place, and whether or not the client or caregiver is assuming responsibility. Instructions to the client to telephone or see the physician must always be included.

5. *Corrections and abbreviations must be clear.* Use standard abbreviations only. Never use White-Out or delete an entry or make any correction that could be misconstrued as a later effort to "doctor" a chart. Draw a line through the mistake, which should still be readable through the line, and initial it. Do not leave blank spaces. If information is to be added out of sequence, mark it "late entry." Do not engage in proxy charting (ie, nurses charting for each other).

6. *Avoid terms such as "maintenance" or "custodial care," as well as "chronic," "stable," or "plateau" to describe a client's condition.* Document the reasons complications might occur or that the client's condition could worsen.

7. *Verify homebound status in the description of the client's condition* and continue to do so at least monthly.

Components of the Home Care Chart and the Initial Visit

A consent form for home care services must be signed by the client or responsible person. Provide information about services in accordance with the Omnibus Budget Reconciliation Act of 1990, which protects the client's right of self-determination. Explain the Patient Bill of Rights (Display 14-9) and the client's responsibilities. Give information about billing, the frequency and duration of services, and the time of the next nursing visit. Inform clients and caregivers how to reach the agency 24 hours a day and how to lodge a complaint, should one arise. Explain the need for advance directives (see Chap. 16).

Record the initial information from the client on an initial database or assessment form, such as the OASIS. List medications on a separate flow sheet for ongoing assessment. Start an initial plan of care, with client input. This plan of care may identify NANDA problem statements to be addressed and may include client-centered NOC outcomes and NIC interventions to reach those outcomes. Some agencies use standardized care plans, including clinical paths, but they are always individualized for each client. Nurses' notes include both flow sheets and a narrative form. The latter is used for special, detailed information and brief summaries. Standardized flow sheets are available for common problems such as diabetes mellitus, congestive heart failure, and depression. If home health aide services are necessary, a separate form is filed on the chart that specifies these duties for a client. If other disciplines are involved in the case, such as physical therapy, that care plan is completed by that health provider. Some agencies have separate forms for interdisciplinary conferences, which must always be documented clearly somewhere on the chart. Of course, current physician's orders must also be filed in the client's chart.

Periodic and Discharge Summaries

These forms must clearly document the reasons a client either needs to continue receiving home care services or is to be discharged. A discharge summary is written if the client has achieved the expected outcomes. If so, the progress should be described in the summary. Another reason for discharge, which is sometimes difficult for the nurse, is that the home situation becomes unsafe or inadequate and intermittent care

---

DISPLAY 14-9
The Client's Bill of Rights: Home Care

1. The client has the right to be informed of his or her rights. The home health agency must protect and promote the exercise of these rights.
2. The home health agency must provide the client with a written notice of the client's rights in advance of furnishing care to the client or during the initial evaluation visit and before the initiation of treatment.
3. The home health agency must maintain documentation showing that it has complied.
4. The client has the right to exercise his or her rights as a client of the agency.
5. The client's family or guardian may exercise the client's rights when the client has been judged incompetent.
6. The client has the right to have his or her property treated with respect.
7. The client has the right to voice grievances regarding treatment or care that is (or fails to be) furnished, or regarding the lack of respect for property by anyone who is furnishing services on behalf of the agency, and must not be subjected to discrimination or reprisal for doing so.
8. The agency must investigate complaints made by a client or the client's family or guardian regarding treatment or care that is (or fails to be) furnished, or regarding the lack of respect for the client's property by anyone furnishing services on behalf of the agency, and must document both the existence of the complaint and the resolution of the complaint.
9. The agency must inform and distribute information to the client, in advance, concerning the policies on advance directives, including a description of applicable state law.
10. The client has the right to confidentiality of the clinical records.
11. The agency must advise the client of the agency's policies and procedures regarding disclosure of clinical records.
12. The client has the right to be advised, before care is initiated, of the extent to which payment for services may be expected from Medicare or other sources and the extent to which payment may be required form the client.
13. The client has the right to be advised of the availability of the toll-free home health agency hotline in the state, the purpose of the hotline, and the hours of operation.

(U.S. Congress [1990]. Omnibus Reconciliation Act of 1990.)

---

is not enough for the client's needs. Discharge may be necessary when a client needs to be rehospitalized or needs to enter an extended-care facility. In this case, the discharge summary may also serve as a referral form to those agencies. Sometimes clients move away, refuse further service, or die. Often discharge becomes necessary when the client no longer needs a skilled service but continues to be helped by the custodial care of a home health aide. These discharges, which require stopping the aide service, can also be difficult for the nurse.

Clinical Paths or Critical Pathways

The use of clinical paths is increasing in home care. Some agencies use the term "critical pathways" or "care maps," but they all mean the same thing. A type of standardized care plan, a clinical path identifies the timing and sequence of interventions for a particular diagnosis. The focus is still on achievement of client outcomes. Specific, essential interventions related to the clinical problem are listed in sequence to achieve the desired outcomes. All health-care professionals involved are included.

Hospitals using clinical paths have experienced cost savings, and the quality of documentation has improved as well. In home care, the use of clinical paths is more challenging because there are so many more variables that can affect the timing and sequence of care and outcome achievement. There are two main motivations for home care agencies to implement clinical paths (Humphrey & Milone-Nuzzo, 1996). First, managed-care contracts are increasingly competitive. These companies are looking for home care agencies that can deliver outcome achievement within a predetermined time at a cost that is competitive with other agencies. This requires progressive, thorough documentation that identifies the steps to achieve the desired outcomes. Second, there is an increased need to look at the client's continuum of care across all settings. Many hospital-based home care agencies are linking the client's hospitalization time with the time of service on home care. If an intermediate setting such as a rehabilitation hospital or an extended-care facility is necessary, that time of service may be included. Third-party payers increasingly require prior authorization for covered services and want to know the total cost required per client, per diagnosis across all care settings. There is talk of future diagnosis-related groups or "lump sum" prepayment approval for each diagnosis or surgical procedure to cover all aspects of care in all settings. Clinical paths could adapt well to such an eventuality because they allow tracking of the continuum of care across more than one setting (see Chapter 12).

The timeline in clinical paths is translated into the number of required visits or weeks of service for a particular diagnosis. Sample clinical paths can be seen in Appendix D. When there is more than one diagnosis, secondary diagnoses are included on the chart on "co-path" forms. A variance is any happening that requires a detour from the clinical path. Variances are not necessarily negative; they include anything that happens that affects the planned care being provided on a visit that may affect the outcome in any way. For example, in a teaching situation, the environmental conditions may be too distracting on a given day and beyond the nurse's control. Or the client or caretaker may be anxious or upset about some unrelated event, making the planned learning impossible on that particular visit. Variances are the way that clinical paths are individualized for a particular client. One objection to clinical paths is that they are said to be too mechanical and not accommodating enough to individual differences and life situations, but documentation of variances can allow for that.

Computer Systems in Home Care

Some nurses use laptop or hand-held computers to enter data in the home; this is called point-of-care documentation. In some systems, the nurse uses a pen or wand to enter data on the screen, avoiding the need for keyboard proficiency. Other systems require nurses to fill out data worksheets in the client's home, and the data are later transcribed onto a computer by clerical staff at the agency office.

The value of computer systems to home care agencies is not limited to clinical documentation. Integrated computer systems can link administrative and financial data with client clinical data. Client confidentiality is maintained by the use of access codes available only to those who need to know. Scheduling, billing, statistics, inventory, payroll, management reports, and total quality management programs are all part of the system. Good, integrated computerization is a valuable step toward greater efficiency and cost savings. Standardized terminology systems with numerical codes, such as NANDA, NOC, and NIC lend themselves well to computerization.

THE NURSE SPEAKS . . .
About Diabetic Teaching

As a nurse working for a large home care agency, I have learned that it's so important to listen to clients to find out what they want to learn and how they want to learn it, instead of following some preestablished plan. One of my clients, Leonard, was a well-known leader in our community and an intelligent man, but he was irrational about his diabetes. His doctor wanted to put him on insulin, but he adamantly refused. Home care was ordered because he had an infected wound on his right foot. He frequently walked barefoot in his house and yard.

Clearly, Leonard did not want me to talk about diabetes. So I taught him diabetic foot care but called it "preventive" foot care. I taught him the ADA diet but called it "foods and the diet you need to heal." Both the diabetic education specialist and the psychiatric-mental health clinical specialist were helpful when I conferred with them. I used a modified desensitization process for Leonard's denial or phobia of his diabetes. I continued dressing his foot wound, which was not healing well.

One day he said, "I think losing your independence is the worst thing that can happen to anyone." I countered with stories about well-known people, starting with Franklin D. Roosevelt, who continued to lead active, productive lives despite chronic health problems. I focused on several well-known persons with diabetes and explained how they managed their diabetes, kept very active, and avoided complications. Later, he was able to use the word "diabetes" for the first time in talking about others. So then I could relate diabetic high blood sugar with nonhealing wounds and infections.

The next day, Leonard was able to personalize and said that he wanted to control "*my* diabetes." So I called his doctor about an order for teaching him self-administration of insulin, use of a glucometer, and other aspects of diabetic care. He learned quickly and was doing both proficiently when his wound healed and he was discharged from home care.

Mary Lou
HOME CARE NURSE

CLINICAL APPLICATION

A Critical Thinking Case Study About a Total-Care Home Care Client

You are the home care nurse for Martin, a 10-year-old boy with an astrocytoma. He is lovingly cared for by his single mother with the assistance of home care. The brain tumor makes the boy subject to grand mal seizures, for which he receives phenytoin

(Dilantin) 200 mg every 12 hours through his gastric tube (G-tube). He also receives dexamethasone (Decadron) 1 mg once daily via the same route. Martin is semiconscious. He seems to respond positively to gentle positioning and quiet talk and music. At the same time, he becomes rigid and groans during procedures he does not like, such as suctioning and catheter changes.

 and Think!

- Prioritize Martin's problems and nursing needs. List the hazards of immobility to which he is subject. What can be done to prevent or minimize each hazard?
- What is your role in regard to Martin's mother?
- What do you think are her needs?
- Who is your client in this situation?

You teach Martin's mother to do various position changes while safeguarding an open airway. Suctioning is difficult for her, but she can do it when necessary. The grand mal seizures are equally difficult for her to watch, but she is learning to deal with them. She masters G-tube feedings and medication administration readily, as well as his bowel regimen. She needs frequent reinforcement and encouragement but manages to provide excellent care with the help of a daily home health aide, who is present for 4 hours each morning, and your nursing visit each afternoon.

Martin came home from the hospital with an indwelling catheter, but one of your goals is to teach his mother intermittent catheterization to prevent the frequent cystitis and problems maintaining patency that occur with an indwelling catheter. At present, she feels overwhelmed with learning his other care and is still very anxious about his G-tube.

Martin is an only child. This allows the mother to devote her full attention to caring for him but also increases her anticipatory grief. She wants to keep him and care for him at home as long as possible. You ask if she would like to talk about her spiritual needs. She immediately says yes and asks you to pray for Martin and for her. She says she has been casual about her religious practices and now has many questions about the meaning of what is happening to her son. You offer to contact a clergyperson of her religious faith to visit, but she says she will do that.

The mother informs you that family members are either far away or disinterested, but that she has several caring friends. You suggest she search for someone whom she can trust to care for Martin so she can go out occasionally with friends, just to talk. She tells you that she has already decided to go out for brunch soon and leave Martin with the home health aide because she is pleased with her care and competency. You teach Martin's mother various stress reduction strategies at each visit, as well as the importance of adequate rest and good nutrition for herself. You explain the relationship of stress and lowered immune status, and she agrees to take better care of herself and attend to her own needs to be able to continue to care for Martin. The mother is also your client, not just Martin.

Early one morning, Martin's mother calls to say that he pulled on his G-tube and there is blood oozing around the stoma. You go there immediately and see dried blood and gastric drainage around the tube. The G-tube has progressed to 3 cm from the skin marker, which is normally 1 cm from his skin. Martin's wrists are tied tightly to the bed side rails, and his wrists are red.

 and Think!

- What has happened?
- What should you do about it, if anything?
- What needs to be done first?
- Then how will you proceed?
- What are the risks for Martin in this situation?

It looks like Martin may have pulled the G-tube sufficiently that it is in the stoma tract. Your concern is that a traumatic dislodgement may have occurred. You need to call the physician and report this and get a mitten restraint order for Martin's hands. However, first you must pad and reapply the wrist restraints properly to avoid constriction. You show his mother how to do this, tying the restraints to the bed-frame rather than the side rails, while explaining quietly to Martin. You also explain to the mother that the loose, padded mittens you hope the doctor will order will prevent Martin from pulling on the tubing again without causing the increased frustration, restlessness, and constriction that can occur when the wrists are tied. Tying Martin's wrists was emotionally difficult for her, so the idea of mittens makes her feel much better.

The physician calls back, orders the mitten restraints, and tells you to remove the G-tube and insert a #16 Foley catheter with a 50-ml balloon into the stoma.

 and Think!

- How would you respond if this G-tube were a percutaneous endoscopic gastrostomy (PEG) tube?
- Where will you get a new #16 Foley catheter?
- What steps will you take in removing the G-tube?
- What is the crucial step?
- What will you do before inserting the new catheter?

A PEG tube is inserted through the esophagus into the stomach with the aid of an endoscope. It is then pulled through a stab wound from the stomach to the exterior wall. An internal disk remains around the tube inside the stomach, and an external skin disk is applied around the stoma opening on the abdomen. These internal and external disks make PEG tubes very secure. PEG tubes are inserted and removed surgically, so you should not try to remove a PEG tube in the home.

Like most home care nurses, you carry a supply of sterile Foley catheters of various sizes in the trunk of your car, along with other supplies. It is most important to drain all the water from the old G-tube balloon before attempting to remove it. Using a Luer-tip syringe, you aspirate through the balloon valve and carefully note the amount of aspirate. In this case, there is little water left in the balloon. This strengthens your suspicion that the old balloon had burst and water had leaked into Martin's stomach. You gently pull out the tube and see that the balloon is indeed empty, confirming your suspicion.

After opening the Foley kit, you change your gloves, using the sterile ones in the kit. You carefully inspect and practice inflating and emptying the new 50-ml balloon before inserting the tube to be sure that it works properly. You cleanse the area around the stoma and lubricate both the stoma and the tube with water-soluble lubricant. You gently feed the tube tip into the stoma but meet resistance. You wait a couple of minutes, talking to Martin soothingly to help relax him. You meet resistance again.

 ## and Think!

- What should you do now?
- Should you remove the tube and call the physician again?
- Should you call your supervisor?
- Should you call 911 and send Martin to the emergency department?

Before doing any of those things, you wait another 3 to 5 minutes, continuing to talk soothingly to Martin. Ask him to take deep breaths. Demonstrate deep breathing to him and try to get him to breathe in synchrony with you. Deep breathing will relax both of you! Then you try once more before calling your supervisor or the physician again. Only if a considerable amount of fresh bleeding occurred from the stoma, and if you could not reach the physician, might you send him to the emergency department.

This time, the deflated balloon glides gently forward through the stoma tract into the stomach. You inflate the balloon with 50 ml of water and verify its location with gastric aspiration.

 ## and Think!

- If no gastric aspirate is obtained, what should you do?
- What could occur?
- What should you do if you feel incompetent to carry out the physician's order but he or she insists that you do so?

If no gastric aspirate can be obtained, you cannot be sure the tube is in the stomach, so you must call the physician. He or she may then order that a portable x-ray machine be sent to the home to check the tube's status. A tube can migrate into the peritoneal cavity if a traumatic tear occurs, such as when Martin pulled the G-tube. Feeding solutions could then cause peritonitis, a serious complication that could be fatal.

If you feel incompetent to carry out any procedure that a physician orders, call and discuss the situation immediately with your supervisor, explaining your rationale. The supervisor will come herself or himself, send another nurse, or call the physician if the orders are outside the realm of nursing.

You finish by looping the tubing on the abdomen and securing it well with tape so that it cannot be pulled out again. You cover the stoma area with a dry sterile dressing. You tell Martin's mother to free his hands from the restraints periodically while she stands at the bedside and can watch him. You remind her that you will send the mitten restraints.

Chapter SUMMARY

Home care nursing practice differs significantly from hospital nursing. Medicare and other third-party payers will reimburse only for nursing services they call "skilled." Their definition of "skilled nursing care" differs somewhat from what nurses know as skilled nursing care. Many registered nurses who are associate degree or diploma graduates work proficiently as home care nurses, although the ideal minimum preparation is a baccalaureate degree. Advanced practice nurses function as specialists, consultants, clinical coordinators, and managers of staff education and quality assurance programs.

This chapter includes instructions on how to do a home visit and explains home health aide functions and equipment used in home care. The nursing process is used as a valuable problem-solving tool. Common client problems seen in home care are listed; diabetes mellitus is the most common diagnosis. Infection control in the home is discussed in detail, as is teaching in home care nursing. Documentation guidelines that meet standards and legal requirements are listed, and point-of-care documentation is described. Initial visit documentation and components of the home care chart and periodic and discharge summaries are described. The value of clinical paths and integrated information systems is discussed.

A list of references and additional readings for this chapter appears at the end of Part 4.

15

Specialized Home Care Services

Key Terms

adjuvant drugs
bereavement counselors
breakthrough pain
coanalgesics
Diagnostic and Statistical Manual IV
dose ceiling zone
enteral therapy
equianalgesic
Groshong
Hickman/Broviac
hospice

Huber needle
infantilize
Infuse-a-Port
infusion therapy
internal flange
Kock pouch
La Leche League
palliative
patient-controlled analgesia
percutaneous endoscopic gastrostomy tube
pejorative

peripherally inserted central catheter
psychomotor retardation
sudden infant death syndrome
Title V
total parenteral nutrition
transdermal route
ventilation therapy
World Health Organization pain ladder

Learning Objectives

1. Describe the hospice philosophy.
2. Explain the criteria for hospice services.
3. List three principles of pain management.
4. Describe coanalgesic and adjuvant drugs.
5. Identify various types of pain and the best treatments for each.
6. Explain factors contributing to the increase in high-technology home care.
7. Describe the three basic modes of high-technology home care in detail.
8. Identify the special problems of pediatric home care.
9. Explain the preventive value of maternal-infant home care programs.
10. List the criteria for psychiatric-mental health home care.
11. Explain the kinds of problems uniquely suited to psychiatric-mental health home care programs.

Home care specialty services include hospice, high-technology home care, pediatric home care, maternal-infant home care, and mental health home care. In some communities, these services are provided in conjunction with general home care services. In other communities, they are provided by separate specialty agencies.

Hospice

One of the fastest-growing, most humane, and most economical health services is hospice. This movement, to help terminally ill clients die comfortably and with dignity, has developed rapidly during the past 20 years. There are almost 2,700 local hospice programs across the United States in all states, providing emotional, spiritual, and hands-on support in home-based and inpatient settings. Some 78% of hospice clients have cancer. Most of the other clients have either heart disease or AIDS, but clients with many medical diagnoses are served.

Palliative, supportive care replaces intrusive, high-technology, futile procedures with physical, spiritual, and psychological comfort to clients and their families. The hospice philosophy was best summed up by Dame Cicely Saunders, founder of the first modern-day hospice in London in 1968: "You matter to the last moment of your life, and we will do all we can, not only to help you die peacefully, but to live until you die."

Hospice neither hastens nor postpones death. It affirms life and regards dying as a normal process that should be as pain-free and as comfortable as possible. Hospice brings hope because it enables clients and families to experience the highest, most rewarding quality of life possible and provides an opportunity for a pain-free, alert, "good" death.

The first American hospice was started in New Haven, Conn., in 1974. From its beginning, the American model stressed hospice as a home service. About 90% of clients live and prefer to die at home. Some hospice clients live and prefer to die in extended-care facilities or hospice centers or as inpatients in hospice-contracted units of hospitals. Heavy use of volunteers as direct patient providers has been part of the hospice model. Of the 115,000 persons involved in hospice care in the United States, about 95,000 are volunteers, giving more than 5 million hours to hospice clients each year. Many hospice volunteers, as well as staff, are registered nurses. Volunteers provide assistance at all levels of their skill but first must complete an extensive training program.

The Hospice Team

The hospice team develops a personalized plan of care that includes clients and families. Serving families' needs is a major consideration in hospice. Even after death, bereavement support is available and frequently provided to families for up to a year. The hospice team meets regularly to refine the plan of care. Hospice nurses help ease the physical symptoms of illness. They are known for their sophisticated knowledge of pain control and comfort measures. Nurses are on call 24 hours, 7 days a week. Special certification is available for experienced hospice nurses who pass a rigorous examination through the National Board for Certification of Hospice Nurses.

The hospice medical director works closely with the client's primary physician and will assume medical care of a client who has no personal physician. The hospice medical director also works closely and supportively with nurses and other members of the staff and volunteers.

Volunteers provide help by sitting with clients, performing errands, helping to write letters, providing a sympathetic ear, providing respite for caregivers, and offering whatever special skills they possess. Nurse volunteers often provide nursing care. Social workers help patients and their families make emotional adjustments. They can be effective in helping families improve communication, locating community resources, and teaching stress reduction techniques. Spiritual care is another major consideration in hospice. Many volunteers receive extra training as spiritual caregivers, supervised by a staff chaplain. Hospice spiritual caregivers serve persons of all religious faiths and those of no faith, respecting each person's beliefs. People often have needs of the spirit that reach beyond religion. Bereavement counselors may be staff members or trained volunteers. Home health aides are other valuable members of the home care team who assist clients with personal care.

Criteria for Hospice Service

According to surveys (Gregory & English, 1994), most clients wait too long to seek help from hospice. One agency recently estimated that on average, a hospice client lives just 23 days after enrolling in the program. Based on 1990 Medicare claims data, clients died an average of 36 days after they enrolled in hospice.

Hospice criteria state that any person will be admitted during the final 6 months of illness when the primary goal is patient comfort and not aggressive treatment. Clients with potentially life-threatening illnesses such as serious heart disease, chronic obstructive pulmonary disease, cirrhosis, AIDS, cancer, Alzheimer's disease, and end-stage kidney disease, should not wait until death is a few weeks away to enroll.

Some clients, such as young AIDS clients, fear that if they enroll in hospice they might miss an opportunity to try a new, promising medication when it is produced. In reality, hospice clients can go off hospice service whenever they want to return to curative therapies. In some cases, curative treatment is approved by hospice if the primary purpose is to provide comfort. One example is an AIDS client who was going blind and was treated as part of a hospice program with intravenous acyclovir to improve his vision and vastly improve the quality of his remaining days.

Sometimes clients or their families do not want to acknowledge that death is coming soon and therefore are not technically eligible for hospice services. Some hospice agencies have developed supportive care services for clients who do not meet the Medicare hospice benefit requirements. Supportive care is funded by donations and fund-raising activities, which volunteers often undertake. Bereavement care is offered under supportive care, as is prehospice care for clients who are not ready to acknowledge and accept hospice services but need the psychosocial and spiritual support of hospice. There is no charge to clients for supportive care. Unfortunately, most hospices do not have enough local financial support to provide supportive care and can provide only the core services.

Cancer Pain Control in Hospice

Because most clients seeking hospice care have cancer, hospice nurses have developed great skill in controlling cancer pain. Clients and their families need to be reassured that most pain can be relieved effectively and safely without oversedation. Almost all cancer pain (more than 95%) can be well managed. However, several recent studies indicate that cancer patients continue to be undermedicated, with their pain poorly managed. A consensus statement from the National Cancer Institute Workshop on Cancer Pain says that undertreatment of pain and other symptoms of cancer is "a serious and neglected public health problem" (National Cancer Institute, 1990).

Pain Assessment

Good pain management is based on a thorough pain assessment. A detailed history, physical examination, and psychosocial assessment should be included. Some nurses and physicians think that pain is objective: according to this misguided approach, if signs of the pain are not objectively evident, no pain is present. In reality, pain is whatever the client says it is. Clients with chronic pain, in particular, may show few signs of distress. The facial expression may be misread as weariness or depression. Autonomic nervous system signs such as sweating, pallor, hypertension, and tachycardia are absent (these are commonly observed with acute pain but are seldom seen in chronic pain). The severity of chronic pain cannot be judged by autonomic and other signs of acute pain such as crying and grimacing.

It is often helpful to have the client keep a log and rate the severity of the pain from 0 to 10, with 10 being the worst possible pain (Fig. 15-1). In addition to intensity or severity, the client should be asked to describe the nature of the pain, the location, and any aggravating or relieving factors. The client's self-report is of primary value.

Sometimes relief of one type of pain leads to greater awareness of another pain. Sometimes new pain develops. These things should trigger another assessment and modification of the treatment plan. The cardinal rule to follow in assessing pain is that pain is whatever the client says it is.

Pharmacologic Pain Management

The pain management program must be carefully individualized to the client because people react so differently to pain and to the medications that treat pain. The World Health Organization's analgesic steps or pain ladder should be used to manage pain (Fig. 15-2). This analgesic step system is a primary principle of pain management. It begins with the simplest and mildest analgesics such as aspirin, acetaminophen, and ibuprofen. Stronger drugs are then added step by step as the pain increases from mild to moderate to severe.

Nothing should be assumed. If analgesic medication has been ordered and the client still has pain, the first thing to determine is whether or not the analgesic is being taken every 4 hours as ordered, or if the client is mistakenly taking the analgesic only as needed. Pain medication for cancer should be taken regularly, not as needed, except for breakthrough pain (intermittent increases in pain that occur spontaneously or in

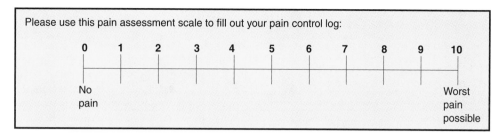

Please use this pain assessment scale to fill out your pain control log:

Date	Time	How severe is the pain?	Medicine or nondrug pain control method	How severe is the pain after one hour?	Activity at time of pain

FIGURE 15-1
Pain management log. (U.S. Department of Health and Human Services [1994]. *Clinical Practice Guideline: Management of Cancer Pain.* Agency for Health Care Policy and Research #94-0592.)

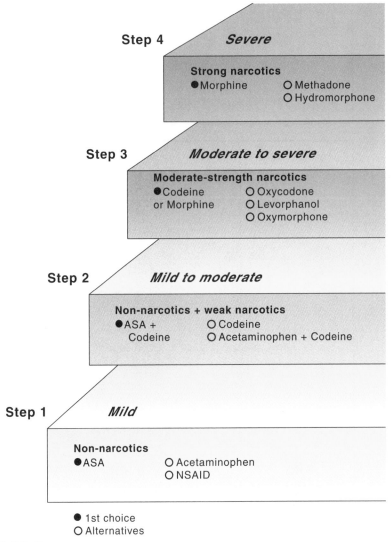

FIGURE 15-2
Analgesic steps (Adapted from the WHO [World Health Organization] Ladder.)

relation to certain activities). It is important to watch for an analgesic's ceiling dose: that is an indication to move up the ladder and add stronger analgesics.

As pain increases, opioids are titrated as needed. At the top of the ladder, morphine sulfate is generally the most effective analgesic for severe pain. It has no ceiling zone. Some clients require very high opioid doses to control their pain. Respiratory depression, a common side effect of opioids, does not seem to be a problem for most of these clients because tolerance develops. However, opioids are not the best analgesic for all types of pain.

A second principle of cancer pain management is the use of coanalgesics and adjuvant medications. Various drugs enhance the effect of opiates, provide independent analgesia for specific types of pain, and treat concurrent problems that exacerbate pain. When increasing the dose of morphine does not control the pain, a careful assessment of the type and location of pain is crucial. Morphine is especially successful in covering "gut" pain but is not as good for bone pain. Bone pain responds to nonsteroidal antiinflammatories such as choline magnesium trisalicylate (Trilisate) or naproxen (Naprosyn). Severe bone pain can sometimes be treated successfully with calcitonin (Calimar) or the bisphosphonates, etidronate (Didronel) or pamidronate (Aredia), according to early clinical trials (USDHHS, 1994). Clients describe bone pain as "achy." Neuropathic pain is described as "burning" or "stabbing" and responds to anticonvulsants such as phenytoin (Dilantin) or carbamazepine (Tegretol). The tricyclic antidepressant amitriptyline (Elavil) is also effective and has been used extensively to treat neuropathic pain. Pressure pain, as from a brain tumor, responds best to corticosteroids (dexamethasone [Decadron] or prednisone [Deltasone]), which provide relief by reducing edema and pressure.

Depression is a major factor that can increase pain perception and should not be ignored. The selective serotonin reuptake inhibitor antidepressants such as fluoxetine (Prozac) or sertraline (Zoloft) work well and have minimal side effects. Elavil is effective, especially if also used for neuropathic pain, but has anticholinergic side effects (constipation, urinary retention, dry mouth, blurry vision, tachycardia). Additional discomfort caused by chronic constipation and distention is prevented if clients are automatically started on a bowel regimen when opiates are ordered. Antiemetic drugs such as phenothiazines and metoclopramide (Reglan) may be added if nausea is a problem. The antihistamine hydroxyzine (Vistaril) helps control nausea, anxiety, and insomnia (USDHHS, 1994).

Long-acting analgesics, along with short-acting analgesics for breakthrough pain, are used for maximum pain control. Controlled-release morphine (MS Contin) is administered every 12 hours. Liquid morphine (Roxanol) or morphine sulfate 10-mg immediate-release tablets are used successfully for breakthrough pain. The oral route is the preferred route for analgesics because it is most convenient and cost-effective. If clients cannot tolerate oral medications, transdermal fentanyl (Duragesic) is an option. Each patch contains a 72-hour supply of Duragesic, which is passively absorbed by the skin. Duragesic is considerably more expensive than long-acting morphine.

In patient-controlled analgesia (PCA), a special pump is set to prescribed dose parameters. Usually there is continuous infusion of opioid medication, plus client-administered boluses of medication to treat breakthrough pain. The infusions are administered intravenously or subcutaneously. PCA can also be administered epidurally. Intraspinal analgesic systems are used only when pain can no longer be managed by other routes. There is no ceiling dose on the amount of analgesics required to keep a hospice patient pain-free.

Nonpharmacologic Pain Management

In moderate to severe pain, nonpharmacologic measures should supplement, not replace, medication. In addition to pharmacologic management, psychosocial, spiritual, and other treatments should be used when caring for clients with cancer pain (Display 15-1). An interdisciplinary panel of clinicians, clients, researchers, and experts in health policy collaborated in producing *Clinical Practice Guideline: Management of Cancer Pain,* published by the Agency for Health Care Policy and Research of the Public Health Service in 1994 (USDHHS, 1994). The following recommendations for nonpharmacologic

---

DISPLAY 15-1
Nonpharmacologic Pain Control Exercises

EXERCISE A: SLOW RHYTHMIC BREATHING FOR RELAXATION

- Breathe in slowly and deeply.
- As you breathe out slowly, feel yourself beginning to relax; feel the tension leaving your body.
- Now breathe in and out slowly and regularly, at whatever rate is comfortable for you. You may wish to try abdominal breathing.
- To help you focus on your breathing and breathe slowly and rhythmically: (a) breathe in as you say silently to yourself, "in, two, three"; (b) breathe out as you say silently to yourself, "out, two, three."

or

- Each time you breathe out, say silently to yourself a word such as "peace" or "relax."
- Do steps 1 through 4 only once or repeat steps 3 and 4 for up to 20 minutes.
- End with a slow deep breath. As you breathe out say to yourself, "I feel alert and relaxed."

EXERCISE B: SIMPLE TOUCH, MASSAGE, OR WARMTH FOR RELAXATION

Touch and massage are age-old methods of helping others relax. Some examples are:
1. Brief touch or massage—hand-holding or briefly touching or rubbing a person's shoulder
2. Warm foot soak in a basin of warm water, or wrap the feet in a warm, wet towel.
3. Massage (3 to 10 minutes) may consist of the whole body or only the back, feet, or hands. If the client is modest or cannot move or turn easily in bed, consider massage of the hands and feet.
    - Use a warm lubricant. A small bowl of hand lotion may be warmed in the microwave oven, or a bottle of lotion may be warmed by placing it in a sink of hot water for about 10 minutes.
    - Massage for relaxation is usually done with smooth, long slow strokes. (Rapid strokes, circular movements, and squeezing of tissues tend to stimulate circulation and increase arousal.) However, try several degrees of pressure along with different types of massage, (kneading, stroking, and circling). Determine which is preferred.

Especially for the elderly person, a backrub that produces relaxation may consist of no more than 3 minutes of slow, rhythmic stroking (about 60 strokes per minute) on both sides of the spinous process from the crown of the head to the lower back. Continuous hand contact is maintained by starting one hand down the back as the other hand stops at

DISPLAY 15-1 *(Continued)*

the lower back and is raised. Set aside a regular time for the massage. This gives the client something to look forward to and depend on.

EXERCISE C: PEACEFUL PAST EXPERIENCES

Something may have happened to you a while ago that brought you peace and comfort. You may be able to draw on that past experience to bring you peace or comfort now. Think about these questions:

1. Can you remember any situation, even when you were a child, when you felt calm, peaceful, secure, hopeful, or comfortable?
2. Have you ever daydreamed about something peaceful? What were you thinking of?
3. Do you get a dreamy feeling when you listen to music? Do you have any favorite music?
4. Do you have any favorite poetry that you find uplifting or reassuring?
5. Have you ever been religiously active? Do you have favorite readings, hymns, or prayers? Even if you haven't heard or thought of them for many years, childhood religious experiences may still be very soothing.

Additional points: Very likely some of the things you think of in answer to these questions can be recorded for you, such as your favorite music or a prayer. Then, you can listen to the tape whenever you wish. Or, if your memory is strong, you may simply close your eyes and recall the events or words.

EXERCISE D: ACTIVE LISTENING TO RECORDED MUSIC

1. Obtain the following:
   * A cassette player or tape recorder (small, battery-operated ones are more convenient)
   * Earphone or headset (this is a more demanding stimulus than a speaker a few feet away, and it avoids disturbing others)
   * Cassette of music you like (Most people prefer fast, lively music, but some select relaxing music. Other options are comedy routines, sporting events, old radio shows, or stories.)
2. Mark time to the music–tap out the rhythm with your finger or nod your head. This helps you concentrate on the music rather than your discomfort.
3. Keep your eyes open and focus steadily on one stationary spot or object. If you wish to close your eyes, picture something about the music.
4. Listen to the music at a comfortable volume. If the discomfort increases, try increasing the volume; decrease the volume when the discomfort decreases.
5. If this is not effective, try adding or changing one or more of the following: massage your body in rhythm to the music; try other music; mark time to the music in more than one manner (tap your foot and finger at the same time).

Additional points: Many clients have found this technique to be helpful. It tends to be very popular, probably because the equipment is usually readily available and is a part of daily life. Other advantages are that it is easy to learn and is not physically or mentally demanding. If you are very tired, you may simply listen to the music and omit marking time or focusing on a spot.

(McCafferey M, Beebe A [1989]. Pain: Clinical Manual for Nursing Practice. St. Louis: Mosby. Reprinted in USDHHS, PHS [1996]. Management of Cancer Pain. AHCPR Publication No. 94-0592.)

pain management are based on the panel's report:

1. Offer cutaneous stimulation techniques (superficial heat and cold, massage, pressure, vibration, transcutaneous electrical nerve stimulation) to alleviate pain.
2. Use distractions and diversional activities. Psychosocial interventions should be introduced early in the course of illness as part of a multimodal approach to pain management. They generally should not be used as substitutes for analgesics.
3. Because of the many misconceptions regarding pain and its treatment, education about the ability to control pain effectively, with correction of myths about the use of opioids, should be included as part of the treatment plan for all clients.
4. Clients and families should be offered the means to contact peer support groups.
5. Pastoral care members should participate in health-care team meetings that discuss the needs and treatment of clients. They should develop information about community resources that provide spiritual care and support for clients and their families.
6. Clients should be repositioned on a scheduled basis during long-term bedrest. Active and passive range-of-motion exercises should be provided. With acute pain, exercise should be limited to self-administered range of motion.
7. Avoid prolonged immobilization whenever possible.
8. Clients who choose to have acupuncture for pain management should be encouraged to report changes in pain problems to their health-care team before seeking palliation through acupuncture.
9. Encourage clients to remain active and to participate in self-care when possible.

High-Technology Home Care

The advent of hospital prospective-payment systems (diagnosis-related groups) resulted in early hospital discharges. This means that many clients are going home while they still require high-technology care. During the early 1980s, various industries began preparing for this eventuality. The durable medical equipment and pharmaceutical industries responded by developing technologies that could be adapted for home care. Portable, user-friendly equipment was developed, along with medications that could be administered at longer intervals. The insurance industry recognized that high-technology care could be administered in the home for a third of the cost of inpatient care and included home care benefits in most of their policies. Home care agencies broadened their policies and educated nurses to work in homes using high-technology procedures.

Although there are many modes of high-technology home care, most services fall into three categories: enteral therapy, infusion therapy, and ventilation therapy. In terms of sophistication of skill and technology, enteral therapy is the simplest and ventilation therapy is the most complex of the three.

Enteral Therapy in Home Care

In enteral therapy, a tube is inserted into the gastrointestinal tract for feedings. If the situation is thought to be very short-term, a nasogastric tube is inserted by the nurse. Long-term situations require the surgical placement of a gastric or jejunostomy tube. Sometimes a large Foley tube is used with an inflatable internal balloon. More often a percutaneous endoscopic gastrostomy (PEG) tube with an internal flange is surgically inserted before the client leaves the hospital. PEG tubes are never removed or inserted by nurses at home, but nasogastric tubes and Foley tubes are often changed by home care nurses.

Feeding solutions are highly concentrated and contain all essential nutrients. Clients with malabsorption syndromes or partial obstructions are commonly fed in this way using either a continuous drip or a bolus method. The nurse must ensure correct tube placement before inserting water, medications, or feeding solution. Close monitoring of the client's fluid and electrolyte balance and ability to tolerate the feedings are important nursing considerations. Documentation must support the necessity for the tube feedings based on the client's primary diagnosis. Some home care clients are on tube feedings for many weeks. Ongoing evaluation of the effects of this form of nutrition must be checked with blood tests and weighing the client. Teaching the client and caregiver effective, safe ways to administer feedings is a basic nursing responsibility in home care. For a clinical example, see the Clinical Application Chapter 14.

Infusion Therapy in Home Care

Some agencies specialize in home infusion therapy, and general home care agencies contract for their special high-technology services when a client needs an infusion. Many general home care agencies are also hiring nurses experienced in starting and managing intravenous infusions in the home. See Appendix E for standardized care plans for home intravenous therapy.

Venous access lines may be either central or peripheral. Port-a-Cath and Hickman/ Broviac, the two main types of central lines, are inserted in the hospital. The Hickman/ Broviac is usually threaded through a major vessel into the superior vena cava to the heart, where it rests just outside the atrium. The other end of the tube protrudes about 10″ from the exit wound, usually on the chest wall. Around the catheter cuff the wound heals in 3 to 10 days, sealing it off. It is kept covered with a sterile dressing. An Infuse-a-Port or Port-a-Cath is similar but is placed under a skin flap subcutaneously, like a pacemaker. A special Huber needle pierces both the skin and the port for access and is held in place by an occlusive dressing (Humphrey & Milone-Nuzzo, 1996).

Peripheral access lines can be used for most therapies. Peripherally inserted central catheters (PICC) are inserted by nurses who have completed special training; nurses cannot legally do this in all states. A PICC is threaded through an antecubital vein to the subclavian vein (peripheral placement) or the superior vena cava (central placement). A Groshong PICC is made of soft silicone rubber tubing and may have a single or double lumen. It contains depth markings and a radiopaque tip and stripe. It has winged connectors, attachable suture wings, and a special three-position valve that inhibits backflow of blood and air embolism. These catheters do not need to be heparinized. Routine maintenance includes catheter irrigation with 5 ml normal saline every 7 days, after intravenous administration of total parenteral nutrition (TPN) or intravenous fluids or medications. The PICC dressing should be changed every 7 days, using sterile gloves. Isopropyl alcohol and povidone-iodine swab sticks are used to cleanse the area, and a sterile gauze or transparent dressing is applied (Fig. 15-3).

Pumps for administration of infusion solutions may be subcutaneously implanted or external. The latter are more commonly used. Many varieties of small, lightweight pumps

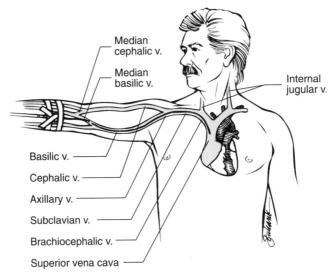

FIGURE 15-3

The venous anatomy of the upper extremity and thorax. Peripherally inserted central catheter (PICC) lines are inserted into the cephalic or basilic veins and advanced to the axillary, subclavian, or brachiocephalic veins or the superior vena cava. (Smeltzer S, Bare B [1996]. *Brunner and Suddarth's Textbook of Medical-Surgical Nursing,* 8th ed. Philadelphia: Lippincott-Raven.)

are available. The type selected depends on the purpose of the infusion and the client's situation. Factors to consider are the length of time and the volume of the infusion, as well as the client's or caregiver's ability to learn to use the pump. Cost and the type of pump covered by the client's insurance are always factors.

TPN requires a teaching program. The client or caregiver needs to learn to set up the infusion, flush the line with heparin (if needed), change the dressing, store the solutions properly, and troubleshoot for complications. Some agencies specialize in providing TPN services.

Mechanical Ventilation in Home Care

Positive-pressure ventilation is most commonly used for clients who cannot breathe on their own. Positive-pressure machines produce forced inspiration followed by passive expiration. Training for home ventilation must begin in the hospital after careful assessment that family or other support personnel will be in attendance 24 hours a day. Sometimes support personnel must include the services of a private-duty nurse. The client's physician and the coordinating respiratory therapist who sets up the equipment must be on call at all times in the event of problems. Criteria for successful home ventilation therapy can be found in Display 15-2.

There is a great deal for caregivers to learn about mechanical ventilation: care of the machine, signs and symptoms of adequate oxygenation, tracheostomy care, suctioning, vital sign monitoring, and signs of infection. The respiratory therapist and machine vendor usually make frequent visits to reinforce teaching and monitor the situation.

DISPLAY 15-2

Summary of Assessment Criteria for Successful Home Ventilator Care

1. The family members and professional staff are competent, dependable, and willing to spend the time required for proper training.
2. The client is willing to go home.
3. The family understands the diagnosis and prognosis.
4. There is evidence of chronic underlying pulmonary abnormalities
5. The client's clinical pulmonary status is stable.
6. The family has sufficient financial and support resources.
7. A psychological consultation with the client and family is made before the client is discharged.
8. The home environment is conducive to accepting the client.
9. The electrical facilities are adequate to operate all equipment safely.
10. The client's environment is controlled, preventing drafts in cold weather and ensuring proper ventilation in warm weather.
11. Equipment cleaning and storage space is available.

(Smeltzer S, Bare B [1996]. Brunner & Suddarth's Textbook of Medical-Surgical Nursing. *Philadelphia: JB Lippincott.)*

Client and caregiver responsibilities are listed in Display 15-3. Sometimes this care is too overwhelming for the client and family to undertake without constant professional help; a private-duty nurse is often the best option.

Pediatric Home Care

There are an estimated 10 million chronically ill children in the United States. Some have developmental delays or disabilities. Some have congenital or hereditary disorders. They are called handicapped, disabled, impaired, retarded, or technology-dependent children. The best and least pejorative of these descriptions is "children with special needs." In 1985, the Crippled Children's Services changed its name to Children With Special Health Needs. This program is funded by Title V of the Social Security Act and is under the administration of the Children's Bureau. Block grants to states with matching funds help finance the care of children with complex medical needs (Wong, 1993).

Ironically, progress has contributed to the increasing number of children with special needs. Medical and surgical advances have enabled premature or very low-birthweight babies to survive in sophisticated neonatal intensive care units. Surgical procedures to correct congenital heart disease and other life-threatening conditions mean that children who would formerly have died are now kept alive, many to live full, productive lives. People with Down syndrome rarely survived to adulthood until this past generation. The increased numbers of automobiles in use in our affluent society means that more children are becoming disabled from auto accidents.

DISPLAY 15-3
Client and Caregiver Responsibilities for Mechanical Home Ventilation

CLIENT CARE

- Monitor visual signs as directed.
- Observe physical signs such as color, secretions, breathing pattern, and state of consciousness.
- Perform physical care such as suctioning, postural drainage, and ambulation.
- Observe the tidal volume and pressure manometer regularly. Intervene when they are abnormal (eg, suction if airway pressure increases).
- Provide a communication method for the client (eg, pad and pencil, electric larynx, talking trash).

VENTILATOR CARE

- Check the ventilator settings twice each day and whenever the client is removed from the ventilator.
- Adjust the volume and pressure alarms if needed.
- Fill humidifier as needed and check its level three times a day.
- Empty water in tubing as needed.

VENTILATOR MAINTENANCE

- Use a clean humidifier when circuitry is changed.
- Keep exterior clean and free of any objects.
- Change external circuitry once a week or more.
- Report malfunction or strange noises right away.

Providing the opportunity for ventilator-dependent clients to return home and to live in familiar surroundings can be a rich, rewarding experience for all. The technical ability now exists to accomplish this. The ultimate goal for the client on home ventilator therapy is to enhance life, not simply to support or prolong life.

(Smeltzer S, Bare B [1996]. Brunner & Suddarth's Textbook of Medical-Surgical Nursing. *Philadelphia: JB Lippincott.)*

As with home care for adults, careful preparation, teaching, and discharge planning must take place before the child leaves the hospital. All needed equipment and services are set up and ready at home before the child is discharged. Ideally, a pediatric home care nurse specialist sets up the plan of care. Community resources should be used and respite care provided for parents if they assume full daily and nightly care of the child.

This is a very difficult adjustment for most parents (Display 15-4). The question of authority comes into play when professionals, such as private-duty nurses, assume much of the care of the child. Some parents have a need to be very controlling in these situations. Some parents are overcome with guilt and are overly permissive so that the

---

DISPLAY 15-4
Key Elements of Family-Centered Care

- Recognizing that the family is the constant in a child's life; the service systems and personnel within those systems fluctuate
- Facilitating parent—professional collaboration at all levels of health care:
    Care of an individual child
    Program development, implementation, and evaluation
    Policy formation
- Honoring the racial, ethnic, cultural, and socioeconomic diversity of families
- Recognizing family strengths and individuality and respecting different methods of coping
- Sharing with parents, on a continuing basis and in a supportive manner, complete and unbiased information
- Encouraging and facilitating family-to-family support and networking
- Understanding the developmental needs of infants, children, and adolescents and their families and incorporating them into health-care systems
- Implementing comprehensive policies and programs that provide emotional and financial support to families
- Designing accessible health-care systems that are flexible, culturally competent, and responsive to family-identified needs

(National Center for Family-Centered Care [1990]. Bethesda, MD: Association for the Care of Children's Health.)

---

children become tyrants. Some parents do not understand the normal developmental changes that take place over time with their child and try to infantilize them. Some parents become burned out with the amount of work required and become neglectful or abusive. All these situations require tremendous skill on the part of the nurse. The whole family is truly the client when a child is chronically ill.

In addition to the high-technology care of enteral feedings, intravenous infusions, and mechanical ventilation previously described, some children are on home apnea monitoring. Premature infants, those at high risk for sudden infant death syndrome, and children who have experienced a life-threatening event during sleep are candidates for apnea monitoring (Humphrey & Milone-Nuzzo, 1996). Parents must learn infant pediatric basic life support before the baby leaves the hospital. Both the nurse and the apnea monitor vendor need to visit often to monitor the situation and reinforce teaching.

Children with cystic fibrosis or other cardiopulmonary dysfunctions often need oxygen in the home. Again, regular monitoring and careful teaching regarding safety precautions with oxygen administration must be supplied by intermittent visits from the home care nurse. Children with end-stage conditions who may be within 6 months of dying should be referred to a hospice. Many services are available to the child and the family at a hospice, and hospice teams develop great skill in helping children and families adjust to death and dying.

Infants sometimes require colostomies for rectal atresia, imperforate anus, or Hirschsprung's disease. Inflammatory bowel disease (ulcerative colitis or Crohn's disease) sometimes requires a colostomy in older children. These colostomies may be temporary or permanent. Occasionally a subtotal colectomy or ileostomy may be performed to cure ulcerative colitis. Then the surgeon fashions a blind pouch called a Kock pouch, which aids in continence of the liquid stools. Whenever possible, an ileoanal pull-through procedure is done to preserve the normal defecation pathway (Wong, 1993). Urinary diversions are necessary for some children with birth defects, neurogenic bladder, or other conditions causing severe ureteral, bladder, or renal damage. As a urinary diversion, a continent Kock pouch reservoir is fashioned from a loop of intestine to form a pouch to collect urine. The pouch contains a nipplelike one-way valve through which a catheter is inserted every few hours to drain the urine (Fig. 15-4). Many home care agencies have enterostomal specialists on their staff to help teach the family or to act as a resource to the primary nurse. They are familiar with all the products and procedures available to prevent skin breakdown and other problems with ostomies.

The acuity of the child and the teaching needs of the family define visit frequency in pediatric home care. Sometimes the primary nurse must persist with the case manager for extra visits if the family has managed-care coverage. Nurses and equipment vendors must be available around the clock. Home health aides are often needed to provide respite, and the nurse should seek other sources of respite care in the community for weekends or evenings. Parents become exhausted and require full service from the agency, including a social worker to help them discuss their many concerns and problems.

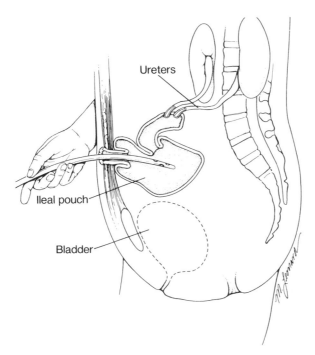

FIGURE 15-4

Continent ileal urinary reservoir (Kock pouch). Urine collects in the pouch and is drained by inserting a catheter through the valve. (Smeltzer S, Bare B [1996]. *Brunner and Sud-darth's Textbook of Medical-Surgical Nursing*, 8th ed. Philadelphia: Lippincott-Raven.)

Maternal–Infant Home Care

The first days at home with a new infant are extremely stressful. Early hospital discharges mean that hospital teaching is cut short, despite the requirement that new mothers be allowed to stay in the hospital 2 days. Learning is reduced because the mother is exhausted, anxious, and still recovering from the birth experience. In our mobile society, the extended family may no longer live nearby to lend support. Many mothers today are single parents or teenage parents. A postpartum nursing visit for all cases is very important for these reasons, and many hospitals are providing them.

In many communities, the health department's public health nurses traditionally make free postpartum visits in actual or potential high-risk maternal-infant situations. The intent is to mobilize needed resources and intervene with health promotion measures as early as possible to prevent the development of serious disease or social problems such as child abuse.

A Normal Postpartum Home Visit

During the visit, perform a complete health history and examination on both the mother and the infant. Assess fundal height, lochia, breasts, episiotomy, and vital signs. Assess the mother's energy level and the amount of sleep she has been receiving. Identify the mother's knowledge and experience, and continue the teaching begun in the hospital. Usually the mother has several questions if she has been at home with the infant for a day or two and may want to discuss problems or potential problems. Provide information about helpful community resources, such as La Leche League if she is breastfeeding.

Check any equipment, such as a breast pump, as well as all medications taken by the mother or infant. Be certain that the mother knows how to proceed if something untoward happens and that she has appropriate telephone numbers and follow-up appointment dates.

Evaluate the environment for safety and hygiene. Assess the mother's bonding with the infant and discuss any issues that need special attention. Assess how the mother holds and talks to the infant and about the infant. Carefully examine the infant, including hydration status, sucking impulse, color, reflexes, bowel and bladder functioning, feeding pattern, vital signs, and height and weight. Be sure to have a physician's order and the mother's signed consent for any procedures performed, such as phenylketonuria testing or light therapy for neonatal physiologic jaundice. Make arrangements for follow-up visits if problems or potential problems exist.

High-Risk Pregnancy Home Care

Home care may be required for various pregnancy complications, such as preterm labor, pregnancy-induced hypertension, diabetes, and hyperemesis gravidarum. The latter may require intravenous replacement therapy at home to maintain adequate hydration. Assess the effects of medications and bedrest. Compliance with a program of bedrest is usually improved when the client is on a home care program. Home care programs in these situations can prevent hospitalization and reduce costs. More importantly, the number of low-birthweight, premature infants is reduced as a result of home care for high-risk pregnant women.

Psychiatric–Mental Health Home Care

Most home care agencies are hiring experienced psychiatric nurses to care for clients with psychiatric diagnoses at home. Increasingly, clients of all ages with mental health problems are referred for home care. Often these clients have one or more medical conditions in addition to their primary psychiatric diagnosis. To be eligible for Medicare or other third-party payments, four criteria must be met:

1. The client must have a psychiatric diagnosis based on the *Diagnostic and Statistical Manual IV*.
2. The client must need the special services of a psychiatric nurse.
3. The plan of care must be under the direction of a psychiatrist.
4. The client must be essentially homebound.

See Display 15-5 for other criteria.

There are many nonphysical reasons why clients might be homebound. Their mental status may make it difficult or even risky for them to leave home. Examples include panic attacks, agoraphobia, risk for suicide or self-harm, intense anxiety, altered thought processes, poor judgment and impulse control, confusion and disorientation, depression with severe psychomotor retardation, vulnerability, and need for constant supervision because of conditions such as dementia or mental retardation. Home care allows clients to remain in their familiar, safe environment and still receive the care they need.

Most of these clients are elderly and depressed. Many have schizophrenia. Others are manic-depressive or have severe anxiety disorders. Various psychiatric diagnoses are seen in home care clients. Medical conditions such as AIDS may compound their problems, and they become isolated and depressed. The elderly often live alone and want to maintain their independence. An estimated 20% to 25% of elderly persons have significant mental health problems, especially depression (Junginger et al, 1993). An estimated 20% of all suicides occur in the elderly population (McBride & Burgerer, 1994). Persons living at home with an exacerbation of schizophrenia frequently become more autistic and respond to hallucinations and delusions instead of maintaining their medication regimen and their human contacts. These people need monitoring and support to keep them out of the hospital.

Agoraphobia is another reason that people become homebound. Panic attacks plague 2% of the general population, more than most people realize. These clients become homebound because of anticipatory anxiety and excessive fears. They cannot seek ambulatory care for their disorders at a clinic or a physician's office. Experienced psychiatric home care nurses can monitor their situation and report back to their psychiatrist.

Psychotropic medication knowledge is quite involved and requires the skill of an experienced mental health nurse. New initiatives in home care provide opportunities for psychiatric nurses to use their special skills out in the community. A master's degree is not required for this role. Registered nurses with 2 years of psychiatric experience in adult or geriatric psychiatric settings can provide reimbursable services. A nurse with a baccalaureate degree requires only 1 year of prior psychiatric experience. A nurse

---

DISPLAY 15-5
Admission Criteria for Home-Based Psychiatric Services

- Be medically stable so as to be an active participant in a goal-oriented interdisciplinary home program
- Present evidence of potential for significant improvement
- Demonstrate significant functional disability resulting from the recent onset or diagnosis of an acute condition or an exacerbation of a chronic condition:
  - Dementia: impairment in ability to recall and retain information
  - Impaired judgment and impulsiveness
  - Behavior that is socially unacceptable or possibly dangerous
  - Disorientation as to place, time, and person
  - Aggressiveness–both verbal and physical–toward others
  - Disturbed thought processes: hallucinations (auditory and visual) or delusions; poor reality testing
  - Suicidal ideation and attempts
  - Severe withdrawal and isolation due to depression
  - Somatic disturbances due to excessive anxiety, such as tachycardia or gastrointestinal dysfunction
  - Overuse and abuse of medication and other substances
  - Severe withdrawal in both a social and emotional respect as a result of mistrust
  - Severe regression in behavior, thought, and relationships (eg, total neglect of basic physical needs)
  - Autistic thinking: illogical interpretation of reality
  - Suspiciousness: fear of others or of leaving home
  - Anxiety: a sense of threat that immobilizes the person to take action
  - Ambivalence: being unable to make life decisions without assistance
  - Phobias: acrophobia and claustrophobia
  - Confusion following surgery, strokes, cancer, hip fractures, and falls
  - Agitation
  - Behavioral or emotional problems associated with the presence of physical illness, drug–drug interactions, resulting side effects, and other toxic reactions

(Spaeksta S, Fitzgerald M [1996]. Home-based psychiatric services. Home Health Care Management & Practice 9[1]:40–48. © 1996, Aspen Publishers, Inc.)

---

with a master's degree in psychiatric or community health nursing requires no additional experience to work in this role. Medicare will reimburse advanced nursing care for therapy as well as assessment and evaluation.

THE NURSE SPEAKS . . .
About Caring for a Client Requiring High-Tech Home Care

Amy was injured at C-1, C-2 in a bus accident when she was 11 years old and became quadriplegic. She spent the following 2 years in the hospital and has been on home care for 3 years with 24-hour nursing care. Amy is intelligent and in many ways reacts like a normal teenager. Her parents tend to infantilize Amy, mainly due to her disability but also because of their culture. They immigrated to the United States from Asia when Amy was a baby. They find Amy's assertiveness and striving for independence deeply disturbing. One example is that Amy insists her hair be washed and styled daily. She asks that her parents buy her contact lenses. She wants frequent manicures and constantly asks her nurses to take her shopping or to the movies. As nurses, we view these behaviors as normal for adolescents. Viewing the family as the client, we seek to interpret Amy's behaviors and help the family deal with her and with their anxiety. Amy tends to manipulate them and play on the guilt they feel regarding her disability.

Amy reclines about 30 degrees in her wheelchair to support her neck. She controls her chair by use of a sip-and-puff device. Amy requires a tracheostomy and a ventilator for survival. The ventilator is a small machine that attaches to the back of her wheelchair. A special valve allows her to speak. Amy attends school and participates in Girl Scouts. If she develops mucus during school, I remove her from the classroom for suctioning. The suction machine is portable. I always carry a sterile suctioning pack with me, plus catheterization equipment. I time Amy's intermittent catheterizations at lunchtime and other breaks to avoid disrupting her school schedule. The evening nurse performs her bowel routine. I am constantly on guard for and respond immediately to any signs of respiratory problems.

The other day, one of those unexpected things happened when I was least expecting it. Amy had a cold, so I especially watched her respiratory status. Suddenly she started to perspire profusely. She complained of a pounding headache. I quickly wheeled her into the hallway and took her vital signs. Her blood pressure was 222/104 mm Hg. I yelled for someone to call 911 as I rushed her into the ladies' room, checked her abdomen for distention, and loosened all her clothing. I gently checked for fecal impaction (minimizing stimulation), and her rectum was empty. I catheterized her and checked her pulse frequently. The paramedics arrived; according to standard routine, they took over and I stepped back, continuing to comfort Amy. Her blood pressure dropped to 110/70 mm Hg and her pulse was 64, because her abdominal distention had been relieved. Therefore, an intravenous infusion was not started, nor did we need to call the physician for an order for emergency antihypertensive medication (which would have been the case had she not responded so quickly). Autonomic dysreflexia had been the last thing on my mind that morning, but one has to be alert for any eventuality when nursing complex cases. Amy may have had a cerebrovascular accident if the dysreflexia had not been treated immediately.

I conferred with the supervisor at my agency about ways to prevent similar episodes in the future. We analyzed and reviewed the daily schedule to see what adjustments might be made to the plan of care to avoid potential autonomic stimulation through abdominal distention and constrictive clothing or even shoes. After conferring with the physician and receiving an order, we decided to add "catheterize with Credé" to the plan. Credé is the application of external, hard, manual pressure over the bladder to empty the bladder completely and avoid residual pockets of urine. We also added a nursing order to the care plan about avoiding tight diapering, clothing, and shoes.

It's not enough to treat the immediate condition. A nurse needs to think about prevention of potential future problems as well.

Betty
VISITING NURSE

CLINICAL APPLICATION

A Critical Thinking Case Study About a Hospice Client in Pain

You are a hospice nurse assigned to assess and admit Carol Adams, age 48, to the hospice program. You find a distraught family awaiting your arrival. Mrs. Adams' husband, Harry, brings you into a large, airy bedroom where Mrs. Adams is sitting up in bed. Four months ago, she was diagnosed with pancreatic cancer. Mrs. Adams seems anxious and exhausted. You introduce yourself, slowly explaining hospice services and what you will be doing during this visit. You notice that Mrs. Adams cringes when she repositions herself in bed.

 and Think!

- How should you proceed?
- What are your priorities?

You stop explaining hospice services and state, "Mrs. Adams, you appear to be in pain."

Mrs. Adams replies, "I'm taking Percocet. Until the weekend, one tablet every 4 or 6 hours helped, but now I need two every 4 hours and I still have pain. I'm awake all night. The pain in my back is so bad that I get out of breath. I didn't think it would get this bad." On further assessment, Mrs. Adams quantifies the pain as a 9 on a scale of 0 to 10 (0 being no pain and 10 being the most severe pain). She adds that she has no allergies to any medications and took morphine in the hospital for 2 days via a patient-controlled analgesia (PCA) pump with good effect. You ask Mrs. Adams permission to call her physician and do so immediately, reporting the increase in pain.

On hearing your pain assessment, the physician orders morphine (Roxanol) 10 mg orally every 4 hours and has her discontinue the Percocet. You teach Mrs. Adams and her husband about Roxanol: the dose, how to administer it, and its side effects. You also teach the importance of taking the Roxanol around the clock and not only as needed for pain.

 and Think!

- Why not just give the Roxanol as needed, rather than around the clock?
- Doesn't that increase the chance that Mrs. Adams will become addicted to morphine?
- Because she had good results using the PCA pump in the hospital, why not use that at home rather than just oral Roxanol?
- Why teach Mr. and Mrs. Adams about the side effects of Roxanol?
- Won't that just frighten them and induce Mrs. Adams to take less medication than she needs?

You explain to them that the best pain control comes with maintaining an adequate, constant blood level of morphine rather than using it only as needed. Potential addiction is not a consideration or a problem in terminally ill clients: less than 1% of hospice clients have become addicted, because need is related to physical pain, not compulsive, psychological dependence. A PCA pump is more complex for the family to use and considerably more expensive than oral Roxanol. It is best to use the simplest, most cost-effective method of pain control as long as it is effective. If it becomes ineffective, more complex measures can be used.

Explaining side effects is very important. Changing to a different narcotic can cause increased lethargy, slight confusion, and occasionally nausea and vomiting. These effects tend to clear up within 48 hours. If the client and family know about them in advance, they are more apt to follow the regimen. Patient education promotes a sense of control and helps combat some of the overwhelming feelings of powerlessness that hospice clients and families often feel.

You explain the physician's order to implement a bowel regimen of Senokot S, one or two tablets daily as needed. On further assessment, Mrs. Adams says that she had been quite constipated but had a bowel movement of small brown pellets yesterday. You instruct her to start the bowel regimen this evening.

 and Think!

- Why is Mrs. Adams receiving Senokot S?
- Specifically, how does it act?
- What is the mechanism that causes Mrs. Adams to be constipated?

Mrs. Adams is obviously exhausted from the pain. You postpone most of the assessment and teaching reinforcement until the next visit. You reassure them that hospice's main goal is to keep her comfortable. You ask Mr. Adams for some background history and other information in the living room. You also meet their two grown daughters, one of whom already went to get the Roxanol and Senokot S, supplied by the hospice program. You tell the family about the availability of 24-hour, 7-day-a-week hospice support, explain hospice services, and tell them you will return the next day.

The following day you find Mrs. Adams a little sleepy but more comfortable. She now rates her pain as a 6, so you call the physician to increase the Roxanol dose to 20 mg. Visits during the next week find Mrs. Adams increasingly comfortable. The pain has subsided, but now Mrs. Adams complains of a constant achiness in her hips. With a diagnosis of bone metastasis, this is not surprising. Again you phone the physician, and he increases the morphine dose.

 and Think!

- What is the purpose of using adjuvant medications when there is no ceiling dose on the amount of morphine that can be used?

You know that morphine is often not very effective in controlling bone pain. You ask the physician if choline magnesium trisalicylate (Trilisate) might be tried, and he orders Trilisate 1 gram orally, three times a day. Within 48 hours, Mrs. Adams remarks that she feels like getting up and about. The Roxanol is switched to long-acting morphine (MS Contin, 60 mg), which she takes every 12 hours. She continues to use the Roxanol for occasional breakthrough pain as needed and continues the Trilisate.

Because Mrs. Adams is more comfortable, she is able to prepare advance directives so that her wishes are carried out should she become confused. She does not want an aide or family member calling 911, because the responding paramedics will then be forced to resuscitate her. A "do not resuscitate" order should be part of the advance directives and must be signed by the physician and available in the home for the responding paramedics.

Mrs. Adams and her family are now ready to receive other services. Mrs. Adams requests that the hospice chaplain visit her to discuss and pray about some of her unresolved questions about dying at such a young age. A hospice volunteer visits once a week to read to Mrs. Adams and give her husband respite. As she weakens, home health aide time is increased and needed equipment, such as a commode and hospital bed, is supplied by the hospice. You stay in close touch with them. The family requests bereavement services and receives some counseling both before and after Mrs. Adams' death. Afterward, they join a bereavement support group for several months.

During the final weeks of Mrs. Adams' life, she was comfortable and alert enough to enjoy her family. The quality of her life had greatly improved and she was able to die with dignity. The family derived great comfort from the knowledge that they were able to care for their loved one at home.

Chapter SUMMARY

Hospice programs are growing rapidly. They seek to enable "good" death and dying by comforting and supporting clients and caregivers. To become eligible for services, clients must be declared to be within 6 months of dying by their physician and no longer pursuing active treatment. Hospice teams include spiritual caregivers and many volunteers who provide direct client services and other assistance. Sophisticated pain control has become a hallmark of hospice care. The analgesic steps and adjuvant and coanalgesic drugs are supplemented by nonpharmacologic pain control measures.

High-technology home care includes enteral therapy, infusion therapy, and mechanical ventilation, as well as other specialized services. Home care nursing assessment should begin in the hospital so that the agency is sure that it can handle the complicated care. Also, the nurse must be thoroughly familiar with all equipment and procedures.

Pediatric home care often involves high technology as well, including apnea monitors. Some hospitals and health departments provide maternal-newborn home visits for normal postpartum assessment and teaching. More often, these visits are done only when problems in the postpartum course have occurred or are anticipated. High-risk pregnancy care is another specialized form of service.

Psychiatric–mental health home care is a growing field, requiring nurses with psychiatric experience. Severe depression, schizophrenia, dementia, agoraphobia, and panic attacks are common problems seen in home care. Psychiatric-mental health nurse clinicians are reimbursed for performing psychotherapy as well as for assessment and evaluation.

A list of references and additional readings for this chapter appears at the end of Part 4.

16

Home Care Legal and Ethical Issues and Improvement of Quality Management

Key Terms

advance directive
artificial life support
artificial nutrition
assisted suicide
benchmarking
beneficiaries
brain death
cardiopulmonary resuscitation (CPR)
chart audits
Choice in Dying
concurrent audits
conditions of participation
continuous quality improvement (CQI)
default mode

"do not resuscitate" (DNR) procedures
durable power of attorney
emergency medical services
euthanasia
Hastings Institute
health-care proxy
incident reporting
instructive directives
liability lawsuits
living will
mission statement
notarized
Omnibus Reconciliation Act of 1990
organ and tissue donation

outcome assessment
participatory management
Patient Self-Determination Act
process assessment
quality assessment
quality assurance
rescinded
retrospective audits
risk management
structure assessment
subpoenaed
surrogate
total quality management (TQM)
United Network for Organ Sharing

Learning Objectives

1. Differentiate between advance directive, living will, instructive directive, health-care proxy, and durable power of attorney.

2. Explain the value of advance directives.

3. Outline the process for developing advance directives.

4. Describe potential problems with "do not resuscitate" procedures in home care.

5. List reasons why not all organ donations can be transplanted.

6. Discuss the pros and cons of legalizing assisted suicide.

7. Differentiate between quality care, quality assurance, quality assessment, quality improvement, and total quality management.

8. Explain how structure, process, and outcome assessments are performed.

9. Describe the value of thorough documentation in total quality management.

10. Define the components of risk management.

11. Discuss the relation between utilization management and the future of a home health agency.

Home Care Legal and Ethical Issues

The same legal issues that apply in other areas of nursing (eg, confidentiality, informed consent, negligence, incidence reporting, and witnessing of documents) also affect home care. Home care nurses are frequently asked to witness legal documents unrelated to home care. Agencies usually discourage nurses from doing so because they may later be called to testify if the document is contested. The issue of abandonment often comes up in home care when a client's insurance has run out or if the safety situation in the home is such that home care services cannot continue. Providing adequate advance notice or suggestions regarding other sources helps negate legal or ethical charges of abandonment.

Advance Directives

Advance directives are written statements that indicate what a person wants or does not want done if in the future he or she becomes unable to make health decisions. Advance directives are valuable tools. They can help protect a client's right to choose care. They can help families by relieving them of the stress and responsibility of having to make difficult decisions on a client's behalf if the client cannot communicate his or her wishes. They help health-care providers by giving guidance for the care desired at the end of life. Without advance directives, the "default mode" is that the equipment goes in, whether it be a feeding tube, an intravenous infusion, or a ventilator. Unfortunately, once started, it is extremely difficult to terminate such lifesaving equipment; it often requires a lengthy legal struggle to obtain a court order to terminate. Courts tend to favor treatment, and families cannot have machines turned off without consent unless the client left clear, convincing evidence of the desire to be allowed to die.

The Patient Self-Determination Act

The federal government in 1990 passed the Patient Self-Determination Act, which is part of the Omnibus Reconciliation Act. This act mandates that all health-care agencies provide information verbally and in writing about the client's right to self-determination. The act states that clients have the right to accept or refuse medical care. Clients also have the right to prepare advance directives in compliance with state law. Nurses must state in the client's chart whether the client has executed advance directives. Clients who are alert can make decisions and communicate about whether or not they want medical care.

The Value and Components of Advance Directives

The advance directive is designed to identify a course of treatment or nontreatment in situations in which the client cannot make decisions or communicate. It is important to consider one's values before creating advance directives. It is not always easy to ask clients to imagine themselves near death and to address certain questions about how they want to die. Nurses encourage clients to talk with health-care providers, family and friends, members of the clergy, or their attorney about their values, such as whether or not they want to prolong life, regardless of the chances of recovery. They ask about religious faith and beliefs about life after death, the desire to die without prolonged suffering, and attitudes about leaving the family with good memories and without difficult burdens.

There are two types of advance directives, which may be called by slightly varied titles in different states: living wills or instructive directions (Fig. 16-1) and health-care proxies, surrogates, or durable power of attorney (Fig. 16-2). These documents can be changed by a competent client at any time. Either type of directive comes into effect if and when the client becomes incompetent to decide or unable to communicate and will not regain that ability. Choice in Dying, the leading volunteer organization devoted to advance directives, offers advance directive forms and information on laws in all states (Display 16-1). Their address is on the resource list in Appendix C and their web site is http://www.choices.org.

Living Wills

Living wills, also called instructive directives in some states, are legal throughout the United States. However, states vary in the manner and format in which they recognize living wills and health-care proxies. It is best to use a living will form specific to the state where the client lives. Home care nurses usually give these forms to clients when they discuss advance directives with them. Living wills allow clients to limit certain life-prolonging measures when there is little or no chance of recovery. Advance directives can also specify instructions about pain relief. Limitations of life-saving measures include:

Cardiopulmonary resuscitation (CPR)
Infusion therapy (intravenous or total parenteral nutrition) providing fluids, nutrients, or medications
Feeding tubes (nasogastric or G-tubes)
Mechanical ventilation
Dialysis, when kidney shutdown has occurred
Medications that are curative, not palliative

It is best to be as specific as possible when writing a living will. Saying, "No extraordinary measures" is not specific enough, because that can be defined differently by different people.

FLORIDA LIVING WILL

Print the date
Print your name

Declaration made this _____ day of _____, 19_____.
I,_____, willfully and voluntarily make known my desire that my dying not to be artificially prolonged under the circumstances set forth below, and I do hereby declare:

If at any time I have a terminal condition and if my attending or treating physician and another consulting physician have determined that there is no medical probability of my recovery from such condition, I direct that life-prolonging procedures be withheld or withdrawn when the application of such procedures would serve only to prolong artificially the process of dying, and that I be permitted to die naturally with only the administration of medication or the performance of any medical procedure deemed necessary to provide me with comfort care or to alleviate pain.

It is my intention that this declaration be honored by my family and physician as the final expression of my legal right to refuse medical or surgical treatment and to accept the consequences for such refusal.

In the event that I have been determined to be unable to provide express and informed consent regarding the withholding, withdrawal, or continuation of life-prolonging procedures, I wish to designate, as my surrogate to carry out the provisions of this declaration:

Print the name, home address and telephone number of your surrogate

Name: _____
Address: _____
Zip Code:_____ Phone: _____

I wish to designate the following person as my alternate surrogate, to carry out the provisions of this declaration should my surrogate be unwilling or unable to act on my behalf:

Print the name, home address and telephone number of your alternate surrogate

Name: _____
Address: _____
Zip Code:_____ Phone: _____

Add personal instructions (if any)

Additional instructions (optional):

I understand the full import of this declaration, and I am emotionally and mentally competent to make this declaration.

Sign the document

Signed: _____

Witnessing procedure

Two witnesses must sign and print their addresses

Witness 1:
   Signed: _____
   Address: _____

Witness 2:
   Signed: _____
   Address: _____

Courtesy of Choice in Dying, Inc.   6/96
200 Varick Street, New York, NY 10014 212-366-5540

FIGURE 16-1
A sample living will. (Choice in Dying, Inc. © 1996. Reprinted with permission.)

Instructions	FLORIDA DESIGNATION OF HEALTH CARE SURROGATE

Print your name

Name_____

      (Last)   (First)   (Middle Initial)

In the event that I have been determined to be incapacitated to provide informed consent for medical treatment and surgical and diagnostic procedures, I wish to designate as my surrogate for health care decisions:

Print the name, home address and telephone number of your surrogate

Name: _____
Address: _____
Zip Code:_____ Phone: _____

If my surrogate is unwilling or unable to perform his duties, I wish to designate as my alternate surrogate:

Print the name, home address and telephone number of your alternate surrogate

Name: _____
Address: _____
Zip Code:_____ Phone: _____

I fully understand that this designation will permit my designee to make health care decisions and to provide, withhold, or withdraw consent on my behalf; to apply for public benefits to defray the cost of health care; and to authorize my admission to or transfer from a health care facility.

Add personal instructions (if any)

Additional instructions (optional):

I further affirm that this designation is not being made as a condition of treatment or admission to a health care facility. I will notify and send a copy of this document to the following persons other than my surrogate, so they may know who my surrogate is:

Print the names and addresses of those who you want to keep copies of this document

Name: _____
Address: _____

Name: _____
Address: _____

Sign and date the document

Signed: _____
Date: _____

Witnessing procedure

Two witnesses must sign and print their addresses

Witness 1:
    Signed: _____
    Address: _____

Witness 2:
    Signed: _____
    Address: _____

FIGURE 16-2
Sample designation of surrogate form. (Choice in Dying Inc. © 1996. Reprinted with permission.)

DISPLAY 16-1
Talking About Choices

- Get the information you need to make informed choices about end-of-life treatments.
- Discuss your thoughts, concerns, and choices with your family and close friends.
- Talk to your doctor about different treatments.
- Obtain copies of advance directives (a living will and a medical power of attorney) for your state.
- Choose a trusted family member or close friend who is willing to be your advocate if you cannot speak for yourself. Appoint this person as your health-care agent.
- Complete the advance directives that follow your state's law.
- Talk to your health-care agent, family, and doctor about your choices. Discuss your choices often, especially when your medical condition changes.
- Keep your completed directives in an accessible place.

(Reprinted by permission of Choice in Dying, 200 Varick St., New York, NY 10014, 212-366-5540; http://www.choices.org)

Health Care Proxies or Agents or Durable Power of Attorney

Naming a trusted person to make decisions about life support or other issues of medical care is important regardless of one's age, because at any time accidents and illnesses can occur that cause total brain injury. A health-care proxy form must be signed and dated in the presence of two witnesses. The proxy or beneficiaries of the client's estate should not act as witnesses. The proxy also must be informed of the wishes stated in the living will. The only statement recommended for this document is, "My agent knows my wishes concerning artificial nutrition and hydration." No other statements are recommended because they might unintentionally restrict the agent's (proxy's) power to act in the client's best interests. If special circumstances arise that may not be covered in a living will, the appointment of a health-care proxy, who can respond flexibly, is very important.

Of the two advance directives, appointment of a health-care proxy is more important than a living will, provided the agent has been well informed of the client's wishes.

What to Do With Documents After They Are Completed

Advance directives should be signed, dated, and witnessed or notarized in accordance with the regulations of the state where the client lives. Copies should be given to the health-care proxy, the family, the physician, and the attorney. The client should carry a wallet card indicating where the advance directive is located. Advance directives should be reviewed regularly and updated if necessary. Copies should be included on medical charts.

"Do Not Resuscitate" Statements and Procedures

Some clients want to include a "do not resuscitate" (DNR) statement with their advance directive. A DNR order indicates that no basic or advanced cardiac life support efforts will be initiated in the event of cardiac or respiratory arrest. This includes chest compressions, artificial breathing, intubation, or emergency medications. The client must be 18 years of age or older and must understand the nature and consequences of life support procedures and the consequences of a DNR order. The client must have the ability to make a reasoned decision or have a health-care proxy. The life-sustaining measures must carry no medical benefit and be futile. A DNR order must be written on the physician's order sheet, demonstrating that the physician concurs with the client's wishes.

Nonhospital DNR Forms

DNR orders have been in existence in hospitals for several years, and since 1995 they have been available for clients receiving home care services (Display 16-2). Clients must be mentally alert and competent when preparing statements about DNR and must have a health-care proxy to act on their behalf when they are no longer able to do so. The physician must be in concurrence with an informed consent and must write the DNR order on the chart. Family members and other caregivers must be informed of the DNR decision. Special DNR home care forms must be used in the 23 states where they are valid.

Occasionally situations occur when a DNR decision is not honored. The physician's order may be rescinded at any time on request and notification of the closest family member or guardian of an incompetent client. Sometimes someone ignorant of the DNR order will call emergency medical services to do CPR when the DNR order is not prominently displayed in the home. Another tragic situation is when a family member calls 911 for oxygen assistance or suctioning. Once the ambulance is called, the paramedics must take the client to the hospital for examination by a physician. This is true of hospice clients as well. Even when DNR orders, living wills, and health-care proxies exist and are shown to the paramedics, they are legally required to transport such clients to the hospital, even for treatments known to be futile. Paramedics can lose their certification unless they transport these clients. This is required because DNR and advance directives are not legally valid in emergencies in the home (Shapiro, 1995). All such clients and their caregivers should be strongly urged not to call the paramedics; they should call the home care or hospice agency instead.

Organ and Tissue Donation

One person's gift of organs and tissues can benefit many people. Heart, lungs, kidneys, eyes, pancreas, liver, skin, bone marrow, and bone can all be harvested from one donor. Because of the great shortage of organ donors, many persons want make this one of their last legacies. Most religions support organ donation. Potential organ recipients are identified on a national computer system coordinated by the United Network for Organ Sharing.

Display 16-2

Do Not Resuscitate Home Care Form

Patient Name: _____

Address: _____

_____

_____

Rescue Squad and/or First Responder to Medical Emergency

D N R
DO NOT RESUSCITATE

You are Authorized to Comply With This DNR Order.

The Above-Named Patient is on Community Hospital's Home Care Program.

This Patient and/or Family and Physician have Deemed that the DNR
Order is Appropriate, Due to the Patient's Terminal Illness and
Expected Death. However, the Patient and Family may Revoke this
Order at any Time and it is Valid Unless Rescinded.

MD_____Date_____
(Signature)

MD Name_____
(Print)

The Home Care Staff has instructed the family to call Home Care with
any questions or problems, 24 hours a day. Please call us prior
to initiating any treatments or transport:

622-8000	8:00 am – 4:00 pm
or	4:00 pm – 8:00 am
622-2000	(ask operator to contact Home Care nurse on call)

ORGAN DONOR CARD

—————————————————————————————————————
PRINT OR TYPE NAME OF DONOR

In the hope that I may help others, I hereby make this anatomical gift, if medically accept-able, to take effect upon my death. The words and marks below indicate my desires.

I give:　　(a) _____ any needed organs or parts
　　　　　　(b) _____ only the following organs or parts

—————————————————————————————————————
Specify the organ(s) or part(s)

for the purposes of transplantation, therapy, medical research or education;

　　　　　　(c) _____ my body for anatomical study if needed.

Limitations or special wishes, if any: _____

A

Signed by the donor and the following witnesses in the presence of each other:

————————————————————————　————————————————————
Signature of Donor　　　　　　　　　　　　Date of Birth of Donor

————————————————————————　————————————————————
Date Signed　　　　　　　　　　　　　　　City and State

————————————————————————　————————————————————
Witness　　　　　　　　　　　　　　　　　Witness

This is a legal document under the Uniform Anatomical Gift Act or similar laws.

For further information consult your physician or

UNOS　PO Box 13770; RICHMOND, VIRGINIA 23225

B

FIGURE 16-3
An organ donor card. (**A**) Front of card. (**B**) Back of card.

Potential organ donors usually carry a donor card in their wallet (Fig. 16-3) or sign their driver's license regarding their intent. It is important to inform the next of kin of this intent, because he or she will probably be asked about organ donation and may refuse. The next of kin must be informed that the donor's body is treated with dignity and utmost respect. The removal of organs is carried out as a regular surgical procedure and does not interfere with customary burial arrangements.

Not everyone's body can be used for organ and tissue donation. Only healthy organs can be transplanted; infections, metastatic cancer, and other conditions such as jaundice, as well as disease of the specific organs needed, may preclude donation. Generally, a healthy young person who suffers brain death is the optimal donor because the other organs and tissues remain healthy if the donor has been on artificial life support systems. Once these support systems have been turned off, the transplantation process must proceed with dispatch to prevent the death of tissues from hypoxia.

Assisted Suicide

Dr. Jack Kevorkian makes the news from time to time because of the controversy surrounding his assistance with suicides. He claims that persons have a right to end their lives when their lives no longer have any quality and are dominated by suffering. He also claims that physicians should assist persons who wish to die, and he demonstrates this conviction by assisting with many suicides. He has been public in his actions in an attempt to challenge the laws that make assisted suicide illegal.

The northern territory of Australia legalized assisted suicide under certain circumstances. Oregon is the only state in the United States that has passed a Death With Dignity Act. This act, approved by public vote, legalizes physician-assisted suicide for qualified clients. However, that decision is being challenged in the courts, so it is not being implemented. In August 1995, a judge ruled that the law violated the equal protection clause of the Constitution's 14th Amendment. Supporters of Oregon's Death With Dignity Act are appealing that ruling. Five other states (North Carolina, Ohio, Utah, Virginia, and Wyoming) are unclear concerning the legality of assisted suicide. New York and Washington have passed laws specifically outlawing assisted suicide (Price & Mauro, 1997). In June 1997, the Supreme Court upheld the right of New York and Washington to ban assisted suicide, indicating that assisted suicide is not a basic right in the United States. At the same time, the right to keep a terminally ill client comfortable by using whatever dose of analgesic is necessary was reaffirmed. In Oregon, citizens again voted in favor of legalizing assisted suicide in November 1997 (Associated Press, 1997).

Assisted suicide is an extremely complex issue with strong arguments on both sides. Assisted suicide simply means that a physician supplies the means for a client to commit suicide. Hospice nurses say that quality of life can be maintained in the final days with good pain management and adequate psychosocial and spiritual support. Good hospice care could make most potential assisted suicides unnecessary. In Nazi Germany, assisted suicide soon led to active euthanasia. At first, people who wanted to die, who were suffering a great deal, and whose lives were "devoid of all quality and meaning" were helped to commit suicide, but with time health-care professionals willingly participated in active euthanasia programs, with less and less emphasis on the client's rights or willingness to die. Soon mentally retarded or physically disabled persons and persons with chronic mental illness were involuntarily killed because the Nazi government decided their lives were "devoid of all quality and meaning."

> In 1941 the psychiatric institution Hadamar celebrated the cremation of the ten-thousandth mental patient in a special ceremony. Psychiatrists, nurses, attendants and secretaries all participated. Everyone received a bottle of beer for the occasion. (Wertham, 1980)

The word "euthanasia" means "a good death" or "mercy killing." Once choice was omitted from the criteria, it was no longer either merciful or good. Nor was it such a big step to proceed to a program of genocide, a program of mass killing. The Nazi program of so-called racial cleansing led to the extermination of millions of persons across Europe.

Of course, active euthanasia is very different from assisted suicide. These examples of the potential corruption of mercy killing might seem extreme, but many people fear corruption of legal assisted suicides in more subtle ways. They may wonder, "Will

Grandma feel subtly pressured to request an assisted suicide when she senses that her care is a burden to the family?''

Others argue that assisted suicide seems to be a natural outflow of the Patient Self-Determination Act of 1990, which gives each person rights regarding his or her body. All experienced nurses know of situations in which patients wanted to end their lives. Sometimes dying becomes an agonizingly long process, even when the client is not suffering pain. Dr. Kevorkian says he always applies certain criteria in selecting his cases to prevent abuse and future corruption.

The Hastings Center on Bioethics has developed guidelines on the termination of life-sustaining treatment and care of the dying. Copies of their report may be secured by contacting the Hastings Institute (see Appendix B).

Quality Management in Home Care

''Quality care'' is a term often heard in the current health-care climate. Quality, like excellence, is difficult to define, but everyone readily recognizes quality or excellence when observing or experiencing it. Accreditation is considered a mark of excellence, indicating that an agency has met stringent criteria set by an independent source such as the Joint Commission on Accreditation of Healthcare Organizations (JCAHO) or the Community Health Accreditation Program (see Chap. 13). Quality assurance programs have been in effect for more than 20 years in many health-care institutions. Usually a small group of personnel are assigned to that task; most of their work focuses on chart audits under the assumption that whatever was done or not done was reflected in the chart. In 1992, the JCAHO changed its terminology: because quality can never be assured, the term ''quality assessment'' was introduced. Since then, most health-care institutions refer to efforts to achieve quality care as ''quality improvement programs.''

Measuring Quality Care

Agencies vary a great deal in the ways they measure quality (Figs. 16-4 and 16-5). Traditionally, three dimensions have been assessed: structure, process, and outcome. Together, they thoroughly measure the quality of care provided by an agency.

1. Studying the *structure* focuses on the framework of the agency, including the organizational structure, staffing patterns, equipment resources, and communication systems. The mission statement, objectives, and employment criteria define the attitudes and purposes of an agency. In assessing quality in structure, what is written in the philosophy is compared with what actually exists in the agency.
2. Nursing practice and skill are assessed in the *process* dimension. Appropriate use of the nursing process is reviewed, as is the work of other members of the home care team, including home health aides. In particular, the relationship between nurses and their clients is studied to learn how much the clients and caretakers are involved in planning and other decisions. Clients and caretakers are sometimes interviewed or mailed a survey. Charts are audited. Thorough documentation is vitally important to the whole quality assessment program.

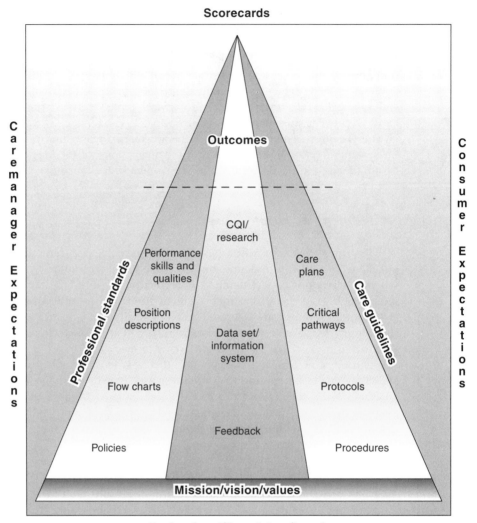

FIGURE 16-4
Organizing framework for quality care. (Peters D [1995]. Outcomes: the mainstay of a framework for quality care. *J Nurs Qual Care* 10[1]:63; © Aspen Publishers, Inc.)

Concurrent audits are performed while the client is still receiving services. Retrospective audits are done with clients who have been discharged. The latter usually provide a more complete picture of the way the nursing process was carried out for a given client; however, concurrent audits allow an opportunity to improve the care for that client if needed.

3. The assessment of outcomes is discussed later in this chapter.

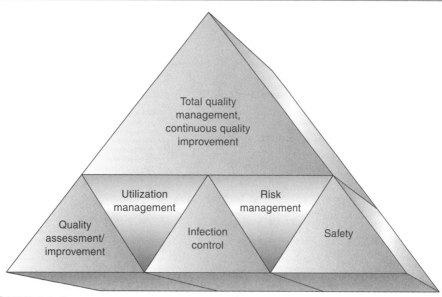

FIGURE 16-5
Integrated quality management. (From Koch MW, Fairly TM [1993]. *Integrated Quality Management: The Key to Improving Nursing Care Quality.* St. Louis: Mosby.)

Performance Appraisal

Each home care nurse's performance and productivity is evaluated periodically by a supervisor. Feedback should be given on an informal and regular basis. When the more formal, written performance evaluation is shared with the nurse, it should contain no surprises. Display 16-3 is an example of a worksheet used to evaluate nursing practice. Display 16-4 shows a productivity measurement classification that identifies the most important elements to be appraised.

Benchmarking is a system used to analyze and measure clinical quality, efficiency, and productivity. Factors such as travel time, client acuity, documentation time, and case administrative tasks all need to be considered in home care. These are useful in making staff assignments and in establishing the number of nurses needed (Gingerich & Zimmerman, 1996).

Chart Audits and Client Surveys or Complaints

Chart audits are valuable because charts contain vital information about all aspects of the client's care. The criteria for quality care are determined beforehand, and the nursing care reflected in the chart is measured against those criteria. A quarterly review of clients' charts is required by the Medicare conditions of participation. Nurses within the agency, both supervisory and staff, perform this quarterly chart review; nurses are careful to avoid reviewing the charts of their own clients. Nursing supervisors are also involved in process assessment with staff on an ongoing basis and when giving periodic

DISPLAY 16-3
Evaluation Worksheet

EXAMPLE OF CRITICAL ELEMENT = PRACTICE MANAGEMENT

Expert in health assessment skills

Skill present?   At what level?

yes   no   1   2   3   4

Organized in approach to time and tasks

Skill present?   At what level?

yes   no   1   2   3   4

Able to analyze a situation and develop an appropriate plan

Skill present?   At what level?

yes   no   1   2   3   4

Able to make independent decisions

Skill present?   At what level?

yes   no   1   2   3   4

Able to deal w/problems in priority order

Skill present?   At what level?

yes   no   1   2   3   4

Able to adjust daily client schedule if unexpected problems occur

Skill present?   At what level?

yes   no   1   2   3   4

Delegates nonnurse tasks to support personnel

Skill present?   At what level?

yes   no   1   2   3   4

For category **Practice Management,** are areas of knowledge and abilities integrated into the visit structure (eg, integrates skills during the visit without wasting time or materials)?

yes   no

Note. 1 = limited skill, 2 = acceptable, 3 = proficient, 4 = expert; use the same format for each critical element of productive practice.
(Benefield L [1996]. Productivity in home healthcare. Home Healthcare Nurse *14[10]:803—812.)*

performance evaluations to staff members. Clients are surveyed informally and formally, and client complaints are studied carefully.

The Importance of Outcome Evaluation and Outcome-Based Care

Measuring the changes in a client's status is called outcome assessment. Client goals are called expected outcomes and are developed and stated in measurable terms. The last stage of the nursing process is evaluation of the expected outcomes. The trend in health care is to look at outcomes as "the bottom line." Managed care is outcome-driven. Clinical pathways are based on the achievement of predetermined outcome steps along the pathway to recovery. For instance, if a diabetic client has not learned to do diabetic foot care, the expected outcome has not been met, regardless of how

DISPLAY 16-4
Productivity Measurement Classification

PRACTICE MANAGEMENT

*Expert in health assessment skills
*Organized in approach to time and tasks
*Able to analyze a situation and develop an appropriate plan
*Able to make independent decisions
*Able to deal with problems in priority order
Able to adjust daily client schedule if unexpected problems occur
Delegates nonnurse tasks to support personnel

KNOWLEDGE/SKILL MAINTENANCE

*Hands-on technical skills in area of practice
*Understands how physical processes of illness and associated complications relate to the client
Able to update technical skills and knowledge of unfamiliar diseases and conditions

WRITTEN DOCUMENTATION

*Completes paperwork tasks to meet Medicare (and other payers) and agency requirements and deadlines

HOME HEALTH-CARE KNOWLEDGE

*Understands rules and regulations governing home health care
*Background in principles of teaching client and family
Knowledge of nutrition teaching

COMMUNICATION

*Good interpersonal communication skills with client and family, staff, and physicians
Uses referrals to other agency services and community resources to meet client needs when appropriate
Able to be a "marketing person" for the agency
Keeps supervisor informed of major changes in clients
Understands the structure of the agency

NURSING PROCESS

Foundation in formulating nursing diagnoses and measurable goals for client care

CLIENT AND FAMILY MANAGEMENT

*Provides clear direction to clients during visits
Deals in realistic and practical ways with situations confronting clients
Activities are planned and implemented based on treatment goals for the client.
Views client as part of a family and community
Encourages client and family independence when necessary
Demonstrates empathy for the client
Recognizes and deals with family concerns related to the client's health problem
During visits, gives time to both psychosocial and physical care
Does not force own values on client and family

*Among most important.
(Benefield L [1996]. Productivity in home healthcare. Home Healthcare Nurse *14[10]:803—812.*)

many times the nurse presented an excellent teaching session about diabetic foot care (process assessment) and regardless of how thoroughly the agency allotted time (structure assessment) or scheduled a diabetic nurse specialist to educate that client. This example demonstrates how all three dimensions (structure, process, and outcome) should be included in an accurate assessment of quality care. Without assessing structure, one might assume that the agency limited the number of visits so that the client could not adequately learn. Without assessing process, one might assume that the nurse did a poor job of teaching. If the client chose not to learn the procedure for some reason beyond the control of the home care agency, the care provided should not reflect poorly on the agency.

Assessments should not be judgmental; rather, they should be a means of data collection. Of course, accountability for outcome achievement is an issue. Once data have been collected, patterns are usually analyzed for facts that signal the need for action or change. For example, in the situation above, a pattern might be noted that the diabetic clients who did not learn to do foot care also had osteoarthritis, which caused them considerable discomfort when they leaned over to do foot care. Therefore, they tended to neglect it and readily forgot how to do it.

Working together on problems such as this leads the home care staff to try to find other ways to enable clients to achieve the needed outcomes. Perhaps a family member or a friend can be enlisted to help, and the client and the nurse can instruct together. This is the most cost-effective way to achieve the goal. If the client has no one to call on for assistance, a home health aide may be assigned to work with the client doing foot care. The assumption here is that a second expected outcome is that this client will take some responsibility for self-care of diabetes.

In *Readings in Community Health Nursing* (1997, p. 279), Spradley and Allender wrote:

> Quality assurance, quality management, and quality improvement are terms used to describe what nurses have always thought they were delivering—a system of quality nursing care. However, this may not always be the case. Another factor, cost of care, is an issue more recently of concern to community health nurses and their agencies. When these two issues are reckoned with, how nursing care is planned, delivered, documented, and evaluated must change. By using a conceptual framework for organizing all the relevant practice components, such as professional standards, protocols, critical paths, and care plans, the delivery of quality care can be measured more effectively.

Total Quality Management

Total quality management (TQM) performance improvement involves the entire agency staff actively working together. Industries with TQM programs demonstrate that this can be an exciting and beneficial process for everyone concerned. It is not a yearly or quarterly event, such as the licensing or certification reviews, but instead is an ongoing, daily process throughout the entire agency. It is a client-centered process that seeks the best possible care to meet client outcomes. All the staff participate. It is a continuing process that includes data collection, analysis, planning, implementation, and evaluation. Planning is prioritized and focused. Data are objective and measurable and are not based on opinion, tradition, or favorite myths. TQM is a system of participatory management. Staff members conduct research and participate in peer review. All nurses and other staff are involved in formulating the agency's mission statement, or at least are aware of it. This climate enables the staff to express opinions freely without fear of repercussions. As they monitor their own work without defensiveness, they share a vision for improvement. This places the responsibility for quality management on each person. The agency provides each staff member with employee education and productivity training.

Major changes within an agency are carefully designed based on an impact study and information from other agencies. The persons most affected are involved in planning the change process. A comprehensive improvement in organizational performance occurs in five steps: designing the process, systematically measuring data, analyzing the data collected, developing a plan for improvement, and then implementing and evaluating the plan. Nurses will recognize this as another use of the nursing process.

TQM or continuous quality improvement (CQI) mean essentially the same thing, except that TQM goes further than CQI. There has been a significant shift in philosophy in the 1990s with the advent of TQM. Instead of an evaluation process that focuses on solving problems that result from errors by staff members, TQM focuses instead on designing systems or processes that improve outcomes, using a positive approach. It is the integrated program and synergistic approach that makes TQM so successful. In a home care agency, that integrated approach would includes infection control, risk management, utilization management, and quality assessment and improvement (Koch & Fairly, 1993). The first component, an infection control program, was discussed in Chapter 14. The process of monitoring an agency's quality for accreditation and licensing purposes was presented in Chapter 13.

Risk Management

Activities that help minimize adverse effects of loss of human, physical, and financial assets are collectively called risk management. Home care agencies must have a policy and procedure in place to identify potential problems or risks to clients or staff and to remove, reduce, or prevent those risks. Risk management is challenging in clients' homes, where the environment is not controlled by the nurse and there is no supervision of care when the nurse is not present. Unsafe or abusive situations or noncompliance situations, in which the client ignores the physician's orders, raise questions of potential liability for health-care providers. Because home care agencies cannot support unsafe situations, sometimes the only thing that can be done is to discharge the client to an extended-care facility or another more supportive, better supervised arrangement.

Incident reporting is the most common way to identify risk. A written description of an actual or potential client injury (or perception by the client or family that an injury has taken place) is called an incident report. Any untoward event or adverse outcome is communicated in writing on the report. A description of the incident, an identification of the cause, and a corrective plan are the three steps in incident reporting (Hughes, 1996). Ideally, the latter will reduce future risk. Incident reports are not filed on the client's charts, where they could be easily subpoenaed in a liability lawsuit. Incident reports are not mentioned in the nurse's notes on the chart where the situation might be recorded. Incident reports legally protect the agency and the nurse because memory of details may be unreliable several months later. All nurses should be strongly encouraged to file incident reports when untoward things happen to clients or staff.

Utilization Management

Utilization management is an important component of TQM. Overuse of services is wasteful and is one of the reasons why health-care costs in the United States are excessively high. Unnecessary services are no longer reimbursed by third-party payers, so the agency must absorb the cost. When this happens frequently, the financial survival of the agency will be in serious danger. However, underuse of services can inhibit achievement of expected outcomes. It is important to provide the exact amount and type of services, equipment, and supplies required. This constitutes quality management.

THE NURSE SPEAKS . . .
About Caring for a Client With Breast Cancer

I work for a hospital-based home health agency. One of my clients, Louise, was a widow with breast cancer. I visited Louise daily for dressing changes because her breast cancer evolved into a 2″ open wound like raw meat. The strong, foul odor from this wound caused social isolation because Louise was embarrassed to have friends visit. She was receiving chemotherapy and was having some adverse effects. Her physician said the cancer was not yet in any vital organs so that Louise could live many months, making her ineligible for hospice. Fortunately, Louise's pain was well controlled.

One of my first goals was to reduce the odor. I had Louise shower with liquid Dial soap, which helped. I conferred with the hospital's enterostomal nurse specialist, who suggested charcoal dressings. I obtained an order for these from the doctor. They reduced the odor a great deal and made all of us much more comfortable.

Louise's only son was in the military. I learned that her deep fear was that she might die before her son's next leave and she would not see him again. "I must talk to him and explain some important things about the past. I'm so afraid I won't see him again. The doctor assures me that it's unlikely because I'm going to live quite a while yet, but I have a strong feeling that I'm going to die soon. I can't get it out of my mind. It keeps me awake at night," she confided."

I decided to contact the Red Cross to see if the son could be brought home early. He was serving on a ship in the Middle East. The Red Cross explained that they would arrange to bring Louise's son home if her doctor would sign a form certifying that the situation were critical. At first the doctor would not do this, saying that Louise was not terminally ill and still had several months to live. I called the doctor again, telling him how much Louise wanted and needed to see her son. I added that the son should visit while Louise is alert, for the sake of both of them. I stressed that Louise believed that she would soon die. The doctor respected that and decided that he could ethically sign the form, certifying an emergency. Within 1.5 days after I took that form to the Red Cross office, the son was home with her! The Red Cross is amazing!

Louise and her son had some wonderful days together, with many long talks. He helped her prepare her advance directives, which she had refused to do earlier. She told me earlier that she was afraid to do so, as if the preparation of advance directives would hasten her death. She added that she had felt she had to stay alive to see her son. A few days later she seemed to let go, went downhill rapidly, and slipped into a coma. Two weeks later Louise died peacefully, with her son at her bedside. He was able to be there to plan and attend her funeral.

Kathy
HOME CARE NURSE

CLINICAL APPLICATION

A Critical Thinking Case Study About Client Safety

You recently transferred from the intensive care unit (ICU) to the home care department in your hospital to get away from the high stress of ICU nursing. You find your role in home care to be quite different, but equally stressful and demanding in a different way.

One day you are assigned to visit Mrs. Dougherty, age 54, who was discharged yesterday with casts on the right arm and leg from fractures of the radius, humerus, and fibula. When you approach the house, three large dogs start barking ferociously, jumping and snarling at the windows. Mr. Dougherty lets you inside when the dogs are controlled. As you enter, your heart sinks: the room is cluttered and filthy, the air is stagnant, and the odor is rank. Mrs. Dougherty is in a bed in the dining room. Walking to her bed, you almost step in dog feces as you try to avoid empty beer cans scattered on the floor. You see cockroaches crawling on the walls. Your first thought is that you must not sit or put your nursing bag down.

 and Think!

- Why should you not set your bag down?
- What are your responsibilities about this environment?
- What can you do about it?

You begin interviewing Mrs. Dougherty while holding your nursing bag. Her husband answers most of the questions for her. When she speaks, she looks at him for approval. He expresses great annoyance because you arrived too early (10 AM), before he'd had a chance to clean up. You explain that you usually call first but they have no telephone. You notice the smell of alcohol on his breath. Mrs. Dougherty is totally helpless with her casted right extremities. She keeps repeating that her husband takes wonderful care of her and he is a wonderful man. Her bed smells of dried urine and there is a bedpan containing urine on the dining-room table.

You explain that you must go get something from your car. You leave your nursing bag in the car lest cockroaches or other vermin get into it. You put in your pockets only the few things you need, plus some paper towels to set things on in the bed if needed. You use hand wipes to clean your hands because the sink is full of dirty dishes and caked food. You take her vital signs, which are normal, and check her right toes and fingers, which are pink and warm. You note several bruises on her body as you complete your examination.

 and Think!

- What can you do to help this client and improve this situation?
- Do you think this situation is safe?

Your referral form says that the client was sent home with the following medications: oxycodone with acetaminophen (Percocet) 1 tablet every 6 hours as needed for pain, clonazepam (Klonopin) 0.5 mg twice daily and 1 mg at bedtime, nizatidine (Axid) 150 mg twice daily, thiamine 1 tablet once daily, and ferrous sulfate 250 mg twice daily. The first two drugs were missing, and Mr. Dougherty says that you must get them for his wife right away because she is in pain. At first the couple insist they never received Percocet and Klonopin. You say you will notify the hospital pharmacy. Mr. Dougherty suddenly remembers that the medications came in a separate pink bag. You both search for the pink bag, but it is not found.

 and Think!

- How are Percocet and Klonopin different from the other medications on your referral form?
- What are the implications of controlled drugs?
- What is the implication for your client?
- What will you do about her pain?
- How can you assess whether or not she has had any Percocet?
- What is the husband's role in all of this?

You assess that Mrs. Dougherty has been quite comfortable during your visit and comment about this. Mr. Dougherty answers that he just gave her aspirin before you arrived. You note that her pupils are constricted and suspect that she did receive some Percocet. You explain that you will return this afternoon after talking the situation over with the doctor.

 and Think!

- What is your assessment?
- Whom should you call first before calling the doctor?
- What other community agency should you contact before calling the doctor?
- What should you do about the housekeeping situation?
- What are the husband's needs, and can you provide for them?

You assess that the environment is just too unsafe for Mrs. Dougherty: no amount of home care services can compensate for the environmental deficits. You suspect an addiction problem with the husband and possibly with Mrs. Dougherty also. You also fear potential abuse of Mrs. Dougherty. Using your car phone, you call your supervisor for guidance because of your relative inexperience with home care situations. Her line is busy, so you call adult protective services and ask if Mr. and Mrs. Dougherty are known to them. They are, but this is the only information they will give you. Reaching your supervisor, you are advised to return to the office to call the doctor and try to arrange for Mrs. Dougherty to be admitted to a long-term care facility while her fractures heal and she is helpless. You notify your other scheduled clients that you will be delayed, and you postpone one client visit until tomorrow.

You are told by your supervisor that you must accept an unclean environment if this is the way these clients habitually live, but you must not help to maintain a client in an unsafe situation. Mr. and Mrs. Dougherty may deny the lack of safety, so you will use your good communication skills when you return to inform them of the plan. They have no telephone and no close neighbors who can give them a message.

You inform the couple that Mrs. Dougherty will be admitted this afternoon to a long-term care facility. Mrs. Dougherty appears relieved, but her husband expresses resistance until informed that their insurance plan will cover the costs until her casts are removed and she is mobile again. It is possible that you will be asked to visit this family again when Mrs. Dougherty is discharged. It is vitally important to continue to be respectful, regardless of your opinion of their lifestyle. If you can build a therapeutic, trusting relationship, the clients may be more open to your suggestions. You might even be able to refer Mr. Dougherty for treatment for his probable addictions and lack of impulse control if they trust you, but you should understand that this is a remote, future possibility. In the meantime, you send your report with recommendations for Mr. Dougherty to adult protective services in the hope that they will be instrumental in getting him to seek treatment.

Chapter SUMMARY

Legal and ethical issues in home care are basically the same as in other types of nursing practice. Abandonment charges may be more common and can be prevented by giving adequate advance notice before home care services are terminated.

Advance directives are important to ensure that clients' wishes are respected regarding high-technology, life-sustaining care near the end of life. Living wills describe the specific services desired or refused. Health-care proxies are agents designated to make decisions if the client cannot communicate. DNR statements and physician orders are important components of advance directives. Some people like to include organ and tissue donation wishes also.

Assisted suicide is a complex ethical and legal issue. Only the state of Oregon has voted in favor of legalizing assisted suicide, and that vote was challenged in the courts. New York and Washington have outlawed assisted suicide. The Supreme Court decided that it is not a constitutional right, so state law prevails.

Various methods are used to measure quality home care. Of the three dimensions used—structure, process, and outcome—the latter is most important, but all have value. Appraisal of nursing care and productivity is part of the process dimension and should be ongoing. Total quality management involves all staff members in the constant improvement of quality care delivered by an agency. Quality management includes quality assessment and improvement, utilization management, infection control, risk management, and safety.

Quality care with cost containment are the watchwords of health care as we enter the 21st century. They are not mutually exclusive: they can be accomplished with nurses playing a vital role in the process.

A list of references and additional readings for this chapter appears at the end of Part 4.

References and Additional Readings

Agee B (1996). How to write clear instructions. *RN* 59(11):26–28.

Ahmann E (1996). *Home Care for the High-Risk Infant*. Frederick, MD: Aspen.

Albrecht M et al (1993). The Albrecht nursing model for home healthcare. *J Nursing Admin* 23(1).

Amenta M (1996). Hospice nursing and managed care. *Home Healthcare Nurse* 14(10):815–816.

Amenta M (1995). The challenge to hospice nurses for the future. *Home Healthcare Nurse* 13(5):7.

American Nurses Association (1992). *A Statement on the Scope of Home Health Nursing*. Washington DC: The Association.

American Health Consultants (1994). *Hospital Home Health*. Atlanta: AHC.

American Psychiatric Association (1994). *Diagnostic & Statistical Manual of Mental Disorders*, 4th ed. Washington DC: APA.

Associated Press (November 5, 1997). Election roundup. Time-News, p. 11A.

Bailey S (1994). Creativity and the close of life. In Corless B, Pillman M. *Dying, Death and Bereavement: Theoretical Perspective and Other Ways of Knowing*. Boston: Jones and Barlett.

Behrendt D (1996). *Clinical Guidelines for Managed Home Care*. Frederick, MD: Aspen.

Benefield L (1996). Component analysis of productivity in home care RNs. *Public Health Nursing* 13(4):233–243.

Benefield L (1996). Productivity in home healthcare: Maintaining and improving nurse performance. *Home Healthcare Nurse* 14(10):803–812.

Berrio M, Levesque M (1996). Advance directives: Most patients don't have one. Do yours? *AJN* 96(8):24–29.

Beschle J et al (1995). Interviews with home health aides caring For people with AIDS. *Home Healthcare Nurse* 13(6):20–24.

Birdsall C, Sperry S (1997). *Clinical Paths in Medical-Surgical Practice*. St. Louis: Mosby.

Bishop E, McNally G (1993). An in-home crisis intervention program for children and their families. *Hosp Commun Psychiatry* 44:182.

Blazek L (1993). Development of a psychiatric home care program and the role of the CNS in the delivery of care. *Clinical Nurse Specialist* 7(4):164–168.

Bobnet N et al (1993). Continuous quality improvement: Improving quality in your home care organization. *J Nursing Admin* 23(2).

Borton D (1997). Isolation Precautions: Clearing Up the Confusion *Nursing 97* 27(1):49–51.

Boyle P (1997). *Getting Doctors to Listen—Ethics and Outcome Data in Context*. Baltimore: Georgetown University Press.

Bradshaw M, Gary G (1993). Patient outcomes measure home health care accomplishments. *Nurs Management* 24(5).

Brent N (1996). Managed healthcare and the home healthcare nurse in the 1990s: Selected legal implications. *Home Healthcare Nurse* 14:100–101.

Brent N (1994). Healthcare reform: Implication for home healthcare nursing and agencies. *Home Healthcare Nurse* 12(1):24–29.

Broussard M, Pitre S (1996). Medication problems in the elderly: A home healthcare nurse's perception. *Home Healthcare Nurse* 14(6):441–443.

Burrell L et al (1997). *Adult Nursing Acute and Community Care*, 2d ed. Stamford, CT: Appleton & Lange.

Callahan M, Kelly P (1992). *Final Gifts: Understanding the Special Awareness Needs and Communications of the Dying*. New York: Poseidon Press.

Canobbio M (1996). *Mosby's Handbook of Patient Teaching*. St. Louis: Mosby.

Carefoote R (1994). Total quality management implementation in home care agencies. *J Nursing Admin* 24(10):31–37.

Carr P (1993). Implications of the implementation of the Patient Self-Determination Act for nurses in the field. *Home Healthcare Nurse* 10:53–54.

Certification of Insurance Rehabilitation Specialists Commission (1993). *CCM Certification Guide— Certification for Case Managers.* Orlando, FL.

Choice in Dying (1996). Medical treatments and your advance directives. *Choices* 5(2). New York: Choice in Dying.

Choice in Dying (1996). Exploring the issue of physician-assisted dying. *Choices* 5(3). New York: Choice in Dying.

Choice in Dying (1996). Dying at home. *Choices* 5(2). New York: Choice in Dying

Clemen-Stone S et al (1995). *Comprehensive Community Health Nursing.* St. Louis: Mosby.

Cody C (1996). Hospice update: The support study. *Home Care Nurse News* 3(1).

Community Home Health Accreditation Program (1993). *Standards of Care for Home Care Organizations.* New York: NLN.

Considine C (1996). Measurement of outcomes: What does it really mean? *Home Healthcare Nurse* 14(6):417–418.

Consumers Union (1996). Medicare HMOs: Luring the elderly. *Consumers Report* 61(10):30–31.

Consumers Union (1996). How good is your health plan? *Consumers Report* 61(8):28–42.

Corbett C, Androwich I (1994). Critical paths: Implications for improving practice. *Home Healthcare Nurse* 12(6):27–34.

Davidhizar R, Shearer R (1996). Using humor to cope with stress in home care. *Home Healthcare Nurse* 14(10):825–830.

Davis E (1994). *Total Quality Management for Home Care.* Gaithersburg, MD: Aspen.

Davis L, Grant J (1994). Constructing the reality of recovery: Family home care management strategies. *Adv Nurs Sci* 17(2):66–76.

De la Cruz F (1994). Clinical decision-making styles of home healthcare nurses. *Image J Nurs Scholarship* 26:222–226.

Dee-Kelly P et al (1994). Managed care. *Nurs Clin North Am* 29(3):471–473.

DeGroot-Kosolcharoen J (1996). Solving the infection puzzle with culture and sensitivity testing. *Nursing '96* 26(9):33–40.

Deming W (1986). *Out of Crisis.* Cambridge, MA: MIT Press.

Demos M (1994). *Risk Management in Health Care* (cassette tape). Tampa: Am Bd Utiliz Review & Qual Assur Physicians.

Deutsche-Cohen M (1996). *Dirty Details: The Days and Nights of a Well Spouse.* Philadelphia: Temple University Press.

Doheny M, Cook C, Stopper M (1997). *The Discipline of Nursing.* Stamford, CT: Appleton & Lange.

Doherty M, Hurley S (1994). Suburban home care. *Nurs Clin North Am* 29(3):483–493.

Donabedian A (1993). *Models of Quality Assurance*, Eighth Annual Symposium on Home Health Care. Ann Arbor: University of Michigan School of Nursing.

Dossey B (1996). Help your patient break free of anxiety. *Nursing '96* 26(10):52–54.

Doughty D (1991). Urinary and fecal incontinence. St. Louis: Mosby.

Doyle R et al (1994). Healthcare Management Guidelines Volume 4: *Home Care and Case Management.* Radnor, PA: Milliman & Robertson Inc.

Drattel A (1996). *The Other Victim.* Santa Ana, CA: Seven Locks Press.

Ellenbacker C, Shea K (1994). Documentation in home health care practice. *Nurs Clin North Am* 29(3):495–506.

Emlet C et al (1995). *In-Home Assessment of Older Adults: An Interdisciplinary Approach.* Frederick, MD: Aspen.

Facente A (1996). Is there life after hospital nursing? *Home Healthcare Nurse* 14(2):117–122.

Fairly T (1994). Caring for chronic pain patients. *Continuing Care* 13(4):14–15.

Fazzi R, Agoglia R (1995). What home care executives should know about managed care organizations: Preliminary results from a national study. *Caring* 14:78–85.

Ferrell B (1996). Managing advanced cancer pain. *Nursing '96* 26(10):28.

Finkelman A (1997). *Psychiatric Home Care.* Frederick, MD: Aspen.

Finn J (1995). Hospice defined: One vision of the future. *Hospice Update: Academy of Hospice Physicians Newsletter* 5(2).

Fischer L (1997). Lessons in home care. *RN* 60(3):55–56.

Fitzpatrick J, Shinners M (1996). How to make assessing as easy as ABC. *Nursing '96* 26(8):51.

Freedman B (1996). Respectful service and reverent obedience: A Jewish view on making decisions for incompetent parents. *Hastings Center Report* 26(4):31–37.

Friedman M (1996). Accreditation and the nurse. *Home Healthcare Nurse.* 14(2):108–110.

Friedman M (1996). Competence assessment: How to meet the intent of the Joint Commission on Accreditation of Healthcare Organization's Management of Human Resources Standards. *Home Healthcare Nurse* 14(10):771–774.

Friend A (1995). Wake-up call for home care providers: Managed care decision-makers tell what they want and what they're willing to pay. *Home Healthline Report* Feb. 13.

Garcia E (1996). Moving change through the system: A model for staff involvement. *MCN* 21(5):219–221.

Gates M et al (1996). Applying advanced directives regulations in home care agencies. *Home Healthcare Nurse* 14(2):127–133.

Gates R, Fink R (1997). *Oncology Nursing Secrets.* St. Louis: Mosby.

Gattera J et al (1994). A retrospective study of risk factors of akathesia in terminally ill patients. *J Pain Symptom Management* 9(7):454–461.

Gilbert N (1994). Home care aides' perceptions of their interactions with community health nurses. *Caring* 13:24–28.

Gingerich B (1996). Home health care reengineered. *Home Health Care Management & Practice* 8(2):1–5.

Gingerich B, Ondech D (1994). *Discharge Planning for Home Health Care.* Frederick, MD: Aspen.

Gingerich B, Ondech D (1995). *Clinical Pathways for the Multidisciplinary Team.* Gaithersburg, MD: Aspen.

Glick D (1994). The relationship between demographic characteristics and nursing problems in home health care. *Public Health Nurse* 11(4):259–267.

Goldberg M (1995). If we're lucky the patient will complain. *AJN* 53.

Goldrick B, Larson E (1993). Wound management in home care: An assessment. *J Commun Health Nursing* 10(1).

Gooldy J, Duncan B (1994). Home care's role in clinical pathways. *J Home Care Practice* 6(2):63–69.

Gorrie TM, McKinney ES, Murray S (1994). *Maternal-Newborn Nursing.* Philadelphia: WB Saunders.

Green K (1996). *Home Health Aide Training Manual.* Frederick, MD: Aspen.

Gregory D, English J (1994). The myth of control: Suffering in palliative care. *J Palliative Care* 10(2): 18–22.

Greifzu S. Grieving families need your help. *RN* 59(9):22–28.

Gurfollino V, Dumas V (1994). Hospice nursing. *Nurs Clin North Am* 29(3):533–548.

Haddad A et al (1993). Teamwork in home infusion therapy. *Home Healthcare Nurse* 11(1).

Hall J et al (1995). Standardized care plan: Managing Alzheimer's patients at home. *Gerontological Nursing* 211(1):37–47.

Hanley E (1997). Hospice services for home care clients. In Zang S, Bailey N. *Home Care Manual.* Philadelphia: Lippincott-Raven.

Harper D (1997). High-tech home care. In Zang S, Bailey N. *Home Care Manual.* Philadelphia: Lippincott-Raven.

Harris M (1994). Home healthcare nursing is alive, well and thriving. *Home Healthcare Nurse* 12:17–20.

Harris M (1996). Medicare managed care. *Home Healthcare Nurse* 14(2):185–187.

Harris M (1997). *Handbook of Home Health Care Administration*, 2d ed. Gaithersburg, MD: Aspen.

Harvey C (1994). New systems: The restructuring of cancer care delivery and economics. *Oncol Nurs Foundation* 21(1):71–72.

Health Care Financing Administration (1994). *Conditions of Participation for Home Health Agencies.* Washington DC: USDHHS.

Health Care Financing Administration (1996). *Your Medicare Handbook.* Baltimore: USDHHS.

Health Care Resources (1996). *Handbook of High-Risk Perinatal Home Care.* St. Louis: Mosby.

Hester L (1996). Coordinating a successful discharge plan. *AJN* 96(6):35–37.

Heximer B (1996). Spontaneous balloon rupture: troubleshooting G-tubes. *RN* 59(7):22–28.

Home Health Care Revenue Report (1995). *Preparing for Capitation in Home Health Care.* Gaithersburg, MD: Aspen.

Home Health Care Update (1995). *Nursing '95* July:57–59.

Hospice Nurses Association (1996). Ethical issues in the hospice admission process. *Fanfare* 9(4):7.

Hospice Nurses Association Standards and Accreditation Committee (1994). *Standards of Hospice Nursing Practice and Professional Performance.* Pittsburgh: Hospice Nurses Association.

Huber H, Spatz A (1994). *Homemaker/Home Health Aide,* 4th ed. Albany, NY: Delmar Publishers.

Huber R (1994). Relationship Between right-to-die and satisfaction with life. *Am J Hosp Palliat Care* 11(5):13–18.

Hughes A (1996). The impact of risk management and the importance of effective incident/complaint reporting. *Home Health Care Manage Prac* 8(2):32–36.

Humphrey C (1994). *Home Care Nursing Handbook.* Gaithersburg, MD: Aspen.

Humphrey C, Milone-Nuzzo P (1996). *Manual of Home Care Nursing Orientation.* Gaithersburg, MD: Aspen.

Hunt R, Zureck E (1997). *Introduction to Community-Based Nursing.* Philadelphia: Lippincott-Raven.

Huston C, Boelman R (1995). Autonomic dysreflexia. *AJN* June.

Idemoto B et al (1993). Implementing the Patient Self-Determination Act. *AJN* 93(1):20–25.

(1995). *Illustrated Guide to Home Health Care.* Springhouse, PA: Springhouse.

Jaffe M, Skidmore L (1997). *Home Health Nursing Care Plans.* St. Louis: Mosby.

Jaffe M, Skidmore-Roth L (1997). *Home Health Nursing: Assessment and Care Planning.* St. Louis: Mosby-Year Book.

Jirovec M, Dornbrook B (1996). The usefulness of the HCFA Form 485 in predicting home healthcare costs. *Home Healthcare Nurse* 14(6):471–477.

Johanson G (1994). *Physicians' Handbook of Symptom Relief in Terminal Care,* 4th ed. Santa Rosa, CA: Sonoma County Academic Foundation for Excellence in Medicine.

Johnson M, Maas M (1997). Nursing outcomes classification (NOC). St. Louis: Mosby.

Joint Commission on Accreditation of Healthcare Organizations (1995). *Accreditation Manual for Home Care.* Oakbrook Terrace, IL: JCAHO.

Jones D, Churchill J (1994). Archetypal healing: Psycho-spiritual relief of pain in the terminally ill. *Am J Hosp Palliat Care* 11(1):26–33.

Junginger J, et al (1993). Prevalence of psychopathology in elderly persons in nursing homes and in the community. *Hospital and Community Psychiatry* 44:381.

Kauffman J (1995). *Awareness of Immortality.* Amityville, NY: Baywood.

Kelly J et al (1993). AIDS deaths shift from hospital to home. *Am J Publ Health* 83:1433–1437.

Kemp C (1995). *Terminal Illness: A Guide to Nursing Care.* Philadelphia: JB Lippincott.

Kennedy G (1995). The geriatric syndrome of late-life depression. *Psychiatr Services* 6(1):43.

Kertesz L (1995). Medicare: The final frontier of HMOs. *Modern Healthcare* 25:76–84.

Klagsbrun SC (1994). Patient, family and staff suffering. *J Palliat Care* 10(2):14–17.

Klebanoff N (1993). Psychosocial home care. In Johnson B. *Psychiatric-Mental Health Nursing,* 3d ed. Philadelphia: JB Lippincott.

Koch M, Fairly T (1993). *Integrated Quality Management.* St. Louis: Mosby.

Kontzamanis E (1997). The role of the nurse. In Zang S, Bailey N, eds. *Home Care Manual.* Philadelphia: Lippincott-Raven.

Kubler-Ross E (1969). *On Death and Dying.* New York: Macmillan.

Larocca E (1994). *Handbook of Home Care IV Therapy.* St. Louis: Mosby.

Lavin J, Enright B (1996). Charting with managed care in mind. *RN* 59(8):47–48.

Leasia S, Monahan F (1997). *A Practical Guide for Health Assessment.* Philadelphia: WB Saunders.

Liaschenko J (1994). The moral geography of home care. *Advancements in Nursing Science* 17(2):16–26.

Lutz B (1996). Total parenteral nutrition in the older patient. *Home Healthcare Nurse* 14(2):123–125.

Mann L et al (1995). Home care management guidelines: Expect a lot from both nurses & patients. *Home Health Line* Jan. 30:4–7.

Marrelli T (1994). *Handbook of Home Health Standards and Documentation Guidelines for Reimbursement,* 2d ed. St. Louis: Mosby.

Marrelli T, Hilliard L (1996). *Home Care and Clinical Paths.* St. Louis: Mosby.

Martin K et al (1993). Home health clients: Characteristic outcomes of care and nursing interventions. *Am J Public Health* 83(12):1730–1734.

Martin P, Strain J (1995). The ethics of artificial hydration and nourishment. *Fanfare* 9(3):16–17.

Maturen V, VanDyck L (1996). Using outcome-based critical pathways to improve documentation. *Home Health Care Manage Prac* 8(2):48–58.

Maturen V, Zander K (1993). Outcomes management in a prospective pay system. *Caring* 12(6).

Matz B, Gary G (1993). Patient outcomes measure home health care accomplishments. *Nurs Management* 42(5).

McBride AB, Burgener S (1994). Strategies to implement geropsychiatric nursing curricula content. *Journal of Psychosocial Nursing Mental Health Services* 32(4):13–18.

McCaffery M, Beebe A (1989). *Pain: Clinical Manual for Nursing Practice.* St. Louis: Mosby.

McCloskey JC, Bulechek GM (1996). *Iowa Intervention Project: Nursing Interventions Classification (NIC).* St. Louis: Mosby.

McClure G (1994). Home health networks, alliances and acquisitions. *Caring* 13:48–53.

McCormick K, Moore S, Siegel R (1994). *Methodology Perspectives: Clinical Practice Guideline Development.* USDHHS PHS.

McHann M (1995). *What Every Home Health Nurse Needs to Know.* New York: Springer.

McKinnon B (1994). Home TPN. *Continuing Care* 13(4):26–29.

Medicare Home Health Statistics (1996). *Home Health Care Digest* 2(9).

Melum M, Sinioris M (1993). Total quality management in health care. *Quality Manage Health Care* 1(4):59–63.

Mendler V et al (1996). The conception, birth and infancy of an early discharge program. *MCH* 21(4):241–246.

Messenger T, Roberts K (1994). The terminally ill: Serenity nursing interventions for hospice clients. *J Gerontological Nursing* 20(11):17–22.

Mignor D (1996). Management and evaluation of a care plan. *Home Healthcare Nurse* 14(6):163–165.

Milone-Nuzzo P (1996). The emergency department and home care: Strange bedfellows. *Home Healthcare Nurse* 14(6):451–452.

Milone-Nuzzo P (1996). A creative way to use nurse clinical specialists in home care. *Home Healthcare Nurse* 14(3):224.

Monahan F, Drake T, Neighbors M (1994). *Nursing Care of the Adult.* Philadelphia: WB Sanders.

Monteiro L (1997). Florence Nightingale on public health nursing. In Spradley B, Allender J. *Readings in Community Health Nursing.* Philadelphia: Lippincott-Raven. Reprinted by permission of the APHA from *Am J Public Health* 75(2):181–186.

Moore R (1997). "OASIS and conditions of participation." Home Care Reimbursement Information Division *Advisory Letter*, Bulletin #970545.

Morrelli T (1997). *The Nurse's Guide to Home Health Care.* St. Louis: Mosby.

Morris R, Christie K (1995). Initiating hospice care. *Home Healthcare Nurse* 13(5):21–28.

Mullahy C (1994). *The Case Manager's Handbook.* Frederick, MD: Aspen.

Murer C (1994). Standardizing quality indicators. *Continuing Care* 13(4):22–25.

National Association for Home Care (1994). *A Provider's Guide to a Medicare Home Health Certification Process,* 3d ed. Washington DC: NAHC.

National Association for Home Care (1994). *Home Care Employers' Guide to OSHA Tuberculosis Requirements.* Washington DC: NAHC.

National Association for Home Care (1994). *Profile of the National Association for Home Care.* Washington DC: NAHC.

National Association for Home Care (1995). *Basic Statistics About Home Care 1994.* Washington DC: NAHC.

National Association for Home Care (1995). *Legislative Blueprint for Action.* Washington DC: NAHC.

National Association for Home Care (1995). *Report No. 639.* Washington DC: NAHC.

National Family Caregivers Association (1994). *Caregiver Member Survey Report.* Kensington, MD: NFCA.

National Family Caregivers Association (1996). *The Resourceful Caregiver.* St. Louis: Mosby Lifeline.

Neal L (1996). The home care client with Alzheimer's disease. *Home Healthcare Nurse* 14(3):175–178.

Nicholas P (1997). Client teaching and learning. In Zang S, Bailey N, eds. *Home Care Manual: Making the Transition.* Philadelphia: Lippincott-Raven.

Noone C et al (1997). Computerized documentation in home care. In Spradley B, Allender J, eds. *Readings in Community Health Nursing.* Philadelphia: Lippincott-Raven.

Ondeck D (1996). Credentialling corner. *Home Health Care Management & Practice* 8(2):79–80.

O'Ryan J (1994). Guidelines for compliance. *Continuing Care* May:40–42.

Parkman C (1996). Delegation: Are you doing it right? *AJN* 96(9):42–48.

Pearson M (1993). The nurse, the elderly caregiver and stress. *Caring* 12(1).

Peters D (1995). Outcomes: The mainstay of a framework for quality care. *J Nursing Quality Care* 10(1):63.

Portnoy F, Dumas C (1994). Nursing for the public good. *Nurs Clin North Am* 29(3):370–376.

Price R, Mauro T (June, 1997). Advocates promise to press the fight. *USA Today,* p. 4A.

Pratt J (1996). Home health care: A dynamic complex field requiring dynamic competent managers. *Home Health Care Management & Practice* 8(2):6–14.

Quinlan J, Ohlund G (1995). Psychiatric home care: An introduction. *Home Healthcare Nurse* Jan–Feb:20.

Ragland G (1997). *Instant Teaching Treasures for Patient Education.* St. Louis: Mosby.

Reynolds C (1996). How to report medical device problems. *Nursing '96* 26(8):24u–24v.

Rhiner M, Ducharme S (1996). Nonpharmacologic measures to reduce cancer pain in the home. *Home Health Care Management & Practice* 8(2):41–47.

Rice R (1995). Home mechanical ventilator management. *Home Healthcare Nurse* Jan–Feb:73.

Rothenberg R, Sedhom L. (1997). The maternal child visit. In Zang S, Bailey N, eds. *Home Care Manual.* Philadelphia: Lippincott-Raven.

Rozovsky F, Rozovsky L (1994). Home health care law. *The Basics of Health Care Risk Management.* Boston: Little Brown.

Salsberry P et al (1993). Home health care services for AIDS patients: One community's response. *J Commun Health Nurs* 10(1).

Schrof J (1997). Easing hurt in small bodies. *U.S. News & World Report* 122(10):60–65.

Senapatiratne L (1996). On the road with a home health nurse. *RN* 59(4):54–57.

Shames K (1996). Harnessing the power of guided imagery. *RN* 59 (8):49–50.

Shapiro P (1995). Refusing treatment at home: A paramedic talks about nonhospital DNR orders. *Choices* 4(1):5.

Shaughnessy P, Chrisler K (1996). *Outcome-Based Quality Improvement: A Manual for Home Care Agencies on How to Use Outcomes.* Denver: Center for Health Policy & Services Research.

Sheldon P (1994). High technology in home care. *Nurs Clin North Am* 29(3):507–519.

Sherman J, Malkmus M (1994). Integrating quality assurance and total quality management/quality improvement. *J Nursing Admin* 24(3):37–41.

Sherven L et al (1995). *Nursing Care of the Childbearing Family.* Stamford, CT: Appleton & Lange.

Shu E et al (1996). Telephone reassurance program for elderly home care clients after discharge. *Home Healthcare Nurse* 14(3):155–161.

Singh P (1995). Managing chronic congestive heart failure in the home. *Home Healthcare Nurse* 13(2):11–13.

Sloan A (1996). Don't resuscitate, lose your job? *RN* 59(8):51–54.

Smeltzer S, Bare B (1996). *Brunner and Suddarth's Textbook of Medical-Surgical Nursing,* 8th ed. Philadelphia: Lippincott-Raven.

Snyder R (1995). Ethical decisions: Home healthcare providers and patients who choose to die. *Home Healthcare Nurse* 13(5):75–77.

Spector R (1997). *Cultural Diversity in Health & Illness,* 4th ed. Stamford, CT: Appleton & Lange.

Spencer C, Wonder D (1996). *Home Care IV Therapy,* 2d ed. Frederick, MD: Aspen.

Spradley B, Allender J, eds. (1997). *Readings in Community Health Nursing,* 5th ed. Philadelphia: Lippincott-Raven.

Spruhan J (1996). Beyond traditional nursing care: Cultural awareness and successful home healthcare nursing. *Home Healthcare Nurse* 14(6):445–449.

Stackhouse J (1994). Death, dying, bereavement and spiritual distress. In Monahan F, Drake T, Neighbors M, eds. *Nursing Care of Adults,* 2nd ed. Philadelphia: WB Saunders.

Stackhouse J (1997). Facilitative verbal responses. In Leasia S, Monahan F, eds. *A Practical Guide for Health Assessment.* Philadelphia: WB Saunders.

Stackhouse J (1998). Knowledge base for death and dying. In Monahan F, Neighbors M. *Foundation for Clinical Practice,* 2nd ed. Philadelphia: WB Saunders.

Stanhope M, Knollmueller R (1996). *Handbook of Community and Home Health Nursing.* St. Louis: Mosby.

Stocker S (1996). Six tips for caring for aging parents. *AJN* 96(9):32–33.

Struk C. Women and children. *Nurs Clin North Am* 29(3):395–406.

Stulginsky M (1993a). Nurses' home health experience: Part I: The practice setting. *Nursing and Health Care* 14(8):402–407.

Stulginsky M (1993b). Nurses' home health experience: Part II: The unique demands of home visits. *Nursing and Health Care* 14(9):476–485.

Stutts A (1994). Selected outcomes of technology-dependent children receiving home care and prescribed child care services. *Pediatr Nurs* 20(5): 501-507.

Surrency G (1997). Medication management in the Home. In Zang S, Bailey N, eds. *Home Care Manual: Making the Transition*. Philadelphia: Lippincott-Raven.

Sutliff D (1996). Tips to improve communication. *Home Healthcare Nurse* 14(3):195-196.

Talbot L, Curtis L (1996). The challenge of assessing skin indicators in people of color. *Home Healthcare Nurse* 14(3):168-173.

Taguay P (1994). Successful information system integration. *Remington Reports* 11.

Tammelleo A (1993). Legally speaking: Staying out of trouble on the telephone. *RN* October.

Taxes and spending (July, 1997). *USA Today,* p. 8A.

Thobaben M (1993). The legal and moral obligations of home care agencies with regard to the new Patient Self-Determination Act. *Home Healthcare Nurse* 10:55-56.

Thomas-Masoorli S (1996). Intravenous therapy handbook. *Nursing '96* 26(10):48-51.

Turley K, Higgins S (1996). When parents participate in critical pathway management following pediatric cardiovascular surgery. *MCN* 21(5):229-234.

Turner T (1994). *Handbook of Adult and Pediatric Respiratory Home Care*. St. Louis: Mosby.

Uhlman M (1995). Seniors find HMOs more appealing. *The Philadelphia Inquirer* Sept. 3, D1.

U.S. Congress. *Omnibus Reconciliation Act of 1990*. Washington DC: U.S. Govt. Printing Office.

USDHHS (1994). *Clinical Practice Guideline: Management of Cancer Pain*. Agency for Health Care Policy and Research Publication No. 94-0592.

USDHHS (1995). *Using Clinical Practice Guidelines to Evaluate Quality of Care*. Agency for Health Care Policy and Research Publication No. 95-0046.

Wagner J (1996). Wandering and fall prevention: New solutions to a perennial problem. *Nursing '96* 26(8):24s-24t.

Warner I (1996). Introduction to Telehealth Home Care. *Home Healthcare Nurse* 14(1):791-796.

Wendt D (1996). Building trust during the initial home visit. *Home Healthcare Nurse* 14(2):92-98.

Wertham (1980). *The German Euthanasia Program*. Cincinnati: Hayes Publishing.

Wills E (1996). Nurse-client alliance: A pattern of home health caring. *Home Healthcare Nurse* 14(6): 455-459.

Wilson HD (1993). Family caregiving for a relative with Alzheimer's dementia: Coping with negative choices. In Wegner, Alexander, eds. *Readings in Family Nursing*. Philadelphia: JB Lippincott.

Wong, D (1993). *Essentials of Pediatric Nursing*. St. Louis: Mosby.

Worley N (1995). Community psychiatric nursing care. In Stuart G, Sundeen S, eds. *Psychiatric Nursing*. St. Louis: Mosby.

Younger J (1995). The alienation of the sufferer. *Advances in Nursing Science* 17(4):53-72.

Zang S, Bailey N (1997). *Home Care Manual: Making the Transition*. Philadelphia: Lippincott-Raven.

Zasler N (1994). TBI rehabilitation program assessment. *Continuing Care* 13(4):30-43.

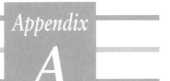

Appendix
A

Death and Dying Customs Among Religious Groups in the United States

	Eastern Orthodox	**Roman Catholic**
Unique Features	Many subgroups. Use of icons. Calendar differs from West. Easter stressed.	Largest group worldwide under central authority of Pope
Care of Dying Clients	Last rites by priest usually mandatory. Do not remove cross. Do not shave males.	Anointment of the sick, Holy Communion, and Reconciliation (confession) important.
Care of Dead	Hands placed in the form of a cross at death	Postmortem care. Funeral directors prepare body for wake.
Organ Donation and Transplantation	Regulations vary with subgroups.	Permitted
Autopsy	Usually opposed	Permitted
Cremation	Usually opposed	Permitted
Passive Euthanasia	Varies: generally should prolong life as long as possible	No extraordinary measures necessary when quality of life is gone
Miscellaneous	Abortion opposed. Infant baptism stressed by Greek Orthodox (not practiced by most Eastern Orthodox groups).	Abortion opposed. Baptism important when death threatens newborns.

	Mainline Protestants	**Evangelical Protestants**	**Fundamentalist Protestants**
Unique Features	From 16th–17th c. Reformation in Europe. Emphasis on Bible, grace, service to others. Most liberal Protestants with formal worship.	More conservative. Emphasis on sharing the Gospel (Billy Graham).	Very conservative, dogmatic, literal interpretation of Bible. Strict lifestyles.
Care of Dying Clients	Clergy visits for Holy Communion, anointment of sick, confession, prayers for healing, Bible reading.	Prayers and Bible reading	Prayers and Bible reading
Care of Dead	Cremation or embalming by funeral director. Closed caskets at funerals or memorial services after burial are common.	Postmortem care, funeral director	Postmortem care, funeral director
Organ Donation and Transplantation	Permitted and valued	Permitted and valued	Varies: generally more restrictive
Autopsy	Permitted	Permitted	Varies: some groups prohibit
Cremation	Common	Permitted	Prohibited by some groups

Continues

	Mainline Protestants	Evangelical Protestants	Fundamentalist Protestants
Passive Euthanasia	Sanctioned	Permitted	Varies with the group
Miscellaneous	Social responsibility and education valued. Cooperate with other churches through the World Council of Churches. Frequently pro-choice regarding abortion.	Cooperate with other churches. Most members are strong opponents of abortion.	Usually exist as independent church congregations without denominational ties. Informal worship. Clergy may be self-ordained. No sacraments. Believe they hold the truth. Do not work cooperatively with more liberal churches. Antiabortion.

Other Church Groups in the United States

Churches	Special Beliefs	Practices	Death and Dying Issues	Miscellaneous
Christian Science	Pain, illness, evil are illusions; only things of the spirit are real.	Avoid medical Rx, psychotherapy, medical tests. Medications usually refused.	Prefer to die at home. No last rites. Autopsies avoided.	Christian Science nurses are listed in the *Christian Science Journal*.
Jehovah's Witnesses	Emphasize Biblical texts in Leviticus	Prohibit intake of blood in any form. Cannot sign informed consent. No oath of allegiance.	Prohibit organ transplants. No last rites or other rituals.	Physicians may need court order to treat children at risk.
Mennonites	Include the Amish. Similar to other evangelical Christians in belief.	19th-century lifestyles. Reject modern machinery. Special dress code. Clean, moral, hard-working farmers. Pacifists but finance wartime relief services.	No extraordinary measures to maintain life. Clergy may anoint the sick. Prefer no autopsy, no cremation. Organ transplant OK, but seldom used.	No health insurance, but conscientious about paying medical bills with help from their community.
Mormons	The Book of Mormon supplements the Bible. The unbaptised dead can be baptised by proxy.	Mormon High Priests are authoritative. Each man must spend 2 years in missionary service. Health prevention highly valued. No coffee, tea, cola, alcohol, or tobacco. Close-knit communities.	Divine healing by laying on of hands. Special white garments worn, not to be removed by nurse. Oppose cremation.	Fast-growing church; second only to Southern Baptists in rate of growth.
New Age	Not an organized religion. Strong influences of eastern thought (Hinduism, Buddhism). Would	Meditation, nontraditional healing practices (holistic). Vegetarians. Astrology, Tarot cards, and crys-	Body should remain untouched at death to allow the soul to pass. (This may eliminate organ donation	Maharishi Mahesh Yogi is an important leader (founder of Transcendental Meditation).

Continues

Churches	Special Beliefs	Practices	Death and Dying Issues	Miscellaneous
	not call themselves a church.	tals used. Health-food stores are centers.	due to time element.) Prefer cremation, natural death, and passive euthanasia.	
Pentecostals	The Holy Spirit is emphasized. Other beliefs vary with denominational affiliation, which may range from R.C. to fundamentalist.	Spiritual healing and speaking in tongues	Stress belief in eternal life. Dying rituals & regulations vary with the church.	The charismatic movement is rapidly growing. Practices vary greatly from church to church.
Quakers (Friends)	Theologically associated with mainline Protestantism with special emphasis on Inner Light inspiration. Pacifism.	No formal liturgy. Quaker meeting is silent meditation. No clergy. Learning & discipline required of each member and individual decisions of conscience. Strong support from each other.	No rituals. Seek information re treatments and actively participate in care. Not apt to resist autopsy. Cremation is preferred. Organ donation, transplants, & passive euthanasia allowed.	Strong tradition of work for social justice. Led fights for abolition of slavery, child labor laws, women's rights, racial equality, and peace.
Seventh-Day Adventists	Old Testament is stressed, esp. Ten Commandments. Believe the dead are asleep until the Second Coming of Christ.	Church held on Saturdays. Vegetarians. No tobacco, alcohol, coffee, tea, or meat. Shellfish allowed.	Practice nonmedication pain control as much as possible. Stimulants refused. Healing prayers by clergy.	Churches sponsor preventive health workshops (eg stop smoking, weight loss).
Unitarian/Universalist	Deists: worship God the Creator. Liberal theology with strong emphasis on humanism.	Dignified worship. Stress education & rational thinking. Liberal religious practices. Value tolerance.	Cremation is preferred. Belief in eternal life is not stressed. Autopsy, organ donation, and transplantation allowed.	Many members support the Hemlock Society, which encourages justifiable suicides and broader euthanasia practices (assisted suicide).

Religious Beliefs and Practices in Death and Dying

	Buddhism	Christianity	Hinduism
Core Beliefs	Religion of enlightenment. Goal to achieve nirvana. Karma-destiny. Subgroups: Zen, Theravada, Mahayana.	Omnipotent, merciful, caring God. Jesus Christ as perfect expression (Son) of God. Biblical authority for guidance. Three major subgroups.	Ancient pantheon of gods. 3 major: Brahma—creator; Vishnu—preserver; Shiva—destroyer.
Lifestyles	8 Paths to nirvana, especially mindfulness and meditation. Cleanliness, beauty, goodness stressed.	Varies with subgroups (fasting, use of alcohol, importance of service to others)	Goal = freedom from bodily desires via yoga, puja, fasting, vegetarianism, no alcohol

Continues

	Buddhism	Christianity	Hinduism
Belief in Life After Death	Reincarnation	Life after death	Reincarnation
Beliefs Regarding Suffering	Pray for healing. May deny pain and refuse analgesics.	Suffering is not God's will and should be resisted.	Destiny for past lives
Dying Rituals	Must stay alert and calm. Monk may chant last rites. Family present.	Vary with subgroup. Holy Communion and Anointing of the sick.	Stay alert through death passage. Rituals by priests.
Physical Care at Death	Important for family to provide physical care	Routine postmortem care by nurses	Only family and close friends should touch the body.
Organ Donation and Transplantation	Seldom opposed	Generally allowed; varies with subgroup.	Problems: Caste beliefs. May need several hours for soul to pass.
Autopsy	Generally allowed	Generally allowed; opposed by some subgroups	Generally allowed
Cremation	Usually preferred	Generally allowed; varies with subgroup	Preferred
Passive Euthanasia (Removal of Life Support)	Generally allowed	Generally allowed; varies with some subgroups	Generally allowed

	Islam	Judaism
Core Beliefs	Allah is the divine being. Mohammed is last and greatest prophet. No images of God permitted.	Jehovah is just, merciful, omnipotent. Jews are the chosen people. Three subgroups: Orthodox, Conservative, Reform
Lifestyles	Must pray 5 times a day facing Mecca. Women segregated. Fasting in Ramadan. No pork, alcohol. "A complete way of life."	Orthodox = strict adherence to Sabbath and kosher traditions. Conservative = varied strictness Reformed = liberal Jews value family, education.
Belief in Life After Death	External life: Heaven and Hell judgment.	Belief in the afterlife
Beliefs Regarding Suffering	Fatalistic; "Allah wills it."	See no value in suffering. Value medical treatment.
Dying Rituals	Confession and seeking forgiveness	Family stays with patient.
Physical Care at Death	Ritual washing by family. Body faced toward Mecca.	Ritual cleansing by burial society. Shomrim stay with body (Orthodox).
Organ Donation and Transplantation	No body part is to be removed (liberals may permit it).	OK with rabbinical permission. Some Orthodox oppose.
Autopsy	Opposed unless mandated by law	Opposed by Orthodox
Cremation	Generally not allowed	Opposed by Orthodox
Passive Euthanasia (Removal of life Support)	Life should be prolonged as long as possible.	Do not believe in artificially prolonging life when no hope of recovery exists.

Addictions, National Nurses' Society on
4201 Lake Boone Trail, Suite 201, Raleigh, NC 27607

Ambulatory Care Nursing, American Academy of
Box 56, East Holly Ave., Pittman, NJ 08071

American Nurses Association
600 Maryland Ave. SW, Washington, DC 20024-2571

Asian/Pacific Community Health Organizations, American Association of
1212 Broadway, Oakland, CA 30305

Black Nurses Association, National
1012 10th Street NW, Washington, DC 20001

Child and Adolescent Psychiatric Nurses, Association of
Philadelphia, PA

Christian Fellowship, Nurses'
P.O. Box 7895, Madison, WI 53707-7895

Emergency Nurses' Association
230 E. Ohio, Chicago, IL 60611

Gerontological Nurses Association, National
7250 Parkway Drive, Hanover, MD 21076

Hastings Center on Bioethics
255 Elm Road, Briarcliff Manor, NY 10510

Hispanic Nurses, National Association of
1501 16th NW, Washington, DC 20036

Holistic Nurses' Association, American
4101 Lake Boone Trail, Raleigh, NC 27607

Home Care, National Association for
519 C St. NE, Washington, DC 20002

Home Healthcare Nurses Association
437 Twin Bay Dr., Pensacola, FL 32534

Hospice Nurses Association
5512 Northumberland Street, Pittsburgh, PA

Indian Health Service/PHS, Office of Human Resources
1616 East Indian School Road, Suite 375, Phoenix, AZ 85016

International Council of Nurses
Box 42, 1211 Geneva, Switzerland

Intravenous Nurses' Society
Belmont, MD

Migrant Resource Program, National
1515 Capital of Texas Hwy S, Ste. 220, Austin, TX 78746

National League for Nursing
350 Hudson, New York, NY 10014

Nurse Practitioners in Reproductive Health, National Association of
2401 Pennsylvania Ave NW, Suite 350, Washington, DC 20037

Nurse-Midwives, American College of
Washington, DC; toll-free 1-888-643-9433

Occupational Nurses, American Association of
50 Lenox Point, Atlanta, GA 30324

Office Nurses, American Association of
109 Kinderkamack Rd, Montvale, NJ 1-800-573-8543

Pediatric Nurse Associates & Practitioners, National Association of
1101 Kings Highway, Cherry Hill, NJ 08034

Politics, Nurses' Coalition for Action in
1030 15th Street NW, Suite 408, Washington, DC 20005

Psychiatric Consultation Liaison Nurses, International Society of
437 Twin Bay Dr, Pensacola, FL 32534

Public Health Association, American (APHA)
1015 15th Street NW, Washington, DC 20005

Public Health Association-Public Health Nursing Section
Archives: Mugar Library, Boston University

Rehabilitation Nurses, Association of
5700 Old Orchard Rd, Skokie, IL 60077

School Nurses, National Association of
16e Route One, P.O. Box 1300, Scarborough, ME 04070-1300

State Boards of Nursing, National Council of
676 N. St. Clair St., Suite 550, Chicago, IL 60611

Student Nurses' Association, National
555 W. 57th St., Suite 700, New York, NY 10019

Substance Abuse, Consolidated Association of Nurses in
303 W. Katella Ave., Orange, CA 92667

Women's Health, Association of, Obstetric and Neonatal Nurses
700 14th Street, Suite 600, Washington, DC 20005-2019

Toll-Free Directory

For toll-free numbers not listed, dial 1-800-555-1212

A

Agency for Health Policy &
Research 1-800-358-9295

AIDS Clinical Trials Information
Service 1-800-874-2572

AIDS National Information
Clearinghouse 1-800-458-5231

Al-Anon 1-800-344-2666

Alcohol and Drug Information Referral
Line 1-800-252-6465

Alzheimer's Association...................... 1-800-272-3900

American Association of Retired Persons
(AARP) 1-800-424-3410

American Board of Medical
Specialties 1-800-776-2378

American Brain Tumor Association ... 1-800-886-2282

American Diabetes Association 1-800-232-3472

American Heart Association 1-800-242-8721

American Liver Foundation 1-800-223-0179

American Parkinson Disease
Association................................ 1-800-223-2732

American Society on Aging 1-800-537-9728

American Society for Deaf Children .. 1-800-942-2732

Arthritis Foundation 1-800-283-7800

B

Birthright 1-800-848-5683

C

Cancer Information and Counseling
Line 1-800-525-3777

Cancer Information Service of the National Cancer
Institute.................................... 1-800-422-6237

Candelighters Childhood Cancer
Foundation............................... 1-800-366-2223

Care Notes & Prayer Notes 1-800-325-2511

Case Management Association 1-800-664-2620

CDC National AIDS Clearinghouse 1-800-458-5231

CDC's National Sexually Transmitted Diseases
Hotline 1-800-227-8922

Choice in Dying................................. 1-800-989-9455

Cocaine Hotline................................. 1-800-262-2463

D

Dial A Hearing Screening Test 1-800-222-3277

E

Eldercare Locator............................... 1-800-677-1116

Epilepsy Foundation of America 1-800-332-1000

G

Gerontological Nursing Association... 1-800-723-0560

H

Health Ministries Association 1-800-852-5613

Health Care Cost Hotline 1-800-225-2500

Hearing Aid Help Line....................... 1-800-521-5247

Hospice Education Institute 1-800-544-2213

Hospice Helpline 1-800-658-8898

I

Insurance Consumers Hotline............ 1-800-942-4242

J

Job Accommodation Network 1-800-526-7234

Job Opportunities for the Blind......... 1-800-638-7518

L

Lupus Foundation of America............ 1-800-558-0121

M

Medicare Handbook and Hotline 1-800-638-6833

N

National Abortion Federation
    Hotline 1-800-772-9100

National Center for the Blind............. 1-800-638-7518

National Center for Youth with
    Disabilities 1-800-333-6293

National Clearinghouse on Family Support/Children's
    Mental Health 1-800-628-1696

National Council on Alcoholism & Drug Dependence
    Hopeline 1-800-622-2255

National Down Syndrome Congress .. 1-800-232-6372

National Down Syndrome Society 1-800-221-4602

National Health Service Corps of the Public Health
    Service 1-800-221-9393

National Health Information Center .. 1-800-336-4797

National Information Center for Children/Youth with
    Disabilities 1-800-999-5599

National Information Clearinghouse for Infants with
    Disabilities 1-800-922-9234

National Institute on Drug Abuse
    Hotline 1-800-662-4357

National Hospice Organization 1-800-658-8898

National Mental Health Association ... 1-800-969-6642

National Organization for Rare
    Disorders................................... 1-800-999-6673

National Rehabilitation Information
    Center 1-800-346-2742

National Retinitis Pigmentosa
    Foundation................................ 1-800-683-5555

National Runaway Switchboard 1-800-621-4000

National Spinal Cord Injury Hotline .. 1-800-962-9629

P

Parish Nurse Resource Center 1-800-556-5368

Pediatric Projects, Inc. 1-800-947-0947

Phoenix Society for Burn Survivors ... 1-800-888-2876

S

Social Security Administration 1-800-772-1213

Spina Bifida Association of America... 1-800-621-3141

U

United Cerebral Palsy Association 1-800-872-5827

United Ostomy Association 1-800-826-0826

United Network for Organ Sharing (UNOS)..............
    ....1-800-24DONOR

V

Veteran Affairs, Nursing Service
    Personnel.................................. 1-800-368-5629

Visiting Nurse Association of
    America..................................... 1-800-426-2547

W

Wellness Reproductions.................... 1-800-669-9208

Y

Y-Me for Breast Cancer 1-800-221-2141

Critical Pathway for a Client with Panic Disorder: Outpatient Treatment

Expected length of treatment: 8 weeks

	Date _____ **Weeks 1–2**	Date _____ **Weeks 3–6**	Date _____ **Weeks 7–8**
Weekly Outcomes	Client will: • Identify initial goals for therapy. • Contract for ongoing treatment. • Participate in treatment plan. • Begin to identify sources of anxiety/panic.	Client will: • Identify ongoing goals for therapy. • Maintain contract for ongoing therapy. • Participate in treatment plan. • Identify strategies to manage anxiety and panic.	Client will: • Describe ongoing strategies to manage panic disorder. • Demonstrate ability to cope with ongoing feelings of panic. • Describe strategies to cope with an inability to cope with stressors.
Assessments, Tests, and Treatments	Psychosocial assessment to include mental status, mood, affect, behavior, and communication. Assist client to explore factors that precipitate panic attacks.	Psychosocial assessment. Assess recent history of anxiety and panic attacks. Explore contributing factors. Discuss effectiveness of cognitive restructuring strategies.	Psychosocial assessment. Assess recent history of anxiety and panic attacks. Explore contributing factors. Discuss effectiveness of cognitive restructuring strategies.
Knowledge Deficit	Orient client to therapy program. Assess learning needs of client. Review initial plan of care. Assess understanding of teaching. Discuss the etiology and management of anxiety and panic disorders. Discuss the physical symptoms of panic and the importance of understanding the meaning of anxiety and panic disorders. Instruct client to maintain journal of anxiety and panic attacks.	Review therapy program and treatment objectives. Review journal of recent panic attacks. Assist client to identify the early signs of anxiety and panic attacks. Discuss strategies to cope with early signs and symptoms of panic attacks, including talking or activity. Discuss additional strategies to cope with panic attacks including expressing anger, positive self-talk, or guided imagery. Teach principles of cognitive restructuring and practice during session.	Review plan of care. Review principles of cognitive restructuring. Assess understanding of teaching.

Continues

	Date _____ Weeks 1–2	Date _____ Weeks 3–6	Date _____ Weeks 7–8
		Teach relaxation techniques and practice during session. Discuss use of exercise to alleviate anxiety/panic. Assist client to explore problem-solving strategies. Assess understanding of teaching.	
Diet	Nutritional assessment. Encourage well-balanced diet from all food groups. Contract with client to avoid stimulants.	Encourage a well-balanced diet from all food groups. Encourage the avoidance of stimulants.	Encourage a well-balanced diet from all food groups. Encourage the avoidance of stimulants.
Activity	Discuss the importance of regular aerobic exercise. Contract for regular exercise program. Sleep pattern assessment. Discuss strategies to provide sleep-enhancing atmosphere for 45 min prior to sleep.	Review ability to begin and continue exercise program. Maintain contract for regular exercise programs. Encourage client to practice relaxation response. Discuss effectiveness of sleep-enhancing strategies.	Review ability to continue exercise program. Maintain contract for regular exercise programs. Discuss effectiveness of sleep-enhancing strategies.
Psychosocial	Approach with nonjudgmental and accepting manner. Observe and monitor behavior. Assist client to understand relationship of unexpressed feelings to anxiety and panic experience. Encourage client to express feelings, thoughts, ideas, and beliefs.	Approach with nonjudgmental and accepting manner. Observe and monitor behavior. Encourage client to express feelings, thoughts, ideas, and beliefs. Provide positive feedback for efforts to incorporate coping strategies into daily life. Assist client to understand relationship of feelings to panic. Assist client to realistically identify strengths and limitations. Explore ways of reframing limitations in a positive manner. Assist client to practice and implement effective coping strategies.	Approach with nonjudgmental and accepting manner. Encourage client to review strategies to manage anxiety and panic.

Continues

Critical Pathway for a Client with Panic Disorder: Outpatient Treatment

	Date _____ Weeks 1–2	Date _____ Weeks 3–6	Date _____ Weeks 7–8
		Assist client to identify potentially stressful situations and role-play coping strategies.	
Medications	Identify target symptoms.	Assess target symptoms. Assess need for medications and refer as indicated. Routine meds as ordered.	Assess target symptoms. Routine meds as ordered.
Consults and Discharge Plan	Family assessment. Establish objectives of therapy with client.	Review with client progress toward therapy objectives.	Review with client progress toward therapy objectives. Make appropriate referrals to support groups.
Variance			

(From *Psychiatric Nursing*, 5th edition, by Wilson and Kneisl. Copyright © 1996 by Addison-Wesley Nursing. Reprinted by permission.)

CLINICAL PATH **CEREBRAL VASCULAR ACCIDENT (CVA), HPN, DYSPHAGIA, TIA**

Patient Name _____ Pt. ID No. _____

ICD-9 Code(s) _____ **436.0, 401.9, 784.5, 435.9**

SOC Date _____ Discharge Date _____

Date Noted	Expected Outcomes	Achieved Y	Achieved N	Achieved Date	Variance Codes	Date Noted	Nursing/Functional Diagnoses	Date Closed
	1. Stable cardiovascular status as evidenced by cardiovascular assessment, per protocol, and blood pressure between ____ and ____ by visit no. ____.						Caregiver role strain, high risk for Outcome(s) no. ____:	
	2. Stable neurological status as evidenced by clinical assessment, per protocol and within desired range, by visit no. ____.						Fluid volume, excess Outcome(s) no. ____:	
	3. Stable functioning of bladder and bowels as evidenced by patient/caregiver understanding of and compliance with home therapeutic regimen by visit no. ____.						Injury, high risk for Outcome(s) no. ____:	
	4. Stable swallowing status, as evidenced by safe swallowing techniques and functional communication by visit no. ____.						Management of therapeutic and medication regimen Outcome(s) no. ____:	
	5. Personal care and hygiene needs stabilized and transferred to patient/family/caregiver by visit no. ____.							
	6. Patient/caregiver demonstrates understanding of and compliance with dietary and hydration regimen as evidenced by clinical assessment by visit no. ____.						Skin integrity, impaired Outcome(s) no. ____:	
	7. Patient/caregiver demonstrates compliance with home therapeutic regimen: medication regimen as evidenced by assessment by visit no. ____.						Thought processes, altered Outcome(s) no. ____:	
	8. Patient/caregiver demonstrates understanding of home safety and exercise program as evidenced by safe ambulation by visit no. ____.						Other: Outcome(s) no. ____:	
	9. Other						Other: Outcome(s) no. ____:	
	10. Other						Other: Outcome(s) no. ____:	
	11. Other						Other: Outcome(s) no. ____:	

(Marrelli TM, Hilliard L [1996]. *Home Care and Clinical Paths*. St. Louis: Mosby.)

CLINICAL PATH **CEREBRAL VASCULAR ACCIDENT (CVA), HPN, DYSPHAGIA, TIA—cont'd**

ICD-9 Code(s) **436.0, 401.9, 784.5, 435.9**

Assessments/Instructions/Interventions	VS No.__	VS No.__	VS No.__	VS No.__	VS No.__	VS No.__	VS No.__	VS No.__	VS No.__
Explain patient rights and responsibilities.									
Assess for home safety management.									
Assess vital signs.									
Assess neurological status.									
Assess hydration and nutrition status.									
Assess coping skills of patient/caregiver.									
Assess patient/caregiver's willingness and ability to provide home therapeutic regimen.									
Assess patient/caregiver's strengths/weaknesses related to therapeutic regimen.									
Assess patient's need for personal care assistance and schedule home health aide, as indicated by visit no. __.									
Refer to: Physical/occupational therapist for home exercise and activities of daily living program (specify visit number).									
Refer to: Speech language pathologist for swallowing safety/communication (specify visit number).									

Continues

413

Refer to: Dietitian for nutritional assessment (especially if receiving tube feedings).

Refer to: Social worker for linkage to appropriate community resources.

Instruct patient/caregiver on home safety._____ on visit no. ____ .

Instruct patient/caregiver on home maintenance program.

Instruct patient/caregiver on medication regimen and compliance (especially note symptoms of medication toxicity).

Venipuncture for ordered laboratory tests

Other:

Other:

Other:

Medical Supplies/Home Medical Equipment Needs

1. Bedside commode

2. Wheelchair/walker

3. Other_____

4. Other_____

Variance codes
1. Patient related
2. Situation related
3. Systems related

Team member signature_____ Initials_____
Team member signature_____ Initials_____
Team member signature_____ Initials_____

Case manager name_____

Patient signature_____
(involved in care planning)

CLINICAL PATH **DIABETES MELLITUS (DM): adult, juvenile, ketoacidosis, PVD**

Patient Name _____ Pt. ID No. _____

ICD-9 Code(s) _____ **250.9, 250.91, 250.11, 250.70**

SOC Date _____ Discharge Date _____

Date Noted	Expected Outcomes	Achieved Y	Achieved N	Achieved Date	Variance Codes	Date Noted	Nursing/Functional Diagnoses	Date Closed
	1. Stable endocrine status by visit no. ____ as noted by blood glucose in range of ____ to ____.						Cardiac output, decreased	
							Outcome(s) no. ____;	
	2. Patient/caregiver demonstrates compliance with treatment regimen, to include dietary and exercise requirements, as well as general health issues by visit no. ____.						Coping, ineffective family/patient	
							Outcome(s) no. ____;	
	3. Patient/caregiver demonstrates understanding and compliance with blood glucose testing, insulin administration, and medication regimens as evidenced by return demonstration by visit no. ____.						Denial, ineffective	
							Outcome(s) no. ____;	
							Knowledge deficit: medication and therapeutic regimen	
							Outcome(s) no. ____;	
	4. Patient/caregiver demonstrates understanding of home safety, general emergency measures related to disease condition, infection control, and proper disposal of contaminated wastes by visit no. ____.						Management of therapeutic and medication regimen, ineffective	
							Outcome(s) no. ____;	
							Nutrition, altered: high risk for body requirements	
							Outcome(s) no. ____;	
	5. Other						Tissue perfusion, altered: peripheral, renal	
							Outcome(s) no. ____;	
	6. Other:						Noncompliance (specify)	
							Outcome(s) no. ____;	
	7. Other:						Other:	
							Outcome(s) no. ____;	
							Other:	
							Outcome(s) no. ____;	

Continues

(Marrelli T, Hilliard L [1996]. *Home Care and Clinical Paths.* St. Louis: Mosby.)

CLINICAL PATH **DIABETES MELLITUS (DM), adult, juvenile, ketoacidosis, PVD—cont'd**

ICD-9 Code(s) _____ **250.9, 250.91, 250.11, 250.70**

Assessments/Instructions/ Interventions	VS No.__	VS No.__	VS No.__	VS No.__	VS No.__	VS No.__	VS No.__	VS No.__	VS No.__	VS No.__	VS No.__
Explain patient rights and responsibilities.											
Assess for home safety management.											
Assess vital signs.											
Assess endocrine status.											
Assess hydration and nutrition status.											
Assess weight.											
Assess coping skills of patient/family/ caregiver.											
Assess patient/caregiver's strengths/ weaknesses related to therapeutic regimen.											
Assess patient/caregiver's willingness and ability to provide home therapeutic regimen.											
Assess patient/caregiver's understanding of disease process and compliance with therapeutic regimen.											
Refer to: Dietitian for nutritional needs and safe allowances.											
Instruct on home safety.											

Instruct on medication regimen and compliance issues.																				
Instruct patient/caregiver on signs of hypoglycemia and hyperglycemia and emergency measures related to those conditions.																				
Instruct patient/caregiver on blood glucose testing.																				
Instruct patient/caregiver on self/caregiver administration of insulin.																				
Instruct patient/caregiver's on home maintenance program (including exercise and correct nutritional allowances). _____ on visit no. _____.																				
Venipuncture for ordered laboratory tests																				
Other:																				
Other:																				
Other:																				

Medical Supplies/Home Medical Equipment Needs

1. Glucometer
2. Insulin syringes/insulin
3. Other____

Variance codes
1. Patient related
2. Situation related
3. Systems related

Case manager name_____

Team member signature_____ Initials_____

Team member signature_____ Initials_____

Team member signature_____ Initials_____

Patient signature
(involved in care planning)

PLAN OF CARE: HOME IV THERAPY

Goals:

Name: _____   **Type of Service:** _____

Diagnosis(es): 1. *Home IV therapy*   **2.** _____

Date	Patient and/or Family Needs and Problems	Unusual Problems	Planned Steps To Meet Needs and Solve Problems	By Whom	Date	Review and Signature
	Hookup and disconnect procedure		Client will be instructed, per procedure, on: • aseptic technique • spiking IV bag and priming tubing • how to access IV line • regulation of fluid rate • heparinization of line • proper securing with tape The client/caregiver must demonstrate proficiency (to the satisfaction of the nurse) in performing and maintaining therapy to initially enroll and to continue in the home care program.			
	Teaching needs: Indications for and concept of home IV therapy		The client will be taught: • the concept of home IV therapy • indications for home IV therapy (e.g., hydration, antibiotics) • benefits of home IV therapy —decreased cost —early return to work and activities of daily living —shorter length of hospitalization —decreased incidence of contracting nosocomial infections			

Continues

Date	Patient and/or Family Needs and Problems	Unusual Problems	Planned Steps To Meet Needs and Solve Problems	By Whom	Date	Review and Signature
	IV site observation and care		Patient will be instructed to keep site dry (no shower, only sponge baths). Patient will be taught to observe site for redness, streaking, swelling, pain and/or leaking at site, and to notify RN. Patient will be taught the side effects of the specific medication that is being administered.			

(Humphrey C, Milone-Nuzzo P [1996]. *Manual of Home Care Orientation*. Gaithersburg, MD, copyright 1996, Aspen Publishers, Inc.)

PLAN OF CARE: HICKMAN CARE

Goals:

Name: _____   **Type of Service:** _____

Diagnosis(es): 1. *Hickman Care* _____   **2.** _____

Date	Patient and/or Family Needs and Problems	Unusual Problems	Planned Steps To Meet Needs and Solve Problems	By Whom	Date	Review and Signature
	Performance of *daily* site care		1. Caregiver will have successfully completed training in Hickman care. 2. Caregiver will be able to demonstrate knowledge of what a Hickman catheter is and of general safety precautions. Hickman catheter care: 　a. Clean work area with alcohol. 　b. Wash hands with liquid soap for 3 minutes. 　c. Gather supplies and open packages. 　d. Remove old dressing and inspect the site for: 　　• leaking of fluids 　　• blood or pus 　　• redness, swelling, or tenderness *Any of the above should be reported immediately to the client's MD or home care nurse.			

Continues

Date	Patient and/or Family Needs and Problems	Unusual Problems	Planned Steps To Meet Needs and Solve Problems	By Whom	Date	Review and Signature
			e. Using peroxide-soaked sterile cotton tip applicator, clean exit site following Hickman catheter care instructions, and apply bandage.			
	Performance of *daily* heparin flush		1. Immediately following daily site care, wash hands. 2. Prepare supplies for flush procedure. 3. Flush Hickman catheter with 2.5 cc of heparin following flush procedure instructions.			
	Performance of *weekly* cap change		1. Once weekly (or more often if indicated) immediately following site care procedure, and preceding heparin flush, change injection cap following cap change instructions. 2. Remove old tape from clamping site and apply new tape. Place tape on a rotating basis, moving from a position close to the skin, outward. Write date on tape.			
	Hickman catheter complications		1. Report immediately any signs and symptoms indicated on signs and symptoms checklist to MD or home care nurse.			

(Humphrey C, Milone-Nuzzo P [1996]. *Manual of Home Care Orientation.* Gaithersburg, MD, copyright 1996, Aspen Publishers, Inc.)

PLAN OF CARE: PORT-A-CATH MAINTENANCE

Goals:

Name: _____   **Type of Service:** _____

Diagnosis(es): 1. *Port-A-Cath Maintenance*   2. _____

Date	Patient and/or Family Needs and Problems	Unusual Problems	Planned Steps To Meet Needs and Solve Problems	By Whom	Date	Review and Signature
	Patient responsibility immediately post-op		Indication for, and explanation of Port-A-Cath will be done by MD and/or nurse.			

Continues

Date	Patient and/or Family Needs and Problems	Unusual Problems	Planned Steps To Meet Needs and Solve Problems	By Whom	Date	Review and Signature
			A. Initially, gauze will be applied post-op (with or without Huber needle inserted in Port-A-Cath, per MD discretion). Dressing will be changed after 24 hours and then every 3 days until incision is healed. B. Patient will be instructed to avoid showering for first 10 days, and that when showering to direct spray on his/her back. Dressing must be changed if it becomes wet or loose. C. Patient will be aware of possibility of swelling around site for up to 2 weeks post-op.			
	Long term		A. Patient will be taught to inspect site for leakage of fluid/infiltration/hematoma, redness, streaking, or tenderness along catheter track. B. If patient is to access Port-A-Cath he/she will be taught per agency procedure specifically hookup, disconnection, and heparinization of Port-A-Cath.			
	Accessing line		Using aseptic technique: A. Set up sterile field, per procedure. B. Using #18g Huber needle and extension tubing, prime with NS, and clamp. C. Clean site, per procedure, with Betadine. D. Palpate Port-A-Cath with one hand, locating center. E. With other hand, push needle perpendicularly through skin into center of device until needle stops. F. Open clamp on extension tubing and infuse solution.			
	Long-term therapy		For continuous or long-term therapy: A. An air occlusive window dressing will be applied.			

Continues

Date	Patient and/or Family Needs and Problems	Unusual Problems	Planned Steps To Meet Needs and Solve Problems	By Whom	Date	Review and Signature
			B. The needle and occlusive dressing will be changed by an RN weekly. C. Line will be primed, per procedure. D. Dressing will be applied, per procedure. E. Dressing will be secured with tape to form a window frame, and extension tubing will be secured on top.			
	Disconnecting line		Using aseptic technique: A. Draw up NS and heparin, per procedure. B. Clean connection with three alcohol wipes between extension tubing and cap, or pump tubing. C. Inject NS and heparin, per procedure. Close clamp. D. Remove dressing. E. With Betadine, cleanse site, per procedure. F. Place thumb and forefinger of one hand on either side of needle, grip hub and pull upward. With other hand, apply pressure to decrease incidence of hematoma.			
	Troubleshooting		A. For spontaneous blood backflow, patient should check connections and tighten, and check pump function. B. Leaking: Check connections and tighten; retape. C. Catheter occlusion: Clamp extension tubing and notify MD/nurse. Instruct patient not to flush. D. For extravasation: Instruct patient to notify MD/nurse. Note needle placement, backflow of blood, catheter disconnection, attempt to aspirate bid. Consider: cracked or separated catheter from Port-A-Cath. E. Withdrawal occlusion: Check needle placement, have patient change position. Consider: thrombosis, cracked or separated catheter.			

Continues

Date	Patient and/or Family Needs and Problems	Unusual Problems	Planned Steps To Meet Needs and Solve Problems	By Whom	Date	Review and Signature
			Instruct patient to notify MD/ nurse with the following signs and symptoms. A. Fever greater than 101° B. Swelling, redness, tenderness or discharge at site, or blood backup in tubing C. Swelling and/or pain in area of collarbone, neck, face, or upper arm D. Prominent veins in neck, face, arm, or chest E. Difficulty swallowing F. Sores in mouth, diarrhea, nausea, or vomiting			

(Humphrey C, Milone-Nuzzo P [1996]. *Manual of Home Care Orientation.* Gaithersburg, MD, copyright 1996, Aspen Publishers, Inc.)

PLAN OF CARE: TPN

Goals:

Name: _____ **Type of Service:** _____

Diagnosis(es): 1. TPN _____ 2. _____

Date	Patient and/or Family Needs and Problems	Unusual Problems	Planned Steps To Meet Needs and Solve Problems	By Whom	Date	Review and Signature
	Observation/ recording and precautions		Need to monitor: • serum electrolytes weekly • urine dipsticks for greater than 1+ glycosuria • weight/nutritional status • vital signs • Hickman catheter site (see care plan) • distended veins in neck, arms, hands secondary to central venous thrombosis • swelling/edema in face, neck, head secondary to infiltration of solution into surrounding tissues			

Continues

Date	Patient and/or Family Needs and Problems	Unusual Problems	Planned Steps To Meet Needs and Solve Problems	By Whom	Date	Review and Signature
	Teaching needs: patient and significant others		The client will be taught: • Check temperature (M-W-F), notify nurse of elevation. Check temperature more frequently if patient feels ill. • Weight/urine dipstick (M-W-F) and document. Check more frequently if patient feels ill. • Importance of balanced diet and adequate alimentation. • Notify nurse of weight gain or loss more than 2 lbs. • Notify nurse of any of the following symptoms: Excessive cramping, gas accumulation, diarrhea, nausea, vomiting, constipation, large urine output, decrease in appetite, if applicable • Teaching and reinforcement of aseptic handwashing technique and maintaining sterility of IV solution delivery system.			

(Humphrey C, Milone-Nuzzo P [1996]. *Manual of Home Care Orientation.* Gaithersburg, MD, copyright 1996, Aspen Publishers, Inc.)

Glossary

abandonment: the unilateral severance of the professional relationship between a health-care provider and a client without sufficient notice, when there is still a need for health care

acquired immunodeficiencey syndrome (AIDS): a chronic, debilitating disease of the immune system caused by the human immunodeficiency virus (HIV)

acupuncture: the piercing of specific body sites with needles to induce pain relief; an ancient form of traditional Chinese treatment for various disorders

adjuvant analgesic drug: a drug that is not primarily analgesic but that research has shown to have independent or additive analgesic properties

advance directive: written directive that allows people to state in advance what their choices for health care would be if certain circumstances should develop, especially when they are unable to communicate logically

advanced practice nurse: registered nurse who has completed graduate study in a specialty area according to specific academic requirements

advocacy: protection and support of another's rights

affective disorders: mood disorders

affective education: teachings that facilitate changes in attitudes, values, and feelings

affective learning: changes in attitudes, values, and feelings

aggregates: people who share some common interest, problem, or goal and in community health practice are considered a unified whole

agoraphobia: type of anxiety disorder characterized by extreme fear and avoidance of places or situations from which escape may be difficult or embarrassing

Aid to Families with Dependent Children (AFDC): a federal and state program to provide financial assistance to needy children deprived of parental support because of death, disability, absence from home, or in some states unemployment. Also called welfare or public assistance.

AIDS dementia: dementia: progressive dementia caused by direct HIV infection of the central nervous system

alternative care modalities: approaches not part of mainstream medical treatment, such as ayurvedic techniques, chiropractic, energy work, healing touch, shiatsu, macrobiotics, homeopathy, rolfing, reflexology, and aromatherapy

ambulatory care: care rendered to clients who come to a physician's office, a clinic, an outpatient department, or health centers of various kinds

American Public Health Association: oldest and largest nongovernmental organization of public health professionals

Americans With Disabilities Act of 1990: a law passed in 1990 to promote the mainstreaming of people with mental and physical disabilities and to protect the rights of the disabled

assisted living facilities: dwellings that provide help with activities of daily living, such as reminders to take medication, assistance with dressing and bathing, and meal preparation

autism: behavior manifested by extreme withdrawal

bacillus Calmette-Guérin (BCG): vaccines that vary in their ability to induce active immunity and thereby prevent tuberculosis. Not routinely used in the United States because of the variability of their success.

basic life support (BLS): cardiopulmonary resuscitation and emergency cardiac care to prevent circulatory or respiratory arrest

beneficence: ethical principle stating that one should do good and avoid doing harm

benzodiazepines: antianxiety medications with addiction potential

bereavement: expected reactions of grief and sadness on learning of the loss of a loved one

biofeedback: training program in which a person learns to influence physiologic responses that are not ordinarily under voluntary control (autonomic) or those for which regulation has broken down because of trauma or disease

bipolar disorder: major mood disorder characterized by episodes of mania and depression

birthing centers: nursing centers staffed by nurse-midwives

blood banks: places where whole blood and certain derived components are collected, processed, typed, and stored until needed for transfusion

Blue Cross and Blue Shield: health-care insurers. Blue Cross covers mainly hospital costs. Blue Shield reimburses health-care professionals.

borderline personality disorder: personality disorder with a pervasive pattern of unstable interpersonal relationships, poor self-image, mood swings, and impulsive behavior

brain death: cessation of brain function

breakthrough pain: intermittent exacerbations of pain that occur spontaneously or in relation to specific activity

capitation: acceptance of a fixed amount of money per enrolled person, per period (usually a year), with agreement to provide some defined set of health-care services to plan members with no additional billing

carcinogenic: cancer-inducing substances that trigger changes in cells resulting in uncontrolled growth

caregivers: persons who provide social and health needs of others

care maps: See **clinical paths**.

case management: method of delivering client care based on client outcomes and cost containment. Components of case management include a case manager for complex cases and the use of clinical paths.

case finding: identification of present or potential health problems by careful, systematic observations of people

case managers: experienced nurses or social workers with a baccalaureate or master's degree who coordinate the total care of clients whose situations are complex and who need a variety of services

Centers for Disease Control & Prevention (CDC): branch of the U.S. Public Health Services whose primary responsibility is the surveillance of disease

certification: a mechanism, usually a written examination, that indicates professional competence in a specialized area of practice

certified home care agencies: home care agencies that have met certain standards and federal regulations so that they are eligible to participate in the Medicare program and be directly reimbursed for services provided

chart audits: official retrospective or concurrent examination of the record of all aspects of client care; used to compare the quality of care provided with accepted standards

chemical dependency: strong, overwhelming preoccupation with and desire to use a drug, experienced as a craving

chlamydia: sexually transmitted disease caused by the organism *Chlamydia trachomatis*; causes infection of the urethra and cervix; may be asymptomatic in the early stages, especially in males

client: person, family, aggregate, or community that is the focus of health-care interventions

clinical paths: synonymous with **care map** and **critical pathway**. A written plan and timetable for a client's care, with a focus on predicted client outcomes.

code of ethics: set of moral rules that apply to people in professional roles

cognitive learning: ability to process information, including remembering, perceiving, abstracting, and generalizing

cognitive-behavioral therapy: teaching the client to process information, correct negative thinking, and substitute hopeful, positive thoughts and behaviors for counterproductive negative thoughts

collaborative practice: advanced practice nurses who work privately with physicians or other health professionals in mutual professional roles

colposcopy: examination of the vagina and cervix with a magnifying instrument; also used for biopsies

combination agency: a public health agency that also includes home care services; may also include hospice services

community: people, location, and social systems

community assessment: process of determining the real or perceived needs of a defined community of people

community health: identification of needs and protection and improvement of collective health within a geographically defined area

community health nursing: speciality of nursing that

addresses the health needs of communities and aggregates, in particular vulnerable populations, as well as sick people in their homes

comorbidity: presence of multiple diseases simultaneously

complementary therapies: interventions that focus on integration of the body, mind, and spirit; may be used in addition to conventional therapies. Examples are relaxation, imagery, and prayer.

compulsion: uncontrollable, persistent urge to perform an act repeatedly to relieve anxiety

conceptual model: set of ideas and assumptions that integrate them into a meaningful configuration

concurrent audits: examination of client records while the client is still receiving care

conditions of participation: federal regulations that provide guidelines for certified Medicare agencies

confidentiality: keeping information private (eg, between client and nurse)

conflict: clash between opposing forces; may be conscious or unconscious, intrapersonal or interpersonal

conscious sedation: light sedation during which the client responds to verbal stimuli and retains airway reflexes

constitutional law: branch of law dealing with the organization and function of government

consultants: experts who provide professional advice, services, or information

continuing care communities: large housing units that offer all levels of living, from totally independent living to the most dependent of skilled nursing care; designed to meet the changing needs of older adults

continuity of care: desirable goal in the delivery of health-care services as the client uses multiple services and providers

contraception: birth control

contracting: process of negotiating a working agreement between two or more parties

control group: in research studies, the persons not receiving the research intervention

cost containment: efforts to keep costs from rising

critical pathway: See **clinical pathways**.

critical thinking: intellectually disciplined process with a composite of knowledge, attitudes, and skills; ability to assess a complex problem, gather facts and underlying assumptions about it, and use problem-solving skills in interventions and evaluations

cryosurgery: exposing tissues to extreme cold to produce areas of cell destruction; used in treating certain tumors and diseased tissues or to stop bleeding

cultural assessment: obtaining information about a culture; specifically, their health-related values, beliefs, and practices

cultural relativism: understanding the values, beliefs, and practices within a particular cultural context and recognizing and respecting these alternative viewpoints

culture shock: state of helplessness, discomfort, and disorientation experienced by people thrust into a different cultural context; can result in misunderstanding and inability to interact appropriately

custodial care: nonskilled care such as bathing, dressing, feeding, and assistance with mobility and recreation

cyberspace: term coined by William Gibson in his 1984 science-fiction novel *Neuromancer* to describe the interconnected world of computers and the society that gathers around them

default mode: value supplied by the system when a user does not specify a command, parameter, or qualifier

defensive medicine: to practice nursing or medicine as if each client is planning a malpractice suit. Leads to ordering an inordinate amount of laboratory and test procedures and charting carefully and defensively.

deinstitutionalization: humanitarian philosophy committed to providing community-based care for the mentally ill; resulted in decreased populations at state mental hospitals and community treatment facilities, as well as the unanticipated homelessness of many mentally ill persons

delegation: assigning someone else work for which one continues to be responsible

deleterious: harmful

delirium: acute temporary disturbance of consciousness with problems of perception, thinking, and memory

delusions: fixed, false beliefs

dementia: permanent gross memory impairment caused by a variety of disorders, mainly Alzheimer's disease and vascular disease in the brain

Department of Health and Human Services (USDHHS): federal government agency responsible for monitoring all health and welfare concerns in the United States

descriptive epidemiologic study: study that examines the amount and distribution of a disease or health condition in a population by person (who is affected?), place (where does the condition occur?), and time (when do the cases occur?)

desensitization: counterconditioning, behavioral technique used to overcome phobias by gradually increasing exposure to the feared stimuli

detoxification: controlled withdrawal from an abused substance

diagnosis-related groups (DRGs): billing classification system used by Medicare; there are 467 diagnoses, with preestablished and fixed reimbursement fees allowed for each.

Diagnostic & Statistical Manual IV (DSM IV): manual published by the American Psychiatric Association

dichotomy: division into two parts

discharge planners: nurses who coordinate a client's transition from one health-care setting to another

DNR orders: "do not resuscitate" orders

dominant values: set of values shared by the dominant or majority culture in a population

dose ceiling zone: highest dose of a medication that can safely be administered

double-blind: neither the researcher nor the research participants know who is in the experimental group and who is in the control group

dually diagnosed: persons with both mental illness and substance abuse, or mental retardation and one of the above

durable power of attorney: also called health-care agent or health-care proxy; this agent has the authority to make health-care decisions when the client cannot

durable medical equipment: hospital beds, wheelchairs, commodes, and other hospital equipment used for home care; reimbursed by Medicare at 80%

dyad: a pair; two people living together, usually husband and wife

dysfunctional families: families in which clear communication is inhibited and in which there is lack of psychological support

electroconvulsive therapy: treatment procedure in which a brief seizure is induced by passing an electric current through the brain

enzyme-linked immunosorbent assay (ELISA) test: a standard screening test for HIV

emancipated minors: minors no longer under their parents' supervision and control. Examples include married teens and teens in the military.

e-mail: electronic mail, a way to send a message via computer

empathy: ability to understand and vicariously experience the feelings and thoughts of others while maintaining one's own identity

employee assistance programs: programs that help an employee when emotional, addictive, or physical illness threatens to interfere with his or her health

empowerment: process of developing knowledge and skills to increase mastery over the decisions that affect one's life

endemic: continual presence of a disease or infectious agent in a geographic area

endogenous reactivation: produced or arising from within

entitlement programs: government programs (Social Security, Medicare, and Medicaid) for which citizens have paid into a fund or paid taxes

entrepreneur: business person who works on his or her own initiative

environmental health: branch of public health concerned with assessing and controlling the impact of people on their environment and vice versa

environmental impact: positive or negative changes on the environment and on the people living in it

epidemic: disease occurrence that clearly exceeds the normal or expected frequency in a community or region

Environmental Protection Agency (EPA): federal agency established in 1970 that is responsible for air, water, and land pollution control

epidemiology: study of the determinants and distribution of health, health conditions, and disease in human population groups

early periodic screening diagnosis and treatment program (EPSDT): a preventive health program for children

equianalgesic: medications having equal painkilling effect; morphine sulfate 10 mg intramuscularly is generally used for opioid analgesic comparisons

equity: providing accessible services to promote the health of populations most at risk for health problems

ergonomics: study of people at work to understand the complex relationships associated with work

escalating costs: constant increase in costs

ethical dilemmas: conflict between moral values; either both choices or neither choice has merit, so there is no clear right and wrong

ethics: discipline that debates what is right and wrong in accordance with personal and professional moral standards and responsibilities

ethnic foods: foods based on heritage; cultures have specific traditional food patterns

ethnocentrism: belief that one's own cultural beliefs and values are best for all

euthanasia: intentional termination of a life of such poor quality that it is not considered worth living. Passive euthanasia is the removal of artificial life-sustaining measures; active euthanasia is "mercy killing."

executive branch of government: chief branch of government empowered to administer the laws and affairs of the state or nation

exogenous: arising from the outside

experimental design: protocol in which investigators institute an intervention or change and then measure the consequences of the intervention, usually with the use of a control group

extended-care facilities: synonymous with nursing homes or long-term care facilities; provide care for persons who need daily care, for chronic conditions requiring either skilled nursing or custodial care

extended family: all persons related by birth, marriage, or adoption to the nuclear family

family assessment: systematic collection and analysis of family data for the purpose of identifying the family's health-related strengths and problems

Family Leave Act of 1993: provides job protection, allowing 12 weeks of unpaid leave to care for a sick family member

family systems theory: theory that the family is a collection of people who are integrated, interacting, and interdependent and the actions of one member affect the actions of other members

fax machines: machines that can send and receive printed material electronically

Federal Register: legal document in which all proposed federal regulations are published

fee-for-service system (FFS): method of reimbursing for medical care; a fee is charged for each service after it is provided

Federal Emergency Management Agency (FEMA): government agency responsible for directing the federal response to disasters

fidelity: keeping one's promises or commitments

forced-choice ranking: selecting the things that have the highest value or rank

free market approach: without governmental restrictions or control

freestanding agencies: agencies not connected to a hospital or other institution

frail elderly: older adults, usually over age 85, who may need assistance in activities of daily living

gag rule: regulation that restricts medical personnel from ordering or informing clients about expensive treatment options or tests

gatekeeper: physician, nurse practitioner, or physician's assistant who decides what tests or specialist's care an HMO member may receive (usually a primary caregiver)

generic: basic

genogram: graphic display of family genealogy (births, marriages, divorces, illnesses, deaths), identifying characteristics (race, religion, occupation), and places of residence

grandiose thinking: exaggerated appraisal of one's worth, importance, power, or knowledge; can assume delusional proportions

G-tube: gastric tube that leads directly into the stomach through the abdomen, usually for feeding

habeas corpus: A writ of habeas corpus gives persons the right to challenge the legality of their detention under U.S. law.

hallucinations: false perceptions in the absence of stimuli; can involve all five senses in the waking state

Hastings Institute: a private organization dedicated to studying bioethics

HAV, HBV, HCV: hepatitis A, B, and C virus

health: state of physical, mental, and social well-being; not merely absence of disease or infirmity

Health Care Financing Administration (HCFA): federal agency responsible for overseeing Medicare

health-care proxy: agent designated by client to make health-care decisions when client is incompetent to do so

health-care rationing: limiting some types of health services to save costs; may jeopardize the well-being of some people

health-care system: all persons, agencies, hospitals, and organizations that deal with health care

health departments: local or state government agencies with responsibility for disease prevention, health promotion, and filling gaps in local services

health fair: community or institutional event designed to provide health education, case finding, and screening

Health Insurance Portability and Accountability Act of 1996: a federal law protecting people from losing their medical insurance for preexisting conditions when they change jobs. It also assigns criminal penalties for transferring funds to other family members to become Medicaid-eligible.

health maintenance organization (HMO): prepaid health plan delivering comprehensive care to members through designated providers. Members must enroll for a specific time, usually 1 year.

health planning: continuous social process in which data about clients are collected and evaluated; the goal is to create a plan to guide change in health-care delivery

health promotion: efforts that help people move closer to optimal well-being or higher levels of wellness

health risk appraisal: process of identifying and analyzing a person's characteristics of health and comparing them with those of a standard age group; allow prediction of a person's likelihood of developing a health problem prematurely

Healthy People 2000: government plan that outlines national health goals and objectives for the year 2000

herd immunity: collective immunity of a group or community; results in failure of a infectious agent to spread because a high proportion of members have developed resistance to the infection

hierarchy: organizational arrangement in pyramid form; authority for decision making is accorded to a few persons at the top, with the least authority given to persons at the bottom

HIV-related dementia: See **AIDS dementia**.

holistic: way of viewing a person as an integrated whole (mind, body, and spirit); reflects the interactive process that occurs in all of us

home care: also called home health care; all the services and products provided to clients in their homes to maintain, restore, or promote their physical, mental, and emotional health. Care can be delivered by an official agency, a hospital-based agency, or a proprietary agency.

hospice: holistic services provided to dying persons and their loved ones to provide a more dignified and comfortable death; aggressive curative treatments are no longer pursued. To be eligible, clients must be declared within 6 months of dying by their physicians.

hospital-based home care: home care agencies that are extensions of hospitals

human immunodeficiency virus (HIV): a retrovirus that attacks the body's immune system; transmitted through sexual contact, sharing contaminated needles and syringes, and transfusion or contamination by infected body fluids

humanistic learning theories: theories that assume people have a natural motivation to learn and that learning flourishes in an encouraging environment

human papillomavirus (HPV): sexually transmitted disease that results in genital warts; a link exists between HPV and cancer

hypothesis: question or supposition proposed to explain an event or guide an investigation

imagery: cognitive-behavioral strategy that uses positive mental images to help produce relaxation and healing

immune globulin: sterile solution containing antibodies from human blood; provides passive immunization for various infectious diseases but lasts only up to 2 months

incidence: all new cases of a disease or health condition appearing during a given time

incident reporting: writing a report about any adverse event or occurrence so that details can be reviewed much later if necessary

indemnity insurance plan: contractual agreement with prepayment of premiums to cover agreed-on expenses or losses—for example, health insurance purchased to pay for health costs

independent practice association: type of HMO made up of physicians in private practice who see HMO members in their offices as well as their other fee-for-service patients

infant mortality rates: rate of death per 1,000 infants (1 month to 1 year old); major indicator of the health of a community

infantilize: to treat as a young child and discourage normal developmental behaviors as a child grows older

infusion therapy: fluids injected slowly into veins for therapeutic purposes

instructive directives: See **advance directives** and **living wills.**

integrated information system: computer systems that link a central database with terminals or personal computers in all departments in the organization

Internet: worldwide group of computer networks that can exchange information

Joint Commission on Accreditation of Healthcare Organizations (JCAHO): the major independent health-care accreditation agency in the United States

judicial laws: laws based on court or jury decisions

Kaiser Permanente: the oldest HMO in the United States

kosher diet: foods prepared and served in accordance with Jewish dietary laws

laissez-faire philosophy: philosophy that power should rest with the people to develop as it will, without government interference

La Leche League: organization whose purpose is to promote breastfeeding

Lamaze program: breathing exercises used to facilitate childbirth and reduce or eliminate the need for analgesia or anesthesia

laptop computers: portable computers

laparoscopic surgery: surgical technique in which an endoscope is inserted into the abdomen to visualize the surgical area; results in a tiny incision and causes minimal surgical trauma to the client

latchkey children: children who come home from school to an empty residence with no supervising adult present

latent infection: an infection that is not yet apparent, often in the early stages

learning readiness: emotional state, abilities, and potential that allow learning to occur

liability lawsuit: suit brought because of a health-care worker's failure to meet an obligation or because of professional conduct that results in client injury

lifestyle behaviors: behaviors associated with daily living such as nutrition, exercise, sleep, play, rest, and work. Use of nicotine, alcohol, and other drugs is commonly included in a lifestyle behavior assessment.

litigation: court action to determine legal issues and the rights and duties between parties in a lawsuit

living will: written advance directive specifying the medical care a person desires or refuses should he or she lack the capacity to consent to or refuse treatment at some point

lobbying: process by which a person or group acts on behalf of others to influence decisions of policy makers

locus of control: feelings about whether a person can control his or her destiny (internal locus) or if his or her destiny is controlled by outside forces (external locus)

long-term care facilities: facilities where persons who are dependent on others for assistance receive nursing care depending on their needs

long-term care insurance: private insurance to pay for care in a long-term care facility or home care

mainstreamed: participating in regular school activities and assigned to regular classrooms

managed care: system of total health care in which costs are minimized and the client prepays for a set period of time (usually 1 year)

managed-care company: a for-profit or not-for-profit health-care organization that offers prepaid care in its system for a given time period (usually 1 year); the goal is to provide quality health-care outcomes to clients at the lowest possible cost, with a strong emphasis on prevention

mandated reportable or notifiable disease: a disease that health-care providers must by law report to state or local public health officials. These diseases are of public interest because of their contagiousness, severity, or frequency.

mandatory policy: required policy

marijuana: illegal substance made from the hemp plant (*Cannabis sativa*); when smoked or consumed, it makes users feel mildly euphoric and relaxed, with more intense sensory perceptions

marketing: planning and implementation of carefully formulated programs directed at target groups to sell products or ideas

massage therapy: manipulating muscles with pressure or various types of strokes to induce relaxation and stimulate circulation. The two most common types of massage are Swedish and shiatsu, which uses acupressure. Reflexology is a type of foot massage believed by adherents to influence many body systems.

Meals on Wheels: local program in which one hot meal and sometimes a second cold meal is delivered each day to elderly people in their homes

measurable outcomes: objective changes in the client's health status that can be measured, tested, or recounted by the client

Medicaid: program that provides joint federal and state payment of health services for the blind, disabled, elderly, and families with dependent children who are medically indigent; covers participants in the Aid to Families With Dependent Children program and the Supplemental Social Security program

medically indigent: people who cannot afford health-care insurance and lack health and medical services

medical savings account (MSA): new form of tax-sheltered savings account set up by clients to be used for health-care costs. Leftover money in the fund can build tax-free until age 65. Clients may also withdraw money early for nonhealth-related expenses, but it is then taxable

Medicare: federal program that provides health insurance for all U.S. citizens who are 65 years or older and certain disabled persons. Part A is hospital and home care insurance; Part B is medical, outpatient care insurance.

medication clocks: charts that show when medications should be taken

meditation: method of achieving a state of deep rest and inner peace with increased alpha waves by focusing on a repetitive name or word

mentally impaired: people with limited ability to function because of significant neurologic, behavioral, or psychological disorders

mental retardation: subaverage intelligence (IQ below 70) with impairments in social skills, communication, or safety

mental status examination: assessment of the client's orientation, thinking, judgment, and mood through the use of structured questions

methadone maintenance program: providing a synthetic narcotic in controlled, decreasing amounts in clinics as a substitute for street heroin to wean adults from their addictions and the need to commit crimes to support their addictions

migrant workers: laborers who work for farmers or ranchers and travel from one job to another throughout the seasons as needed

milestone chart: type of planning chart that establishes when and by whom the planned objectives will be accomplished

mission statements: statement of purpose that defines the reason for the existence of an organization

monoamine oxidase inhibitors: group of antidepressant drugs; must be used carefully because foods containing tyramine or other medications can induce a hypertensive crisis

morbidity rate: relative disease rate; ratio of the number of sick persons to a total given population

mortality rate: relative death rate; the sum of deaths in a given population at a given time

mosaic of cultures: pattern or design made up of distinct cultures

multidisciplinary providers: health-care providers from various disciplines—for instance, nurses, physicians, physical therapists, social workers, respiratory therapists, occupational therapists

multiphasic screening: various screening tests often given to children; includes sensory screenings

multiproblem families: family units that face many problems and may have the resources to solve their own problems

National Committee for Quality Assurance (NCQA): organization that accredits managed-care companies

national health plan: plan that provides health insurance coverage for all citizens through a single-payer system

National Home Caring Council: accreditation agency that focuses on home health aide services

neuroleptic medications: medications used to treat schizophrenia or other disorders characterized by psychosis

neuropsychiatric: newer term that is replacing "psychiatric." It takes into consideration new knowledge about the brain and the strong neurologic basis of psychiatric disorders.

National Institute of Occupational Safety and Health (NIOSH): federal agency responsible for investigating workplace illnesses, accidents, and hazards

noncompliance: failure to use or complete a treatment program

nonmaleficence: avoiding or preventing harm to others as a result of one's choices and actions

nonverbal cues: communication without the use of words; usually more powerful than verbal communication

nuclear family: mother, father, and children living together

Nurse Practice Act: statute that defines the practice of nursing and guides the scope of nursing practice on a state-by-state basis

nursing centers: clinics managed and served by nurse practitioners and other advanced practice nurses who deliver primary health care

nursing homes: extended-care facilities

obsession: persistent, unwanted, intrusive thought that cannot be eliminated by logic

Office of Aging: local agency that often receives state funding; sponsors senior nutrition programs and other services to help the elderly

official public agencies: agencies that are mandated to offer a particular group of services and are supported by tax dollars

Omnibus Reconciliation Act (OBRA) of 1990: law that protects clients' rights of self-determination regarding health care

online: computer term meaning connected to a host system, such as an online service, a bulletin-board system, a public-access site, or the Internet

opportunistic infections: infections that result when one's resistance or body defense system is reduced, as in AIDS

optimal functioning: performing to the best of one's ability

ordinances: local laws

Occupational Safety and Health Administration (OSHA): federal agency charged with setting standards and regulations to improve the health and safety of American workers

outcome criteria: establishment of patient goals to be achieved through a combination of nursing and medical interventions, with client participation

outcome-driven: focusing on changes in a client's health status as a result of care or program implementation

outcome evaluation: quality measure that examines the consequences of a program

outreach workers: workers assigned to locate people with specific health problems (eg, tuberculosis) to increase their access to and compliance with treatment

palliative therapy: therapy performed to relieve or ease pain rather than to cure

pandemic: worldwide outbreak of an epidemic disease

panic attacks: episodes of sudden intense fear or sense of impending doom

paranoia: pervasive distrust and suspiciousness

parish nursing: nursing service provided by churches or hospitals to promote wellness, using a holistic approach, in congregation members

participatory management: system in which workers have input into planning, implementing, and evaluating the work of the organization

particulate respirator masks: masks worn by healthcare personnel working with possible active tuberculosis cases

partner notification program: contact tracing to identify and locate partners of people who have been diagnosed with a communicable disease; the goal is to notify them of the exposure

passive immunity: immunity resulting from antibodies produced and received from others; gives immediate protection but lasts only a few weeks

Patient Bill of Rights: document prepared by the American Hospital Association that defines the provider–client relationship within an organization

Patient Self-Determination Act of 1990: part of the Omnibus Reconciliation Act; states that clients have the right to accept or refuse medical care and that all health-care agencies must notify clients of their rights both verbally and in writing

pejorative: having a negative connotation

performance appraisal: method by which employees are evaluated based on standards of practice and a specific job description

peripherally inserted central venous catheter (PICC): used for the administration of intravenous fluids, blood products, drugs, and parenteral nutrition solutions, as well as the withdrawal of blood samples for testing

PES: parts of a full nursing diagnosis. P is the NANDA problem statement, E is the etiology or related factors, and S is the signs and symptoms that support the diagnosis,

public health nursing: branch of nursing that focuses on the interrelatedness of health conditions, illness prevention, and health promotion, with a focus on the needs of the sick poor

phobias: intense, irrational fears

plaintiff: person who initiates a lawsuit against a defendant and seeks compensation, usually in the form of money

point-of-service (POS) riders: HMO options that allow members to go to specialists and other providers of their choosing for an extra fee

polypharmacy: taking multiple medications

post-traumatic stress disorder: anxiety disorder in which an extremely traumatic event is reexperienced, accompanied by symptoms of autonomic arousal and avoidance of stimuli associated with the trauma

preferred provider organizations (PPOs): organization of physicians, hospitals, and other health-related services that contract with a third-party payer organization to provide comprehensive health services to subscribers on a discounted fee-for-service basis

prescriptive authority: authority granted by some states for advanced practice nurses to prescribe some types of drugs and devices

prevalence: total number of cases of a particular disease or disorder, both newly diagnosed and chronic, in a given area

preventive services: services provided with the goal of avoiding disease or injury or minimizing the consequences

primary care provider: physician (internist or family practice), nurse practitioner, or physician's assistant assigned to or chosen by members when they enroll in a managed-care program

primary prevention: measures taken to prevent illness or injuries from occurring

prior authorization: process of obtaining coverage approval for a service or medication; without this approval, the service will not be covered by the insurance or managed-care company

private-duty nursing: a nurse who cares for one client on a regular basis for several hours daily, either in the home or in the hospital

proactive: taking initiative, rather than reacting to external forces

process evaluation: assessment of how well a group of people or an agency is functioning

progressive muscle relaxation: relaxation exercise in which each muscle group is tensed and relaxed several times

proprietary home care agency: freestanding, for-profit home care agency; services are provided based on third-party reimbursement schedules or by self-pay

prospective-payment system: paying for health-care services in advance based on rates derived from predictions of annual service costs

prospective study: research study design that looks forward in time to find a causal relation

psychoanalysis: form of psychotherapy developed by Sigmund Freud to bring forth insight from the unconscious by free association, transference, and dream analysis

psychobiological revolution: study of biochemical, genetic, and molecular interactions among cognition, emotions, and behavior

psychomotor learning: physical skills that can be demonstrated

psychomotor retardation: slowness of body movements, speech, and thinking

psychosis: mental disorder characterized by delusions, hallucinations, and other disturbed thinking patterns that cause clients to be out of touch with reality

public health: science and art of promoting health, preventing disease, and protecting the public's health through organized community efforts

public health agencies: government-sponsored agencies on a local, state, or national level devoted to promoting and maintaining the health of the population

public health nursing: field of nursing that synthesizes the public health sciences and the theory of nursing to improve the health of persons, families, and communities

pulse oximeter: noninvasive device used to assess arterial oxygenation

quality assessment: monitoring client care to determine the degree of excellence attained

quality assurance: system used to ensure that all products or services are of uniform quality, conform to a predetermined standard, and equally satisfy customers

Reach to Recovery: American Cancer Society program for women recovering from breast cancer

recertification: in home care, the renewal and recertification of services performed every 60 days by the health team if continued services are needed

recidivism: recurrence

referral: process that occurs between agencies or community resources to provide continuity of care for a client

reflection of feeling: communication skill in which the nurse reiterates either the implied message or the content of what clients say about their feelings

regulatory health policy: policy that attempts to control the allocation of resources by directing the agencies or persons who offer resources or provide public service

rehabilitative: efforts aimed at restoring function or minimizing disability

reimbursement payments: payments for services provided, usually from a third-party source

reliability: consistency in a given research variable within a particular population

rescinded: taken back or withdrawn

research: investigation of a problem or phenomenon; includes systematic collection and analysis of data for the purpose of establishing facts, solving problems, or gaining new information

respite care: temporary relief from duties provided to a family or caregiver

retrospective audit: quality assessment process that studies patterns of care over a specified period of time in the past, using record audits and statistical review of trends in services provided

retrospective fee-for-service basis: paying for health-care services after they are received, with a fee charged for each service

retrospective study: study design that looks backward in time to find a causal relation

risk management: recognizing potential liability exposures to prevent financial loss

schizophrenia: mental disorder that lasts at least 6 months, including 1 month of active symptoms with grossly distorted thoughts (delusions), perceptions (hallucinations), and behaviors (autism)

school-based health center: physical or mental health services provided for schoolchildren, located in or near a school

scope of benefits: type and degree of benefits provided by health insurance plans or managed-care companies

screening: detecting disease in groups of asymptomatic, apparently healthy persons

secondary prevention: attempts to detect disease in its early stages so that early diagnosis and treatment can be offered

selective serotonin reuptake inhibitors: antidepressant drugs that enhance the availability of serotonin in the brain

self-determination: right to direct one's own choices

self-efficacy: sense of self-confidence and capability

service providers: persons, agencies, and organizations that provide health and human services

sexually transmitted disease (STD): disease acquired as a result of sexual intercourse with an infected individual

skilled nursing facilities: facilities that offer nursing, medication, and therapy services for a client who does not require acute care but requires ongoing skilled nursing care

smart cards: credit card-like devices that can store up to eight pages of medical data on a computer chip; will help coordinate care for very mobile clients or those who see multiple providers

spirituality: the process of seeking a relationship with the transcendent

state board of nursing: organization in each state that is responsible for licensing professional nurses

statute: legislation declaring, commanding, or prohibiting something

stereotyping: making an assumption about a person based on his or her perceived membership in a group

stigmatize: to characterize or mark as disgraceful

structure assessment: evaluation of an organization's framework

subculture: relatively large aggregate of people within a society who share separate distinguishing characteristics

subpoena: court order for a person to appear at a certain time and place to testify in a matter; certain documents, such as clients' charts, can also be subpoenaed

subsidized care: care paid for with a government grant

sudden infant death syndrome (SIDS): death that occurs during infancy for which there is no definite cause

suffering: state of severe distress associated with events that can threaten the intactness of the person

supplemental security income (SSI): payments to aged, blind, or disabled who have no other resources to bring their income level up to a minimum standard

surrogate: substitute

survey: assessment method that uses a list of questions to collect data for analysis of a specific group or area

taboo: proscribed by the culture as improper and unacceptable

tertiary prevention: interventions provided to help improve health problems to minimize disability and help restore function

third-party reimbursements: payments made to providers of health care by others than the consumer who received the care; examples are Medicare and Medicaid

tort: private or civil wrong by act or omission, not including breach of contract

total parenteral nutrition (TPN): solution of amino acids, carbohydrates, and fatty acids infused into the circulatory system to provide nutrition when the gastrointestinal system is not functioning

total quality management (TQM): management philosophy in which there is continuous emphasis on customer satisfaction. TQM is a comprehensive term referring to the systems and activities used to achieve all aspects of quality care and to maintain continuous client satisfaction.

transcultural nursing: practice in which a nurse is grounded in his or her own culture but has the skills to live and work effectively in a multicultural environment

triage: classification of sick or injured people according to severity during a disaster to ensure the most efficient care

tricyclic antidepressants: the first group of antidepressant drugs developed

triply diagnosed: having three diagnoses; seen frequently among the homeless population who are mentally ill, self-medicate to treat their anxiety with injectable street drugs, and become infected with HIV

unconscionable: not in accordance with what is just or reasonable

unconscious drives: forces that motivate us arising from the part of the mind that is out of personal awareness

universal coverage: health insurance plan that ensures health-care services to all citizens

United Network for Organ Sharing (UNOS): national computer network of potential organ recipients

utilization management: process that seeks to eliminate the overuse of health-care services and thus to decrease the cost of those services

values: lasting, organized set of beliefs of relative worth

values clarification: process used to help people recognize their values and underlying motivations to help them gain self-understanding and guide future actions

variance: outcome or event that differs from expected goals or standards

variations in meaning: Words and concepts mean different things to different people.

vector: nonhuman carrier of disease organisms that can transmit these organisms directly to humans, such as insects or rodents

ventilator: mechanical device for artificial ventilation of the lungs

veracity: telling the truth

visiting nurse: a registered nurse who cares for the sick in their homes

visiting nurse associations: not-for-profit, nongovernmental agencies organized by persons or communities to provide home care services to the sick and their families

visualization and imagery: using one's imagination and positive thinking to reduce stress and promote healing

vital statistics: information that reflects what is going on in a community—for instance, births, deaths, adoptions, divorces, marriages, causes of death

voice mail: computerized system in which the user can send, receive, store, and transfer messages using the keys on a touchtone phone; it has many more capabilities than an answering machine

voluntary health agencies: privately funded and operated organizations existing to meet specific health needs—for example, the American Cancer Society and the American Heart Association

vulnerable population: persons more likely to develop health problems as a result of exposure to risk

web of causation: factors that interact with each other to influence the risk or distribution of health outcomes

welfare-oriented system: system that provides free health care to those who cannot afford it

wellness: dynamic state of health in which persons progress toward higher levels of functioning, thus maximizing their mental, physical, spiritual, emotional, and social potential in their environment

Western blot test: a more reliable test for HIV than the ELISA test; used to verify positive ELISA results

Women, Infant, and Children (WIC) program: supplemental food program administered by the federal Department of Agriculture through state health departments that provides nutritious foods to pregnant women, infants, and children under 5 years with low incomes who are at nutritional risk

worker's compensation: responsibility of employers to compensate workers for wages lost and health care needed because of occupational injury or illness

World Health Organization (WHO): an international health organization sponsored by the United Nations

World Health Organization pain ladder: system of increasing pain medication incrementally as pain worsens; developed by the World Health Organization

World Wide Web: a computer service on the Internet

Index